Hormone Balance

for dummies®
A Wiley Brand

Hormone Balance

by Isabella Mainwaring, CDP, QLS, OCN
Hormone health coach

for dummies®
A Wiley Brand

Hormone Balance For Dummies®

Published by: **John Wiley & Sons, Inc.**, 111 River Street, Hoboken, NJ 07030-5774, www.wiley.com

Published simultaneously in Canada

For general information on our other products and services, please contact our Customer Care Department within the U.S. at 877-762-2974, outside the U.S. at 317-572-3993, or fax 317-572-4002. For technical support, please visit https://hub.wiley.com/community/support/dummies.

Wiley publishes in a variety of print and electronic formats and by print-on-demand. Some material included with standard print versions of this book may not be included in e-books or in print-on-demand. If this book refers to media such as a CD or DVD that is not included in the version you purchased, you may download this material at http://booksupport.wiley.com. For more information about Wiley products, visit www.wiley.com.

Library of Congress Control Number is available from the publisher.

ISBN 978-1-394-30374-8 (pbk); ISBN 978-1-394-30376-2 (ebk); ISBN 978-1-394-30375-5 (ebk)

SKY10097984_020625

Contents at a Glance

Table of Contents

Introduction

It's been incredible to watch hormone health emerge from the shadows and take center stage over the past 15 years. At 13, I found myself grappling with debilitating metabolic, reproductive, and mental health issues, only to be told by specialists that my test results were "normal," my symptoms were "just part of being a woman," or that I'd eventually "grow out of it." (Spoiler: I didn't.) Patients like me, who refused to settle for these dismissive explanations and pushed relentlessly for answers, have helped drive this conversation forward. At the same time, emerging research began highlighting the vital role hormones play in our overall health and longevity. Advances in testing have allowed us to measure and monitor hormone levels with greater accuracy and autonomy than ever before. This collective effort has sparked a much-needed wake-up call, fundamentally reshaping our understanding of hormone health.

My search for answers has revealed that our hormonal apparatus evolved to suit a world far different from the one we live in today. While our ancestors faced physical exertion, intermittent food availability, and natural stressors, modern life presents an entirely new set of challenges: processed foods, sedentary lifestyles, a loneliness epidemic, chronic stress, and environmental toxins. Our hormones are simply ill equipped to handle this new state of affairs.

The consequences of the mismatch between our biology and modern environment are staggering. Chronic hormone-related diseases such as type 2 diabetes, heart disease, and obesity are now leading causes of death globally, with rates of infertility and reproductive conditions such as polycystic ovary syndrome (PCOS) and endometriosis skyrocketing. According to the World Health Organization, heart disease alone claims the lives of around 18 million people each year, while type 2 diabetes affects over 537 million adults worldwide and is responsible for nearly 2 million deaths annually. Both conditions often stem from metabolic dysfunction caused by modern dietary habits and lifestyles. I've come to learn that our hormones are alarm bells, warning us through uncomfortable symptoms that our current way of living is incompatible with our biology.

So, whether you're dealing with specific symptoms, a hormone-related condition, or disease, or you're simply looking to optimize your health and longevity, *Hormone Balance For Dummies* is your comprehensive guide to understanding these alarm bells. This book goes far beyond the mainstream, cookie-cutter advice to dive into the often overlooked and intricate web of biological, psychological, and social root-cause factors such as negative self-talk, generational trauma, unprocessed emotions, poor gut health, processed foods, exposure to toxins that mimic our hormones, and so much more.

Taking the first step toward cultivating a hormone-supportive lifestyle may feel daunting, but once you begin, you'll find it's easier than you think. The physical, emotional, and psychological benefits of supporting your hormones are incredibly rewarding. In fact, these positive habits can become quite addictive because you'll soon find yourself with more energy, capacity, confidence, and clarity than ever.

However, there's no need to overhaul everything in your life all at once. In fact, I recommend starting slow and gradually introducing new, healthy habits at a pace that feels comfortable for you. This isn't a diet or short-term fix; it's a new way of life that you can adapt to gradually. You'll find plenty of guidance in this book on how to create sustainable habits and release those that no longer serve you. For example, one week you may start by swapping out conventional cleaning products for natural alternatives. Then the following week, you could add a short walk after meals to reduce blood sugar spikes.

The key to success with hormone balance is consistency, not perfection. Every small change will add up over time. Modern life hasn't been designed with our optimal health in mind, and it's easy to get swept up in busy schedules. However, illness, a diagnosis, or disruptive symptoms can serve as the wake-up call you need to start prioritizing yourself. Let this book inspire you to gift yourself the opportunity for better health now and in the future.

One of the best things about the *For Dummies* series is that its format is incredibly straightforward and easy to navigate. Whether you're skimming for a quick answer or diving deep into a chapter, you'll find clearly defined sections and plenty of real-world examples that make understanding the complex world of hormones easier than ever.

Foolish Assumptions

When writing this book, I made the following assumptions about you:

- You may have heard of hormone health but likely don't know much beyond what was covered in high school health class. Don't worry — I break down new concepts and terms as they come up.
- You're likely dealing with symptoms of hormone imbalance and are open to seeking solutions. This book offers practical guidance — everything from

where to seek professional help to diet and lifestyle changes you can realistically implement in your daily life.

- Even if you don't have noticeable symptoms right now, you're interested in using the latest science to optimize your physical, mental, and emotional well-being. You're keen to prevent future health issues and maximize your vitality and longevity.

Icons Used in This Book

Throughout this book you'll see the following icons to draw your attention to certain paragraphs.

REMEMBER

This icon highlights key points or essential pieces of information that help you gain a better understanding of hormone balance.

TIP

When you see this icon, it flags practical advice or crucial information for putting hormone balance tips and tricks into practice.

TECHNICAL STUFF

This icon gives you technical information or terminology that may be helpful to level-up your knowledge but isn't necessary to your understanding of the topic.

WARNING

This icon warns against potential problems (for example, common misconceptions that might lead you down the wrong path).

Beyond This Book

This book will always be here for you to refer to, offering guidance and reassurance as you navigate each stage of your hormone journey, so you can adapt your approach as your needs evolve. For more information, you can check out the accompanying Cheat Sheet, which contains important information that you may want to save somewhere, print out and refer to on a regular basis. Go to `www.dummies.com` and search for **Hormone Balance For Dummies Cheat Sheet**.

Don't forget to explore the online appendix, which you can find at www.dummies.com/go/hormonebalancefd. It's full of resources that will help you select healthy foods and safe, natural products for personal care and household cleaning. It outlines key endocrine-disrupting chemicals (EDCs) and processed ingredients to avoid as well as practical steps for minimizing their impact on your body. Each list is designed to empower you to make healthier choices that fit within your lifestyle and budget, prioritizing options that support hormone balance and overall wellness.

Where To Go From Here

This book has been intentionally structured to build a strong foundation of knowledge, helping you understand the intricate, interconnected nature of hormones before diving into specific symptoms and solutions. By guiding you step-by-step through the basics, complex topics, and practical advice, the chapters are designed to equip you with a comprehensive understanding so you can create an effective, personalized hormone balancing action plan. Whether you're starting from scratch, seeking deeper insights on specific issues, or looking for actionable strategies, I encourage you to follow the flow of the book while skipping past sections irrelevant to you. I cross-reference chapters frequently throughout the book, guiding you to other places where you can find additional insights or related information.

REMEMBER

Keeping a positive attitude and finding some humor in hormone imbalances will help you a great deal, which is why the Dummies series continues to present complex topics in a lighthearted, accessible way. At times, you may feel like doing anything but laughing. I know; I've been stuck in the Valley of Despair, too. But scientific research is clear about the benefits of a positive attitude, not only for hormone health but also for achieving successful outcomes and long-term goals. Studies show that people learn and retain information more effectively when humor is part of the process, making the journey to hormone health feel lighter and more enjoyable. In a nutshell, those who laugh are the ones who last!

1

Understanding Hormone Balance and Why It's Important

IN THIS PART . . .

Discover what hormone balance for men and women really means and why it's so critical for long-term health.

Get to know your endocrine (hormone) system and the powerful hormones that regulate everything from stress and sleep to reproduction and metabolism.

Explore the hormone hierarchy and how imbalances in one or two key hormones can trigger a domino effect in your body.

Navigate the stages of hormonal transformation from puberty to menopause or andropause (yes, men's hormones change too!) and learn how these transitions impact your mental and physical health.

Understand the profound link between hormone health and overall health and how imbalances can drive symptoms and diseases you may not have connected to your hormones before.

IN THIS CHAPTER

» Finding out what *hormone balance* means

» Understanding how to detect when your hormones need attention

» Appreciating why maintaining healthy hormones is important

» Clarifying the unique risks of imbalance for men and women across life stages

Chapter 1 Hormone Balance for Life

For thousands of years, Homo sapiens (that's us!) thrived through movement, deep social connections, and striking a delicate balance between short-term survival needs and long-term rewards. Our bodies evolved under conditions of high physical activity, close-knit communities, and a natural rhythm that ebbed and flowed between periods of work and rest. In this environment, our hormones were perfectly tuned to keep us functioning at our best.

Today, our lifestyle looks drastically different, even though our hormonal machinery remains unchanged. Instead of working with the land and moving under the sun, we order groceries online, sit for hours glued to screens, and have traded active, community-centered lives for a world driven by instant gratification and digital connectivity. While these conveniences have certainly made life easier, they've also disrupted the natural rhythms our hormones depend on, leading to imbalances that show up in our energy, mood, fertility, metabolism, and so much more.

This chapter dives into the essentials of hormone balance and why it's vital at every stage of life. You find out how these chemical messengers influence your mind and body, identify signs of imbalance, and discover why investing in your hormonal health is one of the most rewarding choices you can make — helping you feel, look, and live at your absolute best.

Defining *Hormone Balance*

Hormone balance is a dynamic concept that intertwines both the body's natural functions and social or cultural expectations. Physiologically, it refers to a state where hormones covered in this book, such as insulin, cortisol, testosterone, dopamine, and estrogen interact smoothly, supporting mental clarity, energy, stable mood, fertility, metabolic health, and many other processes.

However, because of the public's growing awareness of the power of hormones and the pressure that modern life is putting them under, the concept of "hormone balance" has been shaped over the past decade or so by societal ideals of wellness.

REMEMBER

Real hormone balance is less about achieving the fantasy of a flawless biological state and more about building mind and body resilience. Real balance is a flexible, evolving foundation that supports you through life's demands, pressures, and natural hormonal shifts as you age. Each person's hormonal profile is as unique as a snowflake, with no two exactly alike. This means that what balance looks and feels like for you may be entirely different from someone else because it's shaped by your lifestyle, genetics, personal rhythms, and preferences.

Honoring all experiences

REMEMBER

This book specifically focuses on hormone health for cisgender male and female bodies. Hormone health is deeply individual, and the experiences of transgender and nonbinary individuals are unique and complex, each deserving thoughtful, dedicated exploration. While covering all identities in detail is beyond the scope of this book — which already ambitiously spans the full range of two genders across their lifetimes — my hope is that you'll still find valuable insights and guidance here to support you on your health journey.

Therefore, when I refer to male bodies, I mean AMAB (assigned male at birth), and I mean AFAB (assigned female at birth) when referring to female bodies. These terms help us consider biological aspects while honoring all gender identities. This book has been written with the hope that everyone feels welcome and empowered to explore their unique relationship with their body and its health. For example, some transwomen engage in practices covered in the following chapters, such as "cycle syncing," to connect with feminine energy and honor their gender identity — an inspiring illustration of how public conversations about gender are becoming more sophisticated and inclusive.

Introducing your hormones

REMEMBER

Everyone has a miraculous, self-governing endocrine (hormone) system that is focused 24 hours a day and 365 days a year with helping your body function properly. The endocrine system (which Chapter 2 describes in more depth) produces and releases over 50 different hormones — the body's chemical messengers.

Each hormone has a unique role and works to keep you feeling mentally, emotionally, and physically balanced. From insulin managing your blood sugar levels, to cortisol helping the body respond to stress (physical or psychological), hormones are at the heart of how we experience our health, energy, and resilience daily. They even impact your senses!

While measuring and tracking hormones has been historically challenging due to their fluctuating and often subtle nature, innovations covered in Chapter 14 are now emerging that could transform the way we test and monitor them, offering relief to millions struggling with symptoms and hard-to-diagnose conditions. With these advancements, our understanding of these powerful substances continues to grow, shedding light on their complex roles and methods of communication.

Clarifying the components of balance

In our younger years, a balanced hormone profile supports growth, development, and healthy reproductive capabilities. As we age, our hormonal needs evolve, and balance means preserving energy, muscle mass, bone health and overall wellness to keep us feeling healthy and happy. Key indicators of this balance include stable energy, a positive and adaptable mood, restful sleep, clear skin, and a sense of calm and fulfilment.

Hormone health at any stage is the result of a complex interaction between biological, psychological, and social factors — a dynamic bio-psycho-social system. Therefore, true hormone balance requires a holistic approach that recognizes the intricate connections between your biology, mindset, and social environment.

Biological factors

Hormone health is driven by a complex network of biological processes, including genetics, which can set the stage for specific hormonal patterns or conditions. However, genes alone don't tell the whole story. Lifestyle and environmental factors can alter gene expression through epigenetics, a dynamic process explored throughout this book.

Our hormones also follow natural biological rhythms, which are easily disrupted by poor sleep, excessive screen time, shift work, or chronic stress. These disruptions can lead to metabolic issues, inflammation, and reproductive challenges. For a deeper dive, check out Chapter 2 on hormonal "clocks," Chapter 8 on genetic influences, and Chapter 14 on testing options. Additionally, the body needs to efficiently process and eliminate hormones once they've done their job. Chapter 3 covers this detox process and offers practical ways to support your body's natural cleansing systems.

Psychological factors

Chronic stress, unprocessed emotions, and unresolved trauma can lead to long-term issues such as fatigue, irregular or painful periods, mood disorders, and even hormone-driven diseases. Our sense of purpose and self-worth also play crucial roles in modulating hormones such as dopamine, serotonin, and oxytocin — the "happy hormones" that contribute to our resilience and sense of fulfilment.

Additionally, the addictive pull of short-term rewards from social media, gaming, endless news cycles, or pornography creates dopamine-driven feedback loops that amplify stress and disrupt hormone regulation, particularly in young adults. Chapter 9 explores the critical link between the nervous system and hormone regulation, and Chapter 17 offers practical strategies for managing stress and building long-term resilience.

Social (and environmental) factors

Strong social connections can buffer stress and boost oxytocin release, fostering a sense of safety and belonging. However, the modern epidemic of loneliness is driving up levels of cortisol, undermining our immune function, depleting energy, and eroding overall resilience. At the same time, our environment presents new challenges to hormonal balance; toxic diet and comparison culture, sedentary lifestyles, and exposure to endocrine-disrupting chemicals all contribute to a disrupted hormonal landscape. For instance, urban living often limits access to green spaces and nature, which are essential for supporting mood-regulating hormones and promoting a sense of well-being.

REMEMBER

My point here is that biology, mental health, and environment are deeply interconnected; they form a dynamic system where each part influences the others. Chapters 6, 7, and 11 explore the rising rates of hormone imbalances and delve into how these bio-psycho-social shifts are impacting our hormonal health in profound ways.

A root-cause revolution

Western medicine, as valuable and miraculous as it is, is focused on treating symptoms and disease rather than preventing them. It's mostly curative in focus, rather than preventative, and therefore, often fails to recognize this intricate bio-psycho-social interplay, address the root causes of hormonal imbalances, and view the body as a holistic, integrated entity. Therefore, it's important to engage confidently with healthcare professionals to benefit from sophisticated, evidence-based therapies, while also taking proactive individual steps toward hormone balance.

TIP

Your head might be spinning at this point, but I promise that hormone balance doesn't need to be super complicated. In fact, it can be approached in a straightforward, accessible way by focusing on root causes. The root-cause approach involves identifying and addressing the fundamental factors that impact multiple hormones simultaneously, creating balance more naturally and sustainably.

Part 4 focuses on these core aspects so you can create the conditions for your hormones to regulate themselves, minimizing the need for ongoing intervention.

Knowing When Your Hormones Are Off Balance

Hormone imbalance symptoms are surprisingly common in otherwise healthy individuals. They often serve as the body's early warning signals that something is off. Whether they manifest as fatigue, mood swings, low libido, afternoon energy crashes, irregular periods, or changes in weight, these signals are your body's way of communicating that something may not be right with your delicate endocrine system. Tracking your symptoms regularly (using the guidelines provided in Chapter 15) and familiarizing yourself with what they may mean (covered in various chapters such as 6 and 13) are the most crucial tools in understanding and managing your hormone health.

REMEMBER

Body awareness and symptom tracking are the missing links that connect the data from tests (covered in Chapter 14) with how your body actually feels, helping you fine-tune your treatment, management, or prevention plans. No test will ever be able to offer the full picture without the context of how you feel on a day-to-day basis. So, by keeping a log of your symptoms (you find out how in Chapter 15), you begin to build a map of your body's natural rhythms and responses to your diet, lifestyle, time of the month, or stress. It also helps you identify patterns that might be missed in a one-off doctor's visit or a single lab test.

Stuck with symptoms

No matter the current state of your hormone health, there are so many effective strategies you can put in place to actively manage and, in many cases, reverse your symptoms. If you experience regular discomfort, the first step is to identify and document them. Noting these details, especially when speaking with a medical professional, can help determine whether the symptoms indicate a hormone imbalance or align with the pattern of a more serious, hormone-driven condition or disease.

REMEMBER

This distinction is crucial. Imbalances, conditions, and diseases each require different levels of support. Hormone imbalances can often be addressed with lifestyle changes to diet, sleep, exercise, and stress management that support your body's natural ability to rebalance itself. Hormone-driven conditions, such as polycystic ovary syndrome (PCOS), may require a more targeted approach that combines lifestyle shifts with specific interventions to prevent further progression. Then, hormone-driven diseases, such as type 2 diabetes or thyroid disorders, often require medical intervention, medications, or specialized treatment in addition to lifestyle changes to restore and maintain health.

Hormonally driven conditions

When left unaddressed, hormone imbalances can evolve from pesky symptoms into more persistent conditions such insulin resistance. They happen when hormone levels are consistently too high, too low, or erratic, creating stress within the body's internal systems. Unlike temporary symptoms that may fluctuate (say perhaps, in line with your menstrual cycle), conditions involve chronic patterns that interfere with normal bodily functions and are a sign your body's regulatory mechanisms are struggling to keep up.

For many people, these conditions can initially seem manageable but may gradually impact quality of life as symptoms become more pronounced. For example, high estrogen levels in women might stimulate the growth of fibroids, which are noncancerous tumors in the uterus. Addressing these conditions typically requires a combination of lifestyle changes and, in some cases, targeted medical interventions to support the body's efforts in restoring balance.

Hormonally driven disease

When imbalances and conditions progress further, they can lead to hormonally driven diseases such as type 2 diabetes, hypothyroidism, osteoporosis, and certain hormone-related cancers. They represent much more serious disruptions in the body's systems that require comprehensive, and often medical, support.

REMEMBER

For example, untreated insulin resistance can progress into type 2 diabetes, while prolonged thyroid dysfunction such as Hashimoto's or other thyroid diseases can significantly impact your long-term well-being and require regular monitoring and an ongoing commitment to lifestyle changes to manage symptoms and improve outcomes. While medical support is often essential, lifestyle choices will always play a crucial role in managing these diseases. This combined approach gives the body the resources and stability it needs.

Finding hope and success amid a diagnosis

Receiving a diagnosis isn't the end of your journey. It's the beginning of a path toward transformation and healing. It offers clarity and direction, empowering you to take control of your health. With the right knowledge, support, and lifestyle changes, many symptoms can be managed or even reversed, giving you the tools to improve your physical and mental health.

Maintaining Hormone Balance

While conventional approaches — such as medication for thyroid issues — are undeniably valuable in managing and alleviating symptoms (particularly in acute or severe cases), over recent decades, both the general public and medical professionals have lost sight of the personal power people hold to prevent hormonal imbalances and address root causes simply through daily choices.

In previous generations, people had the luxury of living in relatively nontoxic environments, free from today's barrage of processed foods, toxic 24/7 news cycles and hormone-disrupting chemicals. We need to accept that the landscape has changed. We can no longer afford to be passive about our health, assuming that Western medicine alone will patch things up. Chapters 6, 7, and 11 explore how our fast-paced, convenience-driven lifestyles have led to a reliance on quick fixes — something that offers immediate relief — but the inescapable truth is that the pressures of modern life place significant strain on our bodies. Now, more than ever, taking proactive, informed action is essential for maintaining balance.

Finding motivation

TIP

Finding your "why" for this journey is essential, whether it's the desire for more energy, improved mood, better sleep, boosting fertility, losing weight, or setting yourself up for great health in later life. Your why serves as your North Star — the guiding motivation that keeps you focused and resilient through the inevitable ups and downs of this lifelong journey.

What many of my clients find reassuring to learn is that the human body possesses a remarkable ability to regenerate itself. For example, I shocked my general practitioner by reversing my post-pill PCOS and healing the multiple cysts on my ovaries by staying dedicated to this work. Your body wants to heal and self-repair, you just need to give it the right support. Of course, while not all diseases or more serious conditions can be entirely reversed, some can, and these interventions will certainly help alleviate symptoms and optimize your health.

Taking radical responsibility

What I hope I have been making clear is that your body is not betraying you; it's merely responding to the environment and circumstances in which it has been placed. Yes, modern life has put incredible strain on your hormones. Yes, the available information is often confusing. And yes, it's easy to feel lost in a medical system that often treats your body as a series of isolated parts rather than an interconnected system. However, you have endless opportunities to use the knowledge you'll gain throughout these chapters, listen to your body, identify root causes, and begin making necessary changes.

REMEMBER

Taking radical responsibility for your health isn't about blaming yourself when things go wrong. (You want to reduce stress levels, and blaming yourself won't do that!) It's about owning your power in every situation and seeing obstacles as opportunities to rise rather than as reasons to give up or as evidence that it won't work out for you.

Short- versus long-term measures

Achieving lasting hormone health requires a blend of both short- and long-term strategies. By addressing immediate needs while also investing in sustainable habits, you can create a strong foundation for lifelong well-being:

- **Short-term measures**, such as using birth control for painful periods, taking targeted supplements, or practicing stress-relief techniques, offer quick relief and help manage acute symptoms. While these solutions can make the journey smoother, they're only part of the equation and aren't sufficient for lasting balance on their own.
- **Long-term measures**, such as prioritizing balanced, nutrient-dense meals, committing to quality sleep, resolving past trauma, processing stored emotions, and building muscle mass (all covered in Part 4) are the true pillars of sustainable hormone health. It's this consistent dedication to hormone-supportive lifestyle changes that ultimately fosters resilience and sets the stage for lifelong balance.

Why Hormone Health Matters More Than Ever

WARNING

Unfortunately, existing passively in the modern world is almost a guaranteed recipe for imbalance and disease. We're surrounded by factors that chip away at our hormonal resilience, making issues such as PCOS, thyroid disorders, infertility, low sperm counts, and metabolic diseases more common than ever before. Achieving hormone balance is no longer just a wellness trend or "nice to have." It's a critical necessity and form of self-protection that builds a foundation for long-term vitality and disease prevention both for you and future generations.

Taking control of your hormones means stepping back into the driver's seat of your health, unlocking your full power, confidence, and potential. You deserve nothing less than to be at your best — feeling energized, resilient, and unstoppable.

Long-term risks of imbalances

REMEMBER

Hormonal imbalances have a cascading effect that can compromise long-term health and resilience across a wide range of bodily systems. For instance, autoimmune diseases such as Hashimoto's disease, rheumatoid arthritis, and lupus are closely tied to hormone fluctuations — particularly cortisol, which can intensify autoimmune activity and inflammation.

Metabolic disruptions, especially those involving insulin and leptin, can pave the way for serious conditions like non-alcoholic fatty liver disease (NAFLD), leading to progressive liver inflammation. Cardiovascular health is equally dependent on hormonal equilibrium; imbalances in cortisol and insulin can drive high blood pressure and dyslipidemia (unhealthy cholesterol profiles), which ultimately increase the risk of heart disease.

Chapter 13 explores these issues in greater detail, covering signs and symptoms of chronic inflammation, imbalances, conditions and diseases, guidance on when to seek professional help, and practical advice on choosing the right support for your journey.

Gender-specific risks

For men, imbalances in testosterone and cortisol have a profound impact on overall health. Low testosterone levels may result in a loss of muscle mass, reduced energy, diminished libido, and lower sperm quality, all of which impact vitality and fertility. Chronic elevation of cortisol also raises the risk of cardiovascular problems and metabolic conditions such as type 2 diabetes and heart disease.

In women, fluctuations in estrogen, progesterone, and cortisol present unique challenges. A decline in estrogen, particularly during and after menopause, increases the risk of osteoporosis due to its effect on bone density. Excess estrogen, exacerbated by xenoestrogens (environmental chemicals that mimic estrogen) and poor gut health, can raise the risk of estrogen-dominant cancers and conditions such as fibroids and endometriosis. Low progesterone contributes to menstrual irregularities, mood disturbances, and fertility issues. Chronic cortisol imbalances can lead to weight gain, osteoporosis, and reproductive health disorders such as PCOS.

Balance: A gift that keeps on giving

Maintaining healthy hormone levels requires consistent care and attention. Life changes — such as aging, starting a new diet, landing a promotion, or divorce — can disrupt your hormonal harmony. The key is learning how to tend to your hormones throughout all stages of life, ensuring they remain resilient and adaptable to whatever comes your way to reduce the risk of developing more severe diseases and conditions in the future.

When your hormones are balanced, you feel energized, clear-minded, and confident — ready to fully embrace life and share your unique gifts with the world. The symptoms you may currently face will become valuable guides as you make your way through this book, pointing you toward toward areas of growth and transformation.

IN THIS CHAPTER

» Meeting the major hormones and their jobs around the body

» Exploring how hormones are made and travel to their destination

» Understanding the functions of your endocrine glands and organs

» Getting to know your hormonal "clocks"

Chapter 2

Getting to Know the Endocrine System

Everyone has a miraculous, self-governing hormone system known as the *endocrine system* that is focused on helping your body function properly. Its network of hormones, organs, and glands works 24/7, all year round. In fact, there are more than 50 different hormones that play a vital role in various processes in your body. Yeah, once you dive into the world of hormones it can get overwhelming and confusing pretty fast. But, luckily for us, hormones operate in a hierarchical structure, which means that focusing on a key group of hormones is not only more manageable but often enough to make a significant impact on your overall health. By targeting these core hormones, you can address many foundational aspects of hormone balance, which in turn helps regulate other hormones and bodily processes. Think of it like a positive domino effect, where adjusting these core hormones sets off a chain reaction, helping other hormones naturally fall into balance. It's a targeted approach that simplifies hormone health, empowering you to make meaningful changes without the overwhelm of micromanaging each hormone.

In this chapter, I introduce you to the major hormones in your endocrine system and explain the roles that they play in helping your body maintain homeostasis (balance). You'll get to know what your hormones are made from, the various endocrine glands and organs that build and secrete them, as well as the different biological clocks that turn hormones on or off and up or down to keep everything running smoothly and regulating processes such as sleep, energy, reproduction, and metabolism.

Understanding the Major Hormones and Their Jobs

Hormones are signaling molecules created by endocrine (hormone-producing) glands that travel via the blood and other bodily fluids to arrive at their destinations and affect nearly every process in your body. As chemical messengers, their role is to coordinate and regulate processes by sending signals from the endocrine system to various organs and tissues to ensure that the body functions properly and responds to internal and external signals, such as the sunrise or eating a meal. Most hormones work by telling different organs and systems when to start or stop certain activities. Some hormones even interact with each other.

So, in this section, I introduce you to the body's major hormones and break down our current understanding of their different roles across the body.

Stress hormones: Cortisol and adrenaline

Two of the most well-known hormones are cortisol and adrenaline, which play important roles in your fight/flight/freeze/fawn response. You're probably familiar with feeling your heartbeat increasing before a big sporting event, as you prepare to talk in front of a crowd, or when you experience sexual attraction. These are just some of the reactions in your body driven by these two powerful stress hormones.

TIP

Although it's often seen in a negative light, stress isn't always a bad thing. In fact, in moderate amounts, it can be incredibly beneficial, helping to sharpen your focus and boost energy.

Cortisol

REMEMBER

Cortisol is often referred to as the "primary stress hormone" because of its extremely influential effect on your body. In a nutshell, its job is to keep you alive, healthy, and safe from threats, whether they're real, imagined, or perceived (meaning they may not be objectively dangerous but are interpreted as threats based on past experiences or trauma; read more in Chapter 9). As I explain in

Chapter 3, cortisol is a tier 1 hormone, meaning it's a pretty big deal in the hormone hierarchy! It can be helpful to think of it like a team leader who helps coordinate the other hormones and sets long-term strategies to ensure everything runs smoothly over time. Given cortisol's central role in maintaining hormonal balance, I dedicate significant attention to explaining the different ways it impacts your hormonal health in Chapter 16 and offer practical solutions in Chapter 17. For now, here are some of its key functions:

- **Regulating production of other hormones:** Cortisol helps your body quickly and effectively respond to internal or external changes, threats, or dangers by regulating the production of other hormones, such as melatonin, testosterone, hormones, estrogen, and progesterone. Read Chapter 3 to find out more about how this works.
- **Regulating metabolism:** To ensure that you have enough energy to handle prolonged stress or react quickly to danger, cortisol helps regulate how your body uses fats, proteins, and carbohydrates and influences your blood sugar and insulin levels. Read Chapters 16 and 17 for more details.
- **Impacting inflammation:** During stress, cortisol reduces inflammation by suppressing the immune response, helping to prevent overreactions that could be harmful. However, when you're exposed to prolonged stress and high levels of cortisol, your tissues become less sensitive to cortisol, and inflammation increases.
- **Controlling the sleep-wake cycle:** The secretion of cortisol by the adrenal glands follows a daily rhythm when healthy and balanced, peaking in the early morning to wake you up and gradually decreasing throughout the day to prepare you for sleep.
- **Managing stress:** Cortisol levels increase during stress, providing a burst of energy by increasing blood sugar levels and enhancing your brain's use of glucose. It also suppresses nonessential functions, such as digestion and reproduction, to prioritize your body's immediate survival.

REMEMBER

Adrenaline (epinephrine)

REMEMBER

Whereas cortisol is a team leader, adrenaline is part of the emergency response team. When an immediate threat arises, adrenaline rushes to the scene, acting quickly to address the crisis and mobilize resources. It takes cues from cortisol, ensuring that emergency actions align with the broader needs of the body and together, they ensure that you're ready to handle whatever challenges you may face.

Adrenaline's roles include the following:

- **Increasing heart rate:** Adrenaline ensures that more blood — and therefore more oxygen and nutrients — reaches your muscles and vital organs.
- **Expanding air passages:** It relaxes the muscles around your airways, allowing more air to enter your lungs and increasing oxygen supply to your body.
- **Enlarging pupils:** Adrenaline dilates your pupils, improving your vision and allowing you to better assess the situation.
- **Redistributing blood to muscles:** To prepare you for quick physical action, adrenaline redirects blood from nonessential areas (like your skin and digestive system) to your muscles.
- **Mobilizing energy stores:** It helps your body get quick energy by breaking down stored sugar (glycogen) into glucose in the liver and muscles. It also releases fat from fat cells, giving your body even more fuel to handle stress.

Blood sugar hormone: Insulin

REMEMBER

Insulin is another team leader (read about tier 1 hormones in Chapter 3), but it's widely misunderstood and often demonized in discussions about insulin resistance, type 2 diabetes, weight gain, and conditions such as polycystic ovary syndrome (PCOS). As a powerful and essential hormone for maintaining overall hormonal harmony, insulin deserves closer examination, which is why I delve deeply into its role and regulation in Chapters 16 and 17. For now, the key point to embrace is that when insulin balance is disrupted, your body provides key insights through symptoms, signaling what it may need to restore equilibrium. Let's explore its role in more detail:

- **Regulating blood sugar levels:** When you eat, your food breaks down into glucose, increasing your blood sugar levels. Insulin is released by the pancreas to help transport glucose from the bloodstream into your cells, providing them with energy and lowering blood sugar levels back to a safe range. However, if your body doesn't produce enough insulin, or if your cells become resistant to its effects (a condition known as insulin resistance), blood sugar levels can remain elevated in an unhealthy range. This can lead to metabolic complications, such as prediabetes or type 2 diabetes.
- **Storing and using energy:** Think of insulin as a master planner for energy storage and use. It signals cells to take in glucose to be used for immediate energy or stored for the future. When your body has enough energy, insulin helps store excess glucose in the liver and muscles as glycogen. It also promotes the storage of fat for long-term energy reserves.

- **Regulating metabolism:** Insulin plays a central role in regulating metabolism, but it doesn't work alone. It interacts closely with other hormones, such as cortisol, to control the body's use of fats, proteins, and carbohydrates, ensuring efficient and balanced energy production (refer to Chapter 16 for further explanation). This interaction with cortisol is crucial because cortisol can raise blood sugar levels during stress, while insulin helps to counterbalance this effect by enabling cells to absorb glucose.
- **Promoting cellular growth and repair:** Insulin encourages the absorption of amino acids into cells, which are the building blocks for proteins and are essential for repairing tissues and promoting growth.
- **Influencing other hormones:** Insulin not only helps control blood sugar but also influences other hormones. It works with glucagon, which raises blood sugar, by telling the liver to release stored glucose. This teamwork keeps your blood sugar levels steady all day.
- **Clues about the body's needs:** Imbalances in insulin levels can signal what your body needs — more muscle, more movement, better sleep, or less stress. I talk about how to read your body's signals in Chapters 15 and 16.

TIP

Precursor hormones: Pregnenolone and DHEA

REMEMBER

A "precursor" is something that leads to the creation of something else. Think of it like the dough for a pizza: Before you can have a delicious pizza, you need the dough as the base.

Similarly, precursor hormones are the basic ingredients or the raw materials that your body uses to produce the final, active hormones that perform various functions in the body. By understanding and managing the precursor hormones, you can influence the production and balance of the other active hormones.

Pregnenolone and dehydroepiandrosterone (DHEA) are the two of the most influential precursor hormones that form the foundation for much of the body's hormone production.

Pregnenolone

Known as the "grandmother of all hormones," pregnenolone serves as the starting point for the synthesis (creation) of many other hormones, including DHEA, progesterone, and cortisol. Pregnenolone's other roles include

- **Improving brain function:** Pregnenolone is important for thinking and memory. It protects neurons, which are the cells in your brain that send messages and helps create new connections between them. This keeps your mind clear and sharp.

- **Balancing mood:** By contributing to the production of progesterone and other hormones, pregnenolone helps to stabilize mood and reduce feelings of stress and anxiety.
- **Boosting energy and stamina:** By aiding in the production of other important hormones, pregnenolone contributes to better overall energy levels, increases stamina, and reduces fatigue, making it easier to stay active and alert throughout the day.

Dehydroepiandrosterone

DHEA, which is often called the "mother of all hormones" because it's the daughter of pregnenolone, is the powerful precursor to sex hormones such as estrogen and testosterone. Its other roles include the following:

- **Supporting immune function:** DHEA stimulates the production and activity of immune cells, such as T-cells, which are essential for fighting off infections and diseases.
- **Enhancing mood and energy levels:** By influencing the production of sex hormones, DHEA plays a role in maintaining mood stability and energy levels. Adequate levels of DHEA can enhance the production of serotonin and dopamine, which are often called "happy hormones" and are covered later in this chapter. Additionally, DHEA helps combat fatigue by supporting adrenal function and promoting better stress resilience, contributing to an overall sense of vitality and mental clarity.
- **Promoting muscle and bone health:** DHEA is essential for preventing conditions such as osteoporosis and maintaining muscle mass and bone density as you age. It promotes muscle growth by reducing the breakdown of muscle proteins.

WARNING

Now, you might be thinking that taking a DHEA supplement could be a quick way to support your hormones. However, supplementing with DHEA isn't generally recommended because it can disrupt your body's natural hormone balance and lead to unwanted side effects. Exceptions exist in specific therapeutic contexts, such as hormone replacement therapy (HRT) for menopausal symptoms, where DHEA can sometimes be safely applied under medical supervision. For most people, though, it's much more effective to focus on lifestyle strategies that naturally support healthy DHEA levels — such as stress management, adequate sleep, and regular exercise — as outlined in Part 4 of this book.

Reproductive hormones: Estrogen, progesterone, androgens, and testosterone

REMEMBER

Most people are first introduced to hormones in school during sex education, where they learn about sex hormones as they enter puberty. But what many aren't taught is that these hormones are responsible for so much more than your reproductive health and awkward teenage changes. They influence everything from mood to muscle mass and even how bodies respond to stress! What's fascinating is that these hormones aren't static; they change as you grow and age, adapting to your body's evolving needs. (I go into much more detail in Chapter 4.)

REMEMBER

In the following overview of the reproductive hormones, for simplicity, I will only be focusing on cisgender male and female bodies. I acknowledge that the experiences of transgender and nonbinary individuals are complex and deserve their own dedicated exploration, which is beyond the scope of this chapter. When referring to male bodies, I mean AMAB (assigned male at birth); I mean AFAB (assigned female at birth) when referring to female bodies. These terms recognize the biological aspects of sex assigned at birth while being inclusive of all gender identities.

Estrogen

Although it's often seen as the "female" hormone, estrogen plays important roles in both male and female bodies. To keep things straightforward, I discuss estrogen as a single hormone, even though it actually refers to a group of hormones, including estradiol, estrone, and estriol, each of which has unique functions and varying significance at different life stages.

Estrogen in female bodies does the following:

REMEMBER

- **Regulates the menstrual cycle and reproduction:** Estrogen is crucial for the development and regulation of the female reproductive system and menstrual cycle. It helps prepare the body for pregnancy and ensures that the entire process runs smoothly. Additionally, estrogen can boost libido in women, contributing to sexual desire and overall sexual health.
- **Protects bone health:** Estrogen acts like a structural engineer, ensuring your body's framework (bone density) remains strong and resilient. It helps prevent the breakdown of bone tissue, which is why female bodies experience an increased risk of osteoporosis during menopause, when estrogen levels drop significantly.
- **Improves skin and hair:** It stimulates the production of collagen, a protein that maintains skin elasticity and firmness, keeping your skin looking youthful and radiant. It also helps with the hydration and thickness of your hair, giving it that healthy shine and reducing hair loss.

- **Aids brain function:** Estrogen plays a significant role in cognitive functions, including memory and mood regulation. It supports neuron health (the cells in your brain that send messages) and contributes to mental sharpness and emotional stability. Balanced estrogen levels are linked to better cognitive health and a reduced risk of neurodegenerative diseases such as Alzheimer's and Parkinson's. This is also why many women experience memory issues and "brain fog" during menopause; the decline in estrogen levels can affect brain function and cognitive clarity.

REMEMBER

- **Regulates fat distribution:** Estrogen helps manage body fat distribution in women, reducing the accumulation of fat in the abdominal area and promoting a more balanced distribution of body fat. This contributes to a healthier body composition and reduces the risk of metabolic disorders.

Estrogen in male bodies works alongside testosterone to help maintain healthy libido and sexual function. It also supports bone health, aids brain function, and regulates fat distribution. Low levels of estrogen can lead to reduced sexual desire and erectile dysfunction.

Progesterone

Progesterone is the calming, reliable, behind-the-scenes force that ensures everything runs smoothly. It's diligent and stabilizing, and its presence is crucial for maintaining both mental and physical balance in the body, as well as supporting a healthy pregnancy.

Progesterone in female bodies

- **Regulates the menstrual cycle and pregnancy:** Progesterone helps regulate the menstrual cycle and is essential for maintaining pregnancy. It helps ensure there is a stable and supportive environment for the embryo, reducing the risk of miscarriage in the early stages of pregnancy.
- **Balances mood:** Progesterone is like nature's little chill pill. It has a profound calming effect on the brain by interacting with GABA receptors (a neurotransmitter that acts as your brain's "calm-down" signal, reducing excitability and promoting relaxation). Progesterone reduces anxiety, and improves sleep quality, helping to keep you relaxed and balanced, especially during the luteal phase of the menstrual cycle for women when its levels peak. This can help mitigate premenstrual syndrome (PMS) symptoms, such as mood swings.
- **Supporting thyroid function:** It plays a crucial role in supporting thyroid function, which is essential for regulating your energy balance and metabolism. Its role is to help convert inactive thyroid hormones (T4) into their active form (T3), preventing symptoms of hypothyroidism, such as fatigue, weight gain, and depression.

REMEMBER

- **Breast health:** Estrogen encourages breast tissue to grow while progesterone helps keep this growth in check, ensuring that breast tissue grows and maintains itself properly. This balance reduces the risk of developing noncancerous breast conditions and may also lower the risk of breast cancer.

In male bodies, progesterone:

- **Supports sexual health:** In men, progesterone helps balance the effects of estrogen and testosterone, contributing to overall sexual health. It also plays a role in sperm development by regulating the environment within the testes and maintaining libido.

REMEMBER

- **Prostate health:** By balancing the effects of estrogen and preventing the overgrowth of prostate tissue, progesterone helps keep prostate growth in check and reduces the risk of benign prostatic hyperplasia (BPH), a common condition in older men that can affect urinary function.

Progesterone also influences mood and sleep and aids maintaining a healthy weight, energy levels, and overall vitality, just as it does in women.

Androgens

Androgens are a group of hormones often referred to as "male" hormones, but they are present and important in both men and women. The most well-known and significant androgen is testosterone, but other key players include hormones such as androstenedione and dihydrotestosterone (DHT). In a nutshell, the role of androgens is to help define male characteristics, such as increased muscle mass and facial hair.

REMEMBER

Androgens in male bodies contribute to the following processes:

- **Development of male characteristics:** Androgens play a central role during puberty for shaping physical attributes, such as the growth of facial and body hair, deepening of the voice, and increased muscle mass.
- **Sperm production:** They are essential for the production of sperm, support the development of the testes, and ensure the proper functioning of the male reproductive system, contributing to fertility.
- **Maintenance of muscle mass and bone density:** These hormones are essential for physical strength and structural integrity, which means they play a major role in why men typically have greater muscle mass and stronger bones than women.

- **Libido regulation:** Adequate levels are crucial for maintaining a healthy libido and erectile function.
- **Mood and energy support:** Low levels of androgens can lead to symptoms such as fatigue, depression, and irritability while balanced androgen levels help keep spirits and energy levels high.
- **Metabolism support:** Androgens play a vital role in maintaining a healthy metabolism in men, contributing to muscle mass, fat distribution, bone health, energy levels and glucose regulation.

In female bodies, androgens play the following roles:

REMEMBER

- **Influence sexual desire:** Peaks in androgen levels can enhance sexual desire, particularly around ovulation (more on this in Chapters 4 and 11).
- **Impact hair growth:** While balanced androgen levels contribute to normal hair growth patterns, excessive levels can lead to conditions such as hirsutism (excessive hair growth in areas where men typically grow hair). This is often seen in conditions like PCOS, where elevated androgen levels can cause unwanted hair growth, among other symptoms.

As they do in men, androgens in women help maintain muscle mass and bone density, regulate mood and energy, and support metabolism.

Testosterone

The most famous androgen, testosterone, is a hormone capable of developing "masculine characteristics" in reproductive tissues, like the genital tract, and secondary sexual characteristics such as muscle mass and bone density. I explore age-related changes to testosterone for men in much more detail in Chapters 4 and 11. This section takes a closer look at its role in both men and women.

REMEMBER

In male bodies, testosterone

- **Promotes muscle and bone strength:** Testosterone is like the body's innate form of weightlifting, helping to build and maintain muscle mass and strong bones. This is why men typically have more muscle mass than women and why maintaining testosterone levels is important as you age.
- **Enhances mood and energy:** Low levels of testosterone can lead to feelings of fatigue, depression, and irritability. Think of it as a mood booster that helps keep your spirits high and your energy levels up.
- **Supports libido:** Adequate levels are essential for maintaining a healthy libido and sperm production. Men usually experience a peak in sexual desire in the morning when testosterone levels are highest.

REMEMBER

Testosterone in female bodies maintains muscle and bone strength (although it's present in lower levels than in men), helps to stabilize mood and energy levels, and plays a significant role in sexual desire and responsiveness. Peaks in testosterone levels around ovulation lead to periods of increased desire.

Sleep hormone: Melatonin

Melatonin is produced in response to darkness and signals to your body that it's time to prepare for sleep, but it also has other numerous other roles and benefits:

- **Regulating the sleep-wake cycle:** Melatonin levels rise in the evening, remain high throughout the night, and decrease in the early morning. This pattern helps you fall asleep and stay asleep through the night, promoting restful and restorative sleep.
- **Synchronizing circadian rhythms:** Melatonin helps align your body's internal clock with the external environment, ensuring that both your circadian and infradian rhythms are supporting your daily functions and the proper release of hormones to ensure your long-term well-being.

REMEMBER

TIP

Read more about circadian and infradian rhythms later in this chapter in the "Keeping Time with Your Hormonal 'Clocks'" section.

- **Antioxidant properties:** Melatonin protects your cells from damage, reducing your risk of various diseases.
- **Immune system support:** It enhances the production and activity of immune cells, which helps the defend against infections and illnesses more effectively. This is the reason you often get the advice to "sleep it off" when you're sick.
- **Influencing mood:** Proper melatonin levels help prevent sleep disorders and related mood issues such as depression and anxiety.

REMEMBER

Thyroid hormones: T3 and T4

Thyroxine (T4) and triiodothyronine (T3) play really important roles in regulating your body's metabolism, energy production, and overall growth and development. In fact, they influence nearly every cell in the body. I explore the factors contributing to the rise in thyroid imbalances in Chapter 7, but for now, here are some of these hormones' jobs:

REMEMBER

- **Regulating metabolism:** T3 and T4 regulate your metabolic rate, which influences how quickly you burn calories and how efficiently your body converts food into energy.

- **Producing energy:** These hormones ensure your cells have the energy they need to function correctly by increasing production of the energy currency of cells, ATP (adenosine triphosphate).
- **Promoting growth and development:** They are essential for normal growth and development, particularly in children, and contribute to the development of the brain and nervous system, making them critical during pregnancy and early childhood.
- **Regulating temperature:** By influencing your metabolic rate, thyroid hormones play a role in maintaining your body temperature. They help your body produce heat, ensuring that you stay warm in cooler environments.
- **Promoting heart health:** They help regulate heart rate and blood pressure, ensure that your heart pumps efficiently, and provide your body with the oxygen and nutrients it needs.
- **Maintaining mood and cognitive function:** Adequate levels of T3 and T4 are necessary for maintaining mental clarity, mood stability, and cognitive function.

Growth hormone: Human growth hormone

Human growth hormone (HGH) supports a wide array of processes such as muscle growth, bone strength, cognitive function, mood, tissue repair, and energy regulation (metabolism). HGH levels peak during puberty and gradually decline with age, but it continues to promote healing and maintain body composition throughout adulthood.

WARNING

Doctors often prescribe synthetic growth hormone to help children with impaired hormone levels reach their full height. However, there is also a black-market trade in synthetic HGH, particularly among athletes, bodybuilders, and individuals seeking a more muscular appearance. Despite the popularity of synthetic growth hormone, any perceived improvement in muscle strength is more likely due to other substances, such as steroids. Using synthetic HGH without medical supervision can lead to serious health risks, including heart disease, joint pain, and abnormal growth patterns, please consult with a professional.

Happy hormones: Dopamine, oxytocin, serotonin, and endorphins

REMEMBER

When it comes to feeling happy, fulfilled, and generally well, there are a few key players in the body's chemistry that make it all possible. The collective terms for them is DOSE: dopamine, oxytocin, serotonin, and endorphins.

Dopamine: The reward and pleasure hormone

REMEMBER

Dopamine is a key player in your brain's reward system. It's released during enjoyable activities such as eating, exercising, and socializing, creating a sense of pleasure and reinforcing behaviors that make you feel good. Its release encourages you to repeat actions that bring you pleasure and satisfaction.

Dopamine is so influential on overall health and behavior that it's considered a tier 1 hormone in this book, meaning it holds foundational importance for hormone balance. As explained in Chapter 3 and explored in detail in Chapters 16 and 17, dopamine's regulation affects other hormones in a cascading effect. Therefore, understanding and managing dopamine levels can be a game-changer for achieving and sustaining overall hormonal balance. So, let's take a look at what else it helps with:

- **Motivation and drive:** Dopamine is often referred to as the "motivation molecule" because it drives you to pursue goals and rewards. When you achieve something challenging, the surge of dopamine you experience reinforces your behavior, making you more likely to pursue similar goals in the future.
- **Motor control:** Dopamine is crucial for coordinating smooth and controlled muscle movements. A dopamine deficiency can lead to motor control issues, such as those seen in Parkinson's disease.
- **Mood regulation:** Low levels of dopamine are associated with feelings of apathy, sadness, and depression. By maintaining adequate dopamine levels, the brain can help stabilize mood and promote optimism.

WARNING

Although dopamine is essential for motivation and pleasure, it also plays a role in addiction. Substances like drugs and alcohol and certain behaviors such as gambling and using social media apps can hijack the dopamine system, leading to excessive release and reinforcing the addictive behavior. Understanding dopamine's role in addiction is crucial for developing effective treatment strategies.

Oxytocin: The love and bonding hormone

Oxytocin, often referred to as the love hormone or cuddle hormone, is released in large amounts during activities that foster closeness and connection, such as hugging, cuddling your pet, childbirth, and breastfeeding. It helps create strong social bonds by promoting feelings of love, trust, and empathy.

As a tier 1 hormone, which is discussed in Chapter 3 and explored more deeply in Chapters 16 and 17, oxytocin is far more than a simple "feel-good" hormone. It has profound physiological and psychological effects and influences broader aspects of our health, including stress resilience, emotional regulation, and even physical healing. For example, one of its critical functions is lowering cortisol levels, which helps mitigate the effects of chronic stress and creates a sense of safety and calm in the body.

Understanding and actively supporting oxytocin levels is, therefore, vital for achieving and maintaining overall hormone balance. Its ability to shape how we think, feel, and act solidifies its role as a key player in optimizing our well-being. Let's dive into some of its fascinating roles:

- **Social bonding:** Oxytocin helps to deepen connections between partners, friends, and family members. It promotes feelings of trust and security, making it easier to form and maintain relationships.
- **Wound healing:** Interestingly, oxytocin also plays a role in physical health by promoting wound healing. It reduces inflammation and aids in tissue repair, helping the body recover from injuries.
- **Childbirth and lactation:** During childbirth, oxytocin levels rise, stimulating contractions that speed up delivery of the baby. Post-birth, it helps with the ejection of milk during breastfeeding, ensuring the infant receives adequate nutrition.

TIP

- **Stress reduction:** Oxytocin has a calming effect on the body, reducing stress and anxiety levels. When you're participating in activities that boost oxytocin (such as laughing with friends), it counters the effects of cortisol, promoting relaxation and emotional stability.

Serotonin: The mood stabilizer

While dopamine (which I talk about earlier in this chapter) delivers quick bursts of pleasure, serotonin is the steady, reliable friend that helps you maintain a lasting sense of contentment and emotional stability. Here are some of the other things this mood-boosting chemical is up to behind the scenes:

- **Appetite control:** By creating a sense of satiety (feeling full), serotonin can prevent overeating and support healthy eating habits.
- **Mood regulation:** It reduces feelings of depression and anxiety and promotes feelings of happiness and contentment.

REMEMBER

- **Sleep regulation:** Serotonin is a precursor to melatonin, the sleep hormones I mention earlier in this chapter, which means the more serotonin you have, the better your sleep will be.

» **Cognitive functions:** Optimal serotonin levels are essential for maintaining mental clarity, memory, learning, and focus.

» **Gut health:** What's fascinating is that about 90 percent of serotonin is found in the digestive system, where it regulates bowel movements and function. This connection highlights just how important our gut health is for overall well-being. You can read more on that in Chapter 9.

Endorphins: The feel-good chemicals

Endorphins are the body's natural painkillers, produced by the hypothalamus and pituitary gland in response to pain or stress. In fact, there are about 20 different types of endorphins, with the most researched being beta-endorphin, the one famously linked to the runner's high.

Your body releases endorphins not only during exercise but also when you laugh, fall in love, have sex, and even enjoy a delicious meal. This release of endorphins encourages you to seek out the activities that make you feel good, helping to stabilize your mood, get through painful experiences (such as intense exercise, injury, or stress) and generally enhance your overall well-being.

TIP

You can increase your body's endorphin release by engaging in these activities:

» **Meditating and doing breathwork:** Breathing deeply and focusing your brain calms your mind and eases pain.

» **Receiving acupuncture:** An effective way to release endorphins is with pressure points. Placing fine needles into the skin at specific points around the body (or lying on an acupressure mat at home) triggers the release of endorphins.

» **Playing music:** When you sing, dance, or play instruments, you do more than entertain yourself or others. You also release a rush of endorphins, which research suggests could increase your pain tolerance.

» **Laughing:** A good belly laugh can do wonders for your state of mind. Along with releasing endorphins, laughter boosts serotonin and dopamine.

» **Basking in ultraviolet light:** Ultraviolet light stimulates the release of beta-endorphins in the skin. For those winter months or days spent mostly indoors, using a UV light can be a helpful substitute for natural sunlight to keep those beta-endorphins flowing.

Getting to Know the Different Types of Hormones

To make sure your body can quickly and effectively send hormones wherever needed, they come in all shapes, forms, and sizes — kind of like a postal service offers specialized delivery methods. Hormones' differences allow them to interact with their target cells in just the right way, ensuring the right signals are sent and received so the body can keep running smoothly. After all, you don't want a love letter to be delivered to your boss, right? By understanding how these different hormones are built and delivered, you'll be empowered to give your body the right nutrition and support its needs.

Steroid hormones

Steroid hormones, which are made from a type of fat called cholesterol, are fat-soluble, which means they can easily pass through cell membranes (the cell's walls) and directly target or alter activities in the cell. An example is turning genes on or off to regulate processes like growth, metabolism, or your immune response.

REMEMBER

Cholesterol sadly has a bad reputation due to media coverage and health campaigns that focus on the dangers of high cholesterol — particularly its role in heart disease. However, it's important to remember that without cholesterol, your body can't produce these essential hormones: cortisol, testosterone, estrogen, progesterone, androgens, and precursor hormones pregnenolone and DHEA. A balanced diet is key to hormone health, so don't skip egg yolks and red meat!

Peptide and protein hormones

These hormones are made from chains of amino acids, the building blocks of proteins. Since they're water-soluble, they can't just waltz through cell membranes. Instead, they bind to receptors on the cell's surface. Think of the cell receptor as a lock and the hormone as the key. When the right key fits into the lock, it opens the door, triggering a specific response inside the cell. The hormones in this group are insulin, HGH, oxytocin, and thyroid-stimulating hormone, which regulates the production of T3 and T4.

TIP

There are 20 amino acids, and 9 of them are considered essential because your body can't produce them on its own. This is why it's important to eat a variety of protein-rich foods. Don't worry! I include a handy list for you in the online appendix at `https://www.dummies.com/go/hormonebalancefd`.

Amino acid–derived hormones

This type of hormone is like the solo artist of the hormone world, made from a single amino acid instead of a whole band like the group in the preceding section. Depending on their nature, they can be either water-soluble or fat-soluble, meaning some can sneak into cells, whereas others stay at the door. For instance, adrenaline (or epinephrine) knocks and binds to receptors on the cell's surface, but thyroid hormones like T3 and T4 have VIP access and can stroll right in to do their job.

The amino acid–derived hormones are adrenaline, T3 and T4 thyroid hormones, melatonin, dopamine, and serotonin.

Glycoprotein hormones

These hormones come with a special accessory — a carbohydrate! This little addition impacts how they travel and communicate in the body in a few important ways. For example, the attached carbohydrates can boost the hormone's stability in the bloodstream, acting like a shield that keeps it from being broken down too quickly. Plus, they help the hormone make a great first impression when it tries to connect with a cell's receptor.

TIP

That's why including healthy carbs such as whole grains, legumes, nuts, and seeds in your diet is key to making sure your body can produce these glycoproteins effectively.

The hormones in this group may not be the headliners, but they're still important! Here, I give you a quick introduction to their roles, but you can learn more about them in Chapter 11.

The glycoprotein hormones are

REMEMBER

- **Thyroid-stimulating hormone (TSH):** This one regulates the production of thyroid hormones T3 and T4.
- **Luteinizing hormone (LH):** This superstar in the reproductive system triggers ovulation in women and stimulates testosterone production in men.
- **Follicle-stimulating hormone (FSH):** This hormone is essential for reproductive health, promoting the growth of ovarian follicles in women and aiding sperm production in men.

Eicosanoids

Eicosanoids are like the body's fast-acting superheroes, derived from fatty acids and usually staying close to home rather than taking a grand tour through the bloodstream. These quick responders don't stick around for long, which is perfect for their mission: making sure inflammation is kept in check, fighting off infections, and helping the central nervous system react swiftly to any unexpected disruptions. They might not be as famous as the key players such as insulin or testosterone, but eicosanoids are the unsung heroes of your body's health squad. Without these specialized "first responders," your body would struggle to tackle injury and illness effectively.

TIP

Good sources of fatty acids in your diet include getting omega-3 fatty acids from salmon, mackerel, and sardines and omega-6 fatty acids from nuts, seeds, and poultry.

Reviewing the Function of Your Endocrine Glands and Organs

Let's hit pause on the hormones for a moment and zoom out to explore the wider endocrine system — the network that produces, stores, and releases these hormones. This system includes both primary glands and supporting organs.

Primary glands

Think of glands as specialized factories that work to produce and release important substances such as hormones, enzymes, and other vital fluids. If a gland's main job is hormone production, it's known as a *primary gland.*

The primary glands include the following:

- **Pituitary gland, the master gland:** The pituitary gland is your body's hormone conductor. It's a pea-shaped structure located at the base of your brain. Its main function is to instruct other glands to produce hormones while it produces HGH, prolactin (the hormone responsible for milk production, which I talk about in Chapter 4), LH, and FSH, and a few other hormones.
- **Thyroid gland, the butterfly gland or thermostat:** The thyroid gland, which is located in your neck, earned its nickname by being shaped like a butterfly. It controls the metabolic "temperature" of your body to ensure that everything runs smoothly and efficiently, and it produces hormones such as T3 and T4 to

regulate metabolism, body temperature, energy, heart rate, growth, and development.

- **Adrenal glands, the alarm system:** These two small, triangular glands sit atop the kidneys and produce a variety of hormones, including cortisol, DHEA, aldosterone (which regulates blood pressure), adrenaline (epinephrine), and some androgens. Although the adrenal glands produce small amounts of estrogen and testosterone, their main role is managing metabolism, immune responses, libido, and the stress response, all under the direction of the hypothalamus (see the next section) and pituitary gland, which I mention earlier in this list.
- **Pancreas, the glucose manager:** The pear-shaped pancreas is located behind your stomach. It helps regulate blood sugar/glucose by producing insulin, glucagon (which raises blood sugar when needed), and somatostatin, which helps balance these hormones.
- **Gonads (ovaries and testes), the reproductive coordinators:** The gonads, which are located in the pelvic region, produce reproductive hormones such as estrogen, progesterone, and testosterone.

Secondary organs

Organs, which are a group of tissues that work together, are more complex structures than glands. Because they have primary duties beyond hormone production, they're labeled "secondary." But don't let the name fool you. The following secondary endocrine organs are still crucial players in keeping your body in top form:

REMEMBER

- **Hypothalamus, the control center:** From its location in the brain, the hypothalamus is the control center that links the nervous system to the endocrine system via the pituitary gland. The hormones it produces regulate the pituitary gland to control the release of TSH and HGH. Essentially, the hypothalamus is the master regulator that ensures your body maintains balance.

TIP

- **Fat tissue (adipose tissue), the surprising one:** Fat tissue isn't just a place where your body stores energy; it's also an active endocrine organ that produces leptin (for regulating appetite), adiponectin (for glucose metabolism), and estradiol (a type of estrogen). This is why managing a healthy body fat percentage supports balanced hormone levels.
- **Pineal gland, the sleep regulator:** The pinecone-shaped pineal gland lives deep in the brain, where it produces melatonin, the sleep hormone.
- **Thymus, the immune training camp:** The thymus, located in the upper chest, is like the training camp for the immune system, particularly during

early life. It produces thymosin, a hormone that stimulates the development of T-cells, which are essential for immune response.

- **Gastrointestinal tract, the nutrition manager:** The gastrointestinal (GI) tract produces several hormones that aid in digestion and appetite regulation. For example, gastrin stimulates stomach acid production, ghrelin promotes hunger, and secretin helps regulate water and pH levels in the intestines. Additionally, peptide YY and cholecystokinin (CCK) signal satiety, helping to regulate food intake.
- **Heart, the blood pressure regulator:** Your heart produces atrial natriuretic peptide (ANP), a hormone that helps regulate blood pressure by promoting sodium and water excretion through the kidneys.
- **Kidneys, the oxygen monitors:** The kidneys, which are on either side of your spine below the rib cage, produce erythropoietin (EPO), a hormone that stimulates red blood cell production, and renin, which plays a key role in blood pressure regulation.
- **Liver, the detoxifier:** Located in the upper-right abdomen, the liver filters out and breaks down toxins, including excess hormones and substances that mimic hormones (more on that in Chapter 3), preventing them from causing hormonal imbalances, inflammation, or other health issues.

Keeping Time with Your Hormonal "Clocks"

Now, you might be thinking, "But how do all of these different hormones know when to turn on or off and adjust up or down?" This is where your body's biological clocks come into play. They are tightly linked and greatly influence each other.

Circadian rhythms: The 24-hour clock

TIP

You have a 24-hour internal clock in your brain that regulates many of your daily bodily processes such as digestion, body temperature, sleep, elimination, and the production of certain hormones. It's called the circadian rhythm, and it responds to light changes in your environment.

Here's a glimpse at how the circadian rhythm impacts hormones:

- **Regulation of sleep-wake cycle:** As shown in Figure 2-1, melatonin, which is produced in response to darkness, signals your body that it's time to sleep by rising in the evenings. Cortisol levels peak in the morning to wake you up and gradually decrease throughout the day.
- **Impact on metabolism:** Insulin also follows a circadian rhythm, meaning your body processes glucose more efficiently earlier in the day. As I explain in much more detail in Chapters 16 and 17, breakfast really is the most important meal!
- **Mental and physical performance:** HGH secretion peaks during deep sleep which is why adequate sleep is the best way to support muscle repair, immune function, and your overall well-being.

TIP

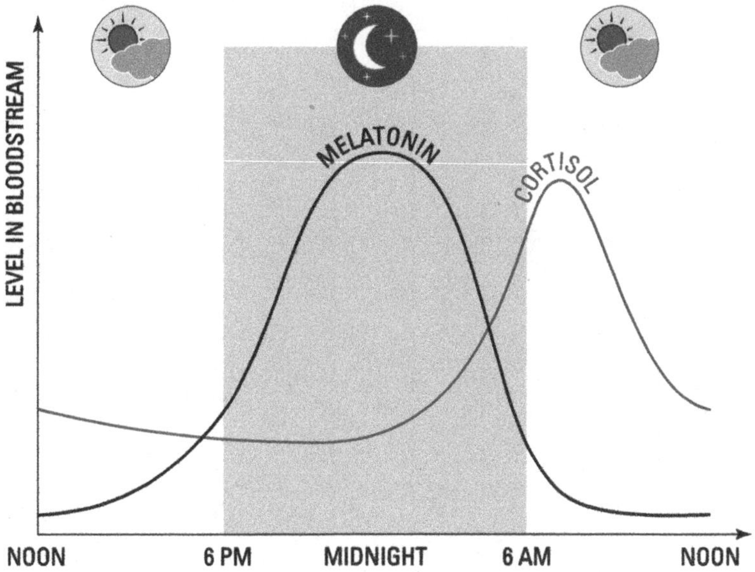

FIGURE 2-1: The circadian rhythm.

Infradian rhythm: Beyond 24-hour clock

REMEMBER

Women and those who menstruate have a second biological clock that kicks in at puberty and continues until menopause. Infradian rhythms are not unique to humans, however; you also see them nature, such as when bears hibernate during winter, birds migrate seasonally, and deer and other mammals breeding.

In humans, this rhythm is tied to the monthly menstrual cycle, which typically lasts 28 days and includes four distinct phases: menstruation, the follicular phase, ovulation, and the luteal phase. However, the infradian rhythm affects far more than just reproductive health. Just as the circadian rhythm governs daily bodily functions, the infradian rhythm influences brain chemistry and physiology, offering different strengths and gifts at various times throughout the month.

REMEMBER

Ignoring this natural rhythm can have significant consequences, from period and fertility issues to major physical and mental health challenges. For more on how to sync your life with your cycle, see Chapter 11.

IN THIS CHAPTER

» Understanding how hormones work together as a team

» Supporting the breakdown and safe elimination of hormones

Chapter 3
Meeting the Hormone Hierarchy

Have you ever considered how an orchestra works? Each instrument, from the violin to the flute, plays its unique part, yet they all come together to create a harmonious symphony. The orchestra has a hierarchy, with the conductor leading, the section leaders guiding their groups, and each musician contributing to the overall performance. This is very much like how hormones function in our bodies. Each hormone has its specific and unique role, but they all work together in a complex hierarchy to maintain balance and health.

In this chapter, I explain the intricate and cooperative nature of hormones. I deconstruct the hormone hierarchy for you to demonstrate how an imbalance in one hormone can set off a chain reaction — much like one out-of-tune instrument in an orchestra can disrupt the entire performance! You will gain insight into the chemistry that allows hormones to send messages between the brain and body to keep you healthy and begin to understand the importance of making sure your hormones are properly broken down and disposed of after they have finished their jobs. Importantly, you'll discover why it's crucial to avoid pesky "hormone-mimicking" chemicals and how they both mess with your hormone balance and your natural detoxification process.

Understanding the Cooperative Nature of Hormones

Hormones are not solitary actors; they function within an elaborate network where each hormone is an influencer and is influenced by others. This intricate interplay is essential for maintaining the body's internal balance, known as *homeostasis*. Just as an orchestra depends on each musician playing their part to execute a beautiful performance, your endocrine system (hormonal system) relies on the precise coordination of hormones to regulate physiological processes effectively.

Some of the key players, such as dopamine and oxytocin, go beyond their physiological roles and significantly influence mood, motivation, and social bonding. Just like an orchestra relies on the violin's melody or the percussion's rhythm to set the tone and pace, these hormones shape the emotional and behavioral "tempo" of the body. When they're out of sync, the entire performance — your hormonal balance — can feel chaotic or disjointed and it can be harder to stick to your healthy routine and habits.

Breaking down the hormone hierarchy

To understand how hormones work together, you need to understand the concept of the hormone hierarchy, which is illustrated in Figure 3-1. This hierarchy categorizes hormones based on their functions, interdependencies and how they shape your decision-making, mood, and behavior.

Your body has more than 50 hormones at work, but I focus on the most influential ones that play pivotal roles in regulating your health, emotional landscape, behavior, decision-making, and well-being, starting with the tier 1 hormones.

Tier 1: Foundational hormones

At the base of the hierarchy (refer to Figure 3-1) are the foundational hormones, which are crucial for the overall stability of the hormonal system and your body's ability to maintain homeostasis. Because these hormones directly affect the entire hormonal hierarchy (primary regulators) or your ability to maintain balance via the decisions you make (supportive modulators), they need to be prioritized in your hormone-balancing efforts to ensure the proper functioning of other hormones (refer to Chapter 2 for more detailed descriptions):

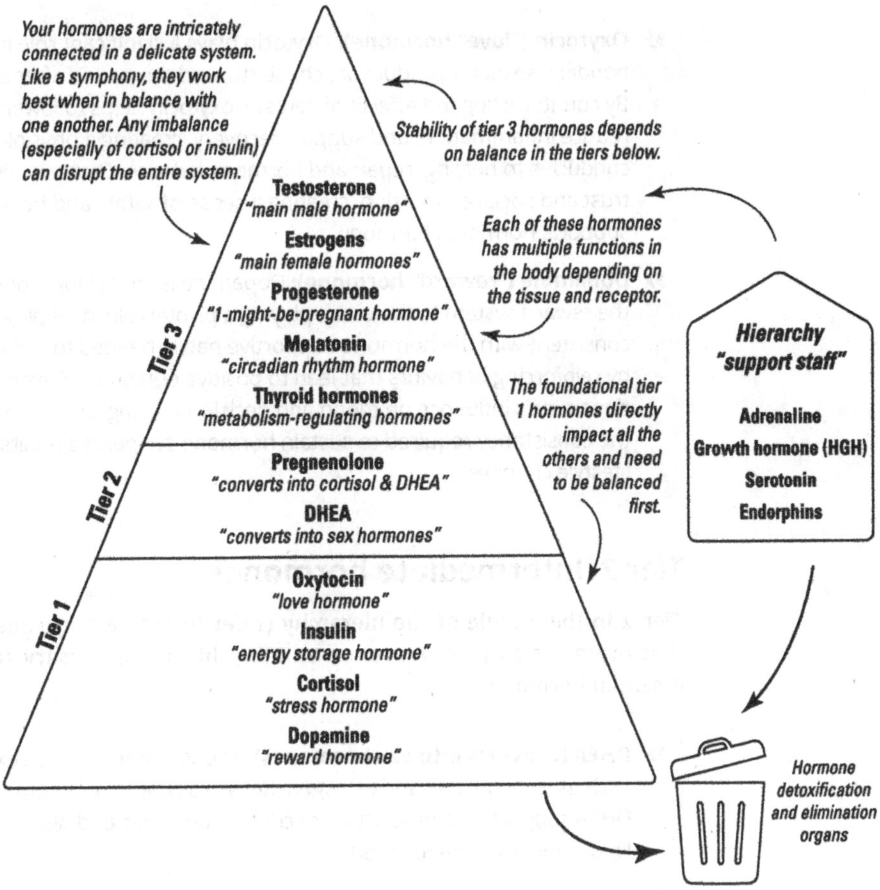

FIGURE 3-1: The hormone hierarchy.

- **Cortisol ("stress" hormone):** Known for its critical role in the body's stress response, cortisol is essential for managing metabolism, reducing inflammation, and maintaining stable blood sugar and insulin levels. However, when cortisol levels are chronically elevated or depleted, it can suppress reproductive hormones, impair thyroid function, and disrupt insulin regulation, leading to widespread hormonal imbalances.
- **Insulin ("energy storage" hormone):** Critical for regulating blood sugar levels, insulin allows cells to absorb glucose for energy or stores it for later use. Dysregulation of insulin can disrupt cortisol levels and promote chronic inflammation, creating a ripple effect that destabilizes the hormone hierarchy. Insulin's effects also extend to fat storage, appetite control, and metabolic health, making its proper regulation a linchpin for balancing the hormonal hierarchy.

- **Oxytocin ("love" hormone):** Oxytocin plays a significant role in social bonding, sexual reproduction, childbirth, and the period after childbirth. By counteracting the effects of cortisol, oxytocin helps to lower stress levels, reduce inflammation, and support recovery, creating a physiological state conducive to healing, repair and hormone balance. Oxytocin also enhances trust and social connection, creating a sense of safety and belonging that supports hormonal harmony.
- **Dopamine ("reward" hormone):** Dopamine is crucial for motivation and the reward system in the brain, playing a pivotal role in helping you stay consistent with the hormone-supportive habits needed to achieve your goals by reinforcing behaviors that lead to positive outcomes. Beyond motivation, dopamine's influence on mood and decision-making can make or break the consistency required to sustain hormone-supportive habits and lifestyle changes.

Tier 2: Intermediate hormones

Tier 2 in the middle of the hierarchy (refer to Figure 3-1) consists of hormones that often act as precursors, or building blocks, necessary for creating other essential hormones:

- **DHEA (converts into sex hormones):** This is a precursor to sex hormones such as testosterone and estrogen. Known as the "grandmother hormone," DHEA supports the production of critical hormones and plays a role in energy, libido, and immune function.
- **Pregnenolone (converts into cortisol and DHEA):** Known as the "mother hormone," pregnenolone is the precursor to many other hormones, including cortisol, DHEA, and progesterone. It influences your stress response, reproductive health, and overall hormonal balance.

Tier 3: Specialized hormones

At the top of the hormone hierarchy (refer to Figure 3-1) are the specialized hormones. These are heavily influenced by and dependent on the balance of the lower tiers. If your levels of tier 1 (particularly cortisol and insulin) and tier 2 hormones are off, then your tier 3 hormone levels will certainly pay the price:

- **Thyroid hormones ("metabolism-regulating" hormones):** These hormones, including T3 and T4, regulate the body's metabolism, energy generation, and overall growth and development.

» **Melatonin ("circadian rhythm" hormone):** Melatonin is essential for regulating sleep-wake cycles, and it helps maintain the body's internal clock and promotes healthy sleep patterns.

» **Progesterone ("I-might-be-pregnant" hormone):** Progesterone plays a key role in the menstrual cycle, pregnancy, and embryogenesis.

» **Estrogens (main female hormones):** These hormones are crucial for sexual and reproductive development, primarily in women.

» **Testosterone (main male hormone):** Testosterone, which is essential for the development of male reproductive tissues, also promotes secondary sexual characteristics and overall health in both men and women.

Hormones outside the hierarchy

To ensure that everything runs smoothly, some hormones work outside the hierarchy. You can think of them as the "support staff," but being outside the hierarchy doesn't make them any less important:

» **Adrenaline (part of the "stress" hormones group):** Works alongside cortisol in the body's immediate stress response, preparing the body for fight-or-flight actions

» **Growth hormone (HGH):** Stimulates growth, cell reproduction, and cell regeneration in humans, playing a pivotal role in human development

» **"Happy" hormones:** Serotonin and endorphins:

- **Serotonin:** Helps regulate mood, appetite, and sleep
- **Endorphins:** Act as natural painkillers and mood elevators

Falling dominoes: Why one hormone imbalance usually leads to another

I know, not *another analogy*, but please bear with me because this one is going to help explain the most effective approach to balancing your hormones.

Imagine setting up a line of dominoes: Each piece is standing upright, aligned perfectly, ready to cascade at the touch of a finger. The moment one domino falls, it knocks into the next, setting off a chain reaction.

In the world of hormones, a similar scenario unfolds when an imbalance occurs. As described in the "Understanding the Cooperative Nature of Hormones" section earlier in this chapter, hormones operate within a finely tuned structure where each one influences and is influenced by others. This interdependence means that a disturbance in one hormone can cause imbalances in others, much like a toppling line of dominoes. Because your tier 1 hormones are the primary regulators of many physiological processes, imbalances in tier 1 can create a domino effect, disrupting the entire hormonal system.

In this section, I bring this to life with some examples.

Tier 1: Cortisol

Cortisol plays a critical role in managing your body's response to stress and has a direct physiological effect on the entire hormonal hierarchy — for example, when stress becomes chronic, cortisol levels remain elevated, leading to a host of issues. Think of it like a bully in the playground that's not letting the other kids (hormones) play:

- **Impact on tier 1 hormone insulin:** When your body goes into a stress response and elevates your cortisol levels due to a threat you've perceived, it dumps glucose into your bloodstream to make sure you have the energy to fight or flee the situation. It's pretty clever really, but over time, this constant demand on the pancreas to produce more insulin can lead to *insulin resistance* — a condition where cells become less responsive to insulin. The result is further hormonal imbalance and an increased risk of conditions like type 2 diabetes, which affects women's reproductive health by causing irregular menstrual cycles, infertility, and elevated levels of male hormones.
- **Impact on tier 2 and 3 sex hormones:** Cortisol competes with sex hormones for the same tier 2 precursor, pregnenolone. When cortisol is high, it diverts resources away from the production of sex hormones such as estrogen, progesterone, and testosterone, leading to imbalances that affect reproductive health, mood, and overall well-being. The consequences can include missing, painful or irregular periods in women or reduced libido, erectile dysfunction, and decreased muscle mass for men.
- **Impact on tier 3 thyroid hormones:** Chronic stress and high cortisol can impair thyroid function, leading to hypothyroidism. This condition slows down metabolism, causing symptoms like fatigue, weight gain, and depression, which further complicate hormonal balance.

Tier 1: Insulin

Frequent spikes and crashes in blood sugar levels, often referred to as blood sugar roller coasters (covered in more detail in Chapter 17), can lead to the development of insulin resistance:

- **Impact on tier 2 hormones:** When insulin resistance develops, it can exacerbate imbalances in sex hormones. For instance, elevated insulin levels can increase the production of androgens (male hormones) in women, worsening conditions like PCOS. This imbalance can lead to further complications, including hair loss, acne, and weight gain.
- **Impact on tier 3 hormones:** Insulin resistance can also influence thyroid hormone production. The thyroid gland needs to work harder to regulate metabolism, which can result in the development of early signs of hypothyroidism. Symptoms like chronic fatigue, difficulty losing weight, and depression can emerge, adding layers of complexity to the hormonal imbalance.

REMEMBER

Your endocrine system is a nearly perfect machine that works hard to keep you alive and thriving, but it needs your support. Focusing on tier 1 hormones creates a stable foundation that supports the entire hormonal hierarchy and enhances your ability to make hormone-supportive decisions, ensuring that your body produces the right amount of hormones at the right time. This is called the root-cause approach, which is covered in Part 4.

Revealing the chemistry of hormone communication

Your endocrine system uses hormones to send messages over long distances between the brain and various parts of the body. This system mainly works through a complex interaction between the brain and endocrine glands.

The hypothalamus, a region in the brain, plays a critical role in the hormonal communication network. It produces releasing and inhibiting hormones that influence the pituitary gland. This gland, often referred to as the "master gland," releases hormones into the bloodstream that affect other endocrine glands throughout the body. These glands then produce hormones that regulate various physiological functions. (Read more about the pituitary in Chapter 2.)

This regulation mechanism is known as a *feedback loop*. Feedback loops are how the endocrine system maintains homeostasis (balance) in the body. If an endocrine gland senses that there is too much of a specific hormone, it initiates changes to decrease the production of that hormone. Conversely, if there is not enough of a hormone, the gland increases production. You can think of it as your body's attempt to self-regulate and self-correct.

How the body uses hormones to communicate

After hormones produced by glands in the endocrine system travel through the bloodstream to reach their target cells or organs. Once they arrive, they bind to specific receptors on or inside these cells, triggering a response. Here's how the process works:

1. **Synthesis:** Hormones are manufactured by endocrine glands in response to specific stimuli. For instance, the adrenal glands produce cortisol in response to stress.
2. **Transport:** Hormones are released into the bloodstream. Some hormones, like steroid hormones, require carrier proteins to travel efficiently through the blood. These carrier proteins ensure that hormones reach their target cells intact and in the right concentrations.
3. **Receptor binding:** Once hormones reach their target cells, they bind to specific receptors, much like a key fitting into a lock. These receptors can be located on the cell surface or inside the cell. The binding of a hormone to its receptor is a crucial step that determines the specificity of hormonal action.
4. **Signal transduction:** The binding of a hormone to its receptor activates intracellular (within a cell) signaling pathways. This process translates the hormonal signal into a specific cellular response. For example, when cortisol binds to its receptors, it triggers pathways that help the body manage stress.
5. **Feedback mechanisms:** To maintain balance and prevent overproduction or underproduction of hormones, the endocrine system relies on feedback mechanisms. One of the most well-known feedback loops is the hypothalamic-pituitary-adrenal (HPA) axis (see Figure 3-2), which governs the body's response to stress and the production of cortisol. But feedback loops also control other essential behaviors and body functions such as sexual function, emotions, eating, drinking, growth, reproduction, energy use, and metabolism.

How hormones communicate with each other

In addition to the direct communication between hormones and their target cells, hormones also interact with each other to regulate various body processes and make sure the body responds appropriately to changing internal and external environments, as described here:

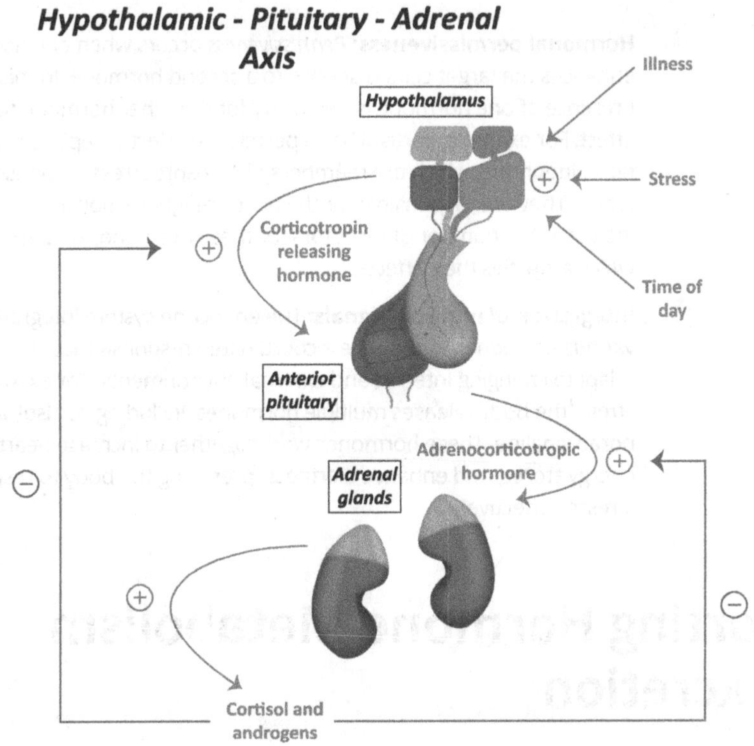

FIGURE 3-2: The HPA axis feedback mechanism.

joshya/Adobe Stock Photos

1. **Hormonal synergy and antagonism:** Hormones can work together *synergistically* or *antagonistically* to produce a combined effect greater or lesser than the sum of their individual effects:

   - **Synergistic interaction** occurs when two or more hormones work together to produce an amplified response. For example, glucagon and epinephrine both promote the breakdown of glycogen to glucose in the liver, and their combined effect is greater than the sum of their individual actions.
   - **Antagonistic interaction** occurs when one hormone opposes the action of another. For example, insulin and glucagon have opposite effects on blood sugar levels; insulin lowers blood sugar, whereas glucagon raises it.

2. **Hormonal cascades:** A series of hormonal activations where one hormone stimulates the release of another hormone, which in turn stimulates the release of yet another hormone. This sequential process involves multiple levels of hormone secretion, leading to a final physiological response.

3. **Feedback loops:** Feedback loops are crucial for maintaining hormonal balance. These loops can involve multiple hormones that regulate each other's levels.

4. **Hormonal permissiveness:** *Permissiveness* occurs when one hormone enhances the target cell's response to a second hormone. In this scenario, the presence of one hormone is necessary for the other hormone to exert its full effect. For example, cortisol has a permissive effect on epinephrine and norepinephrine, which are members of cortisol's stress response "support team." They are responsible for the fight-or-flight response, and cortisol increases the number of receptors for these hormones on target cells, which amplifies their effects.
5. **Integration of multiple signals:** The endocrine system integrates signals from various hormones to produce a coordinated response that allows the body to adapt to changing internal and external environments. For example, during stress, the body releases multiple hormones, including cortisol, adrenaline, and noradrenaline. These hormones work together to increase heart rate, mobilize energy stores, and enhance alertness, preparing the body to respond to the stressor effectively.

Supporting Hormone Metabolism and Excretion

When hormones finish their jobs, it's time for them to retire and make room for the new guys! They need to be broken down and removed from the bloodstream so they don't accumulate and lead to imbalances. When your hormones don't successfully break down or leave your body, your body's signaling systems can become confused, and various health issues can result. For example, inadequate clearance of cortisol can contribute to chronic stress, fatigue, and impaired immune function.

What happens when hormones "finish" their job?

TIP

The liver is the primary organ responsible for metabolizing hormones. It converts hormones into water-soluble forms that can be easily excreted by the kidneys or through bile into the intestines. Supporting liver function through a healthy diet and lifestyle is vital for effective hormone metabolism. This includes limiting alcohol consumption and consuming foods rich in antioxidants, vitamins, and minerals, which aid the liver's detoxification processes.

TIP

After the liver has broken down hormones, the kidneys help remove the metabolites. Metabolites are the byproducts or waste products of this breakdown process. Think of it like a factory where raw materials (hormones) are used to make products, and the leftover scraps (metabolites) need to be disposed of. The kidneys play a crucial role in this disposal by filtering the metabolites out of the blood and excreting them through urine. Drinking plenty of water and supporting kidney health with proper nutrition and lifestyle choices are crucial for maintaining effective hormone excretion. More detailed action steps for supporting these organs are provided in Chapter 17.

The threat of "hormone mimicking" chemicals

In just 70 years, nearly 100,000 new chemicals have been released into the environment, and more than 85 percent of these have never been tested for their health effects in humans! An Emory University–led study published in *Nature Communications* in 2023 even found that measurable levels of PFAS chemicals (human-made chemicals often referred to as "forever chemicals" because they are incredibly resistant to breaking down in the environment and in the human body) were present in blood samples from newborns shortly after birth — meaning the babies had been exposed to the chemicals while still in utero. They also found that exposure to these chemicals may have disrupted the balance of certain processes in the newborns, such as the growth of tissues and the functioning of hormones.

While we have very little scientific knowledge about what happens when these chemicals combine in our bodies, the emerging research clearly suggests that many of them are threatening our health and that of future generations. One of the biggest areas of impact is on our hormones.

REMEMBER

Endocrine-disrupting chemicals (EDCs) are prevalent in the plastics in food containers; perfume, make-up and other personal care products such as toothpaste, bodywash, shampoo, and conditioner; herbicides, pesticides, and hormones used to grow food; in water supply systems as a result of contamination from agriculture and manufacturing; and in the flame retardants in clothes, cars, and home furnishings; and in cigarette smoke (including second- and thirdhand smoke). These EDCs mimic humans' natural hormones, and, in doing so, scramble the messages cells give to each other to make the body very confused!

WARNING

The chemicals can have an impact, from minor to major, on many different hormones, but most frequently, they mimic estrogen. These mixed estrogen messages can cause the imbalances behind most of the hormonal conditions women experience and can cause serious diseases, including diabetes and cancer.

When pregnant people are exposed, they may even interfere with critical developmental stages in the baby in utero, increasing babies' risks of developing birth defects and increasing their long-term risks of being overweight and developing hormonal problems, even including diabetes and cancer!

In men, EDCs can disrupt the endocrine system by mimicking or blocking androgens (male hormones) such as testosterone. For example, phthalates, commonly found in plastics and personal care products, have been shown to reduce testosterone levels. This disruption may lead to a range of health issues, from decreased sperm count and fertility problems to an increased risk of testicular cancer. Additionally, EDCs can contribute to the development of conditions like obesity and diabetes by interfering with the body's natural hormone regulation.

We also know that hormone-disrupting chemicals persist in the environment for decades or longer. DDT, for example, a pesticide that was banned in the United States in 1972, can still be found not only in the soil but also in the blood of those born even after its use was discontinued.

REMEMBER

Your daily choices can have an enormous impact on reducing your daily toxin exposure. In the online appendix at `www.dummies.com/go/hormonebalancefd`, I provide a list of common EDCs and where they're found so that you can assess the products in your environment and take steps toward reducing your exposure.

Support for your "detox" organs

You may already be aware of the threat of toxins and have heard about various detox programs (or even have tried one). Conventional medicine and wellness critics often criticize these detoxes, sometimes with good reason: Unfortunately, many aren't based on sound and safe principles and can even be quite harmful and stressful on the body. However, did you know that *metabolic detoxification* (the body's natural process of eliminating toxins and waste products) is entirely different from the popular concept of detox? It refers to the crucial, everyday process your body performs to "self-clean."

So while the threat of toxins is real and should be taken seriously, your body is also incredibly resilient and has a natural detoxification process managed by several key organs: the liver, kidneys, lungs, skin, and lymphatic system. These organs collaborate to filter and eliminate toxins, waste products, and other unwanted substances. Supporting these organs is crucial for maintaining optimal health, balancing hormones, and ensuring your body efficiently handles detoxification.

REMEMBER

When your body's pathways of elimination become congested, it often leads to a progression of symptoms. The first signs typically emerge in the large intestine, manifesting as constipation, diarrhea, irritable bowel syndrome (IBS), or bloating. If these issues aren't addressed, the liver may become overburdened, leading to symptoms such as food sensitivities, allergies, pain under the right rib cage (especially after eating a rich meal or consuming alcohol), excessive sweating, and foul body odor, particularly from the armpits or feet. Eventually, the lymphatic system and skin may also be affected, resulting in conditions such as acne (cysts, whiteheads, blackheads), rosacea, eczema, dandruff, an oily scalp, and persistent body odor. In this section, I give you action steps specific to each detox organ so you can optimize your body's natural detox process!

The liver: Your primary detoxifier

The liver is often referred to as the body's primary detoxification organ. So if you have a hormone imbalance, you need to support your liver. It performs numerous functions, including breaking down toxins, metabolizing drugs, and converting waste products into less harmful substances that can be excreted. Following are some suggestions for supporting your liver health:

- **Eat liver-friendly foods:** Incorporate foods rich in antioxidants and nutrients, such as garlic, onions, broccoli, and leafy greens.
- **Limit alcohol, caffeine, recreational drugs, and processed foods:** Consuming these things can overwork the liver and hinder its ability to detoxify efficiently.
- **Consider supplements:** Milk thistle and turmeric are known for their liver-supporting effects, but please speak to your healthcare provider before starting a new supplement regimen.

The large intestine

Once the liver metabolizes hormones, they are often excreted into the bile, which is then released into the small intestine during digestion. As the digested material moves through the intestines and into the large intestine, the hormone metabolites are subject to further processing by gut bacteria. To support your large intestine, do the following:

- **Eat insoluble fiber:** Foods rich in insoluble fiber include whole grains, nuts, seeds, and the skins of fruits and vegetables.
- **Eat a probiotic- and prebiotic-rich diet:** Probiotics are beneficial bacteria that support gut health. They're in fermented foods like yogurt, kefir, sauerkraut, and kimchi. Prebiotics, on the other hand, are fibers that feed the

beneficial bacteria, and they're in foods like garlic, onions, leeks, asparagus, bananas, and whole grains. Together, probiotics and prebiotics help maintain a healthy balance of gut microbiota.

The kidneys: Filtering your blood

The kidneys play a vital role in filtering blood and removing waste products through urine. Here are some ideas for supporting your kidneys:

- **Eat a balanced diet:** Reduce your intake of foods high in sodium (such as pizza, breads, and sandwich meats) and eat plenty of fruits and vegetables.
- **Monitor blood pressure:** High blood pressure can damage kidney function over time.

The lungs: Breathing out toxins

Your lungs expel carbon dioxide and other toxins through your breath. To support lung health, try the following things:

- **Avoid pollutants:** Minimize exposure to air pollution, vaping, and tobacco smoke. (Remember, even passive smoking is harmful!)
- **Exercise regularly:** Physical activity helps improve lung capacity and function.
- **Practice deep breathing:** Techniques such as diaphragmatic breathing can enhance lung efficiency.

The skin: Your largest detox organ

The skin eliminates toxins through sweat. Do the following to keep your skin healthy:

- **Maintain good hygiene:** Regular cleansing and exfoliation helps remove toxins from the skin's surface.
- **Use natural skincare products:** Avoid products with harsh chemicals that can damage the skin and are full of pesky EDCs!
- **Sweat regularly:** Engage in activities like exercise, hot yoga, baths, or sauna sessions to promote sweating.

The lymphatic system: Clearing cellular waste

The lymphatic system is like the body's waste disposal and recycling service. It's responsible for collecting garbage (cellular waste and toxins) from all the neighborhoods (tissues and organs). Here's how you support it:

- **Stay active:** Regular movement (especially jumping or rebounding on trampolines!) stimulates lymph flow.
- **Practice dry brushing:** This technique can help stimulate the lymphatic system while also exfoliating the skin.
- **Massage therapy or acupressure mats:** Lymphatic drainage massages and lying on acupressure mats both enhance and stimulate lymph flow.

Additional approaches

Beyond supporting specific organs, there are several strategies to enhance overall detoxification:

- **Eat a nutrient-dense diet:** Focus on whole foods rich in vitamins, minerals, and antioxidants.
- **Stay hydrated:** Adequate hydration is essential for detoxification. Adults should aim to drink at least eight glasses (about 2 liters) of water per day to help the kidneys and other organs flush out toxins effectively.
- **Reduce stress:** Chronic stress can impede detoxification processes. Practice stress-relief techniques such as meditation, yoga, or mindfulness. Chapter 17 is full of tips on how to manage your "stress hormones"!
- **Get adequate sleep:** Sleep is essential for the body's repair and detoxification processes. Aim for seven to nine hours of quality sleep each night.
- **Limit toxin exposure:** Reduce your exposure to environmental toxins such as pesticides, heavy metals, and industrial chemicals. Refer to the online appendix at `www.dummies.com/go/hormonebalancefd` for a complete list of EDCs to avoid.

IN THIS CHAPTER

» Understanding women's hormonal journey from girlhood to menopause and beyond

» Mapping men's dynamic hormonal transitions throughout life

Chapter 4

Understanding Sex Hormone Transformation

From a very early age, children start noticing the differences between biological "boys" and "girls" and encountering all sorts of stereotypes driven by our sex hormones — for example, teenage boys are moody and quiet or girls cry more often.

Think of this chapter as the ultimate upgrade to your high school sex ed class: a crash course that goes beyond the basics and equips you with everything you need to know about how and why your hormones evolve to guide you through the mental, physical, and emotional transformations that define every stage your life. This chapter explains the different phases of sex hormone transformation throughout life for both women and men — because puberty is just the beginning of the ride. Whether you're dealing with the drama of teenage mood swings, the ups and downs of pregnancy, or the subtle (and not-so-subtle) shifts of andropause and menopause, there's a lot going on behind the scenes.

Reviewing the Stages of Female Hormonal Transformation

From the first stirrings of puberty to the transformative experience of pregnancy and through the profound changes of menopause, women undergo a series of complex hormonal shifts that shape not only their physical health but also their emotional and mental landscapes. Historically (before we discovered hormones), these life stages were symbolized by three archetypes: the Maiden, representing youth and new beginnings; the Mother, embodying fertility and nurturing; and the Crone, symbolizing wisdom and life's culmination. Understanding these stages is helpful because it empowers you to embrace the natural ebb and flow of your hormones and see womanhood as a continuous process of renewal, adaptation, and growth.

In this section, we explore the various hormonal shifts and changes a woman can undergo in her lifetime, setting the stage for subsequent chapters that expand on how to maintain hormonal balance throughout life.

Preteen and teenager

During early childhood, sex hormones like estrogen, progesterone, and testosterone are present but at very low levels. This is a period of relative hormonal stability, where growth and development are mainly controlled by other hormones such as like human growth hormone (HGH) and thyroid hormones. But in the preteen years, seemingly out of nowhere, the roller coaster begins.

Preteens: The beginning of hormonal awakening

As young girls approach the preteen years (usually ages 8 to 10), their bodies start preparing for puberty. The brain initiates this process by sending signals to the hypothalamus and pituitary gland, which release luteinizing hormone (LH) and follicle-stimulating hormone (FSH). These hormones travel to the ovaries, prompting the production of estrogen.

Teenage years: Puberty hits

Once a girl reaches her teenage years (traditionally 11 to 14, but more on that in a moment), levels of estrogen, progesterone, and other reproductive hormones dramatically increase, triggering the full onset of puberty. This surge in hormones leads to the development of secondary sexual characteristics, such as breast development, the growth of pubic and underarm hair, and the start of menstruation. These changes are distinct from *primary sexual characteristics*, which include the reproductive organs themselves (like the ovaries, fallopian tubes, and uterus) that have been present since birth but become fully functional during puberty. This first period, known as menarche (pronounced: MEN-ar-kee), marks the young woman's official entrance into her reproductive years and Maiden archetype.

REMEMBER

Moving forward, estrogen and progesterone will work together along with various other reproductive hormones such as LH and FSH to regulate the menstrual cycle, preparing the body for potential pregnancy each month. Chapter 12 covers much more about the menstrual cycle. For now it's important to remember that a girl's body may not initially follow a consistent schedule or rhythm for her periods. The average cycle (the number of days from the start of a woman's period to the start of the next) lasts about 28 days, but it's common, especially in the first two years after a young woman starts getting her period, to skip periods or to have irregular periods.

REMEMBER

It's also normal for the number of days a young woman menstruates to vary. It could be two to seven days, and there could be spotting or "breakthrough bleeding" (light bleeding that can occur at various times during the cycle — either before or after the heaviest portion of the period or even mid-cycle — due to fluctuating hormone levels). That's because the level of hormones that the body makes can be different from one cycle to the next as it tries to establish its new rhythm. Think of it like a car engine warming up: Sometimes it sputters a bit before settling into a smooth, consistent hum.

These hormonal shifts are also the driving force behind growth spurts that seem to happen overnight during the teenage years. And of course, we can't forget mood swings. Thanks to rising estrogen, adolescence can be one of the most unpredictable (and memorable) times of life! Puberty, in a way, is like the hormone rollercoaster of menopause in reverse — imagine navigating it without emotional maturity and healthy coping mechanisms!

Reproductive years and preserving your fertility

As young women transition from the teenage years into adulthood, their bodies reach full maturity, and the menstrual cycle settles into a regular rhythm (if their hormones are balanced). During this phase, growth stabilizes, and mood fluctuations become more predictable as the body finds its hormonal groove.

While the reproductive years are defined by a woman's fertility, a time when the possibility of pregnancy is at its peak, they aren't just about the physical ability to conceive or preserving fertility. They're also about exploration and fulfillment, whether that means developing the emotional and psychological readiness to start a family, build a career, or pursue personal and professional growth. This phase generally spans from the early 20s to the mid-30s, though fertility can start to decline slightly in the late 20s and more noticeably after 35.

This is important to keep in mind, especially as more women are choosing to have children later in life. For instance, back in 1970, the average woman in the U.S. had her first baby at around 21 years old. However, federal data from April 2024 showed that by 2022, the average age for first-time mothers had risen to just over 24 — a record high for the country. Several factors are driving this trend, including concerns about childcare, the pursuit of financial stability, and career priorities. Men are also increasingly reflecting on when and whether to start families.

REMEMBER

As a result, anxiety around fertility and aging is increasing. Contrary to the widespread belief that fertility "drops off a cliff" for women at 35, the decline is actually more gradual. Although fertility does start to decrease around age 30, with a more noticeable decline by the mid-30s, the downward slope is not as abrupt as many fear. For instance, a 2016 U.S. study published in *Fertility and Sterility* found that the chance of pregnancy after 12 months was 87 percent for women aged 30 to 31, 76 percent for those aged 36 to 37, and 54 percent for women aged 40 to 41. Most women do eventually conceive; it may just take longer than expected.

In response to these concerns, many women are turning to egg freezing as a way to preserve their fertility. Although egg freezing has not been considered experimental since 2012, it remains a comparatively new technology, and much about its long-term success is still unknown. Current research suggests that the success rate for a live birth using frozen eggs varies, with younger women generally having higher success rates. However, we still lack comprehensive data on how many women actually succeed in having a baby using their frozen eggs because most women who have opted to freeze their eggs have not yet returned to use them.

TIP

The truth is, taking care of your hormones throughout your reproductive years is one of the most powerful ways to enhance your chances of conceiving naturally or improve the outcomes of fertility preservation methods like IVF and egg freezing. It also prepares you for a smoother experience during perimenopause and menopause! By following the advice in this book about maintaining a healthy lifestyle, managing stress, and being mindful of your body's hormonal rhythms, you can create a solid foundation for fertility, whether you choose to start a family, simply want to feel good, or are trying to prevent diseases like cancer or osteoporosis.

WHY GIRLS ARE HITTING PUBERTY YOUNGER THAN EVER

Young girls have been hitting puberty and experiencing their first periods younger and younger over the last few decades, and a new research shows that in the U.S., the trend isn't slowing down. Zifan Wang and her team at Harvard University gathered data from more than 71,000 individuals in the U.S. who had experienced at least one menstrual cycle. Their findings, published in 2024, showed that those born between 2000 and 2005 typically had their first period at 11.9 years old, which is noticeably earlier than the 12.5 years average for individuals born between 1950 and 1969.

Alarmingly, researchers with the Harvard T.H. Chan School of Public Health's Apple Women's Health Study found that this trend was strongest among Black, Asian, and other people of color and those of low socioeconomic status. In fact, Black girls have been shown to be more than twice as likely as white girls to start puberty early. Some Black girls are experiencing the onset as early as 5 years old.

This trend is concerning because research shows that menstruating before age 12 is linked to an increased risk of conditions like heart disease and certain cancers. For example, a paper published by a group of researchers from the Collaborative Group on Hormonal Factors in Breast Cancer showed that those who begin menstruating between ages 11 and 12 have an almost 10 percent greater risk of breast cancer, on average, than those who start at age 13. These young girls are also impacted psychologically, with increased feelings of loneliness, embarrassment, or feeling "different." If these symptoms are observed, it's very important to determine the cause (whether early puberty or a disease-driven cause such as a hormone-producing tumour) so proper care can be provided.

Scientists have suggested that the increasing rates of childhood obesity are a major factor because menstruation generally starts once a certain level of body fat is reached. Research also shows that stress plays a role because it can elevate androgens and estrogen, potentially triggering menstruation. Another possible factor is exposure to the endocrine-disrupting chemicals (EDCs) discussed in Chapter 3, which are found in certain plastics, pesticides, and consumer products like toothpaste, deodorant, receipts, perfume, and makeup. While the precise role of EDCs in puberty timing remains uncertain, these chemicals have the potential to block, mimic, or disrupt normal hormonal functions, which could influence the timing of puberty.

To lay a strong foundation for the well-being of future generations of girls, early hormone health education will be vital, as will establishing hormone-supportive habits at a young age (which are all topics covered in Part 4 of this book).

Pregnancy and post-pregnancy

Pregnancy is one of the most transformative experiences any human will undergo, both physically and emotionally. As soon as the magic of conception happens, a whirlwind of hormones kicks into high gear, setting the stage for your body to support the growing life inside you. Estrogen (specifically a type called estradiol) is the superstar, helping your uterus expand and nurturing your baby's development. Progesterone is the nurturer, ensuring that your uterine lining is cozy and preventing any premature contractions. Then human chorionic gonadotropin (hCG), the "pregnancy hormone," is the signal flare — making sure your body knows to keep producing progesterone during the early stages of pregnancy, even though it might make you feel a bit queasy and tired in the process. (For more tips on successfully setting yourself up to become pregnant, check out Chapter 12.)

WARNING

Importantly, research shows that the mother's lifestyle during pregnancy and the father's health at conception can both affect the baby's hormones through changes in how the baby's genes are expressed, a process known as *epigenetic imprinting.* For instance, factors such as trauma, diet, stress, and exposure to toxins or EDC's can influence the baby's genes related to hormone control, which may impact the child's development and health. Chapter 6 explores this further in more detail.

After pregnancy, your body undergoes one of the most dramatic hormonal shifts it will ever experience. Key pregnancy hormones such as hCG, progesterone, and estradiol, which were riding high during pregnancy, suddenly plummet as your body no longer needs those elevated levels. This drop is significant — possibly the largest hormonal drop any human can experience — and it's a big reason why the postpartum period can feel so overwhelming.

WARNING

While your hormone levels will eventually stabilize, you may never be exactly the same hormonally as you were before having a baby, and the time it takes to return to a new "balance" or "normal" is different for each woman. Typically, it can take several months to a year for your hormones to stabilize after childbirth, and factors such as breastfeeding influence this timeline because prolactin (the hormone responsible for milk production) remains elevated while you're nursing. This is why it's important to be mindful of the societal pressures to "snap back" quickly after childbirth. Unrealistic expectations can lead to unnecessary stress and misguided health decisions. It's crucial to give your body the time it needs to heal and adapt.

TIP

Becoming a mother isn't just a life event; it's a complete metamorphosis that rivals puberty in scope and impact called *matrescence*. Research shows that pregnancy hormones significantly change your brain, challenging the common belief in "baby brain." Instead of clouding your mind, these changes enhance your cognitive abilities and adaptability, fine-tuning your brain to be more efficient and deeply connected to your new role. (Maternal brain scans are wildly different from nonmaternal scans.) The profound shifts in your brain's reward system and sense of self that you experience are there to help you bond with your baby and embrace the expanded identity that comes with motherhood.

Perimenopause and menopause

REMEMBER

Perimenopause marks the beginning of the last major hormonal transformation in a woman's life. This phase, which often begins in a woman's 40s (though it can start earlier), is like your body's gentle — or sometimes not-so-gentle — reminder that the reproductive years are coming to an end. During perimenopause, estrogen and progesterone levels begin their gradual decline, leading to a range of symptoms such as irregular periods, mood swings, and those infamous hot flashes.

Unlike the steady rhythm of your hormones during your reproductive years, entering perimenopause is like switching from a smooth, predictable highway to a winding mountain road. Your once-consistent ebb and flow of hormones becomes a series of sharp turns and sudden drops, with your body shifting gears unexpectedly and perhaps uncomfortably. Perimenopause is a natural evolution in the cycle of your sex hormones and is covered in more detail in Chapter 12 along with practical strategies for managing symptoms.

So, if perimenopause is the winding mountain road, then menopause is the summit. The marker of menopause is when a woman has gone 12 consecutive months without a menstrual period. It's the official end of your reproductive years. By this stage, estrogen and progesterone have settled into a lower, steady state, and your periods have stopped.

Post-menopause

Today, as in ancient times, women in this stage of life (the Crone archetype) hold a unique power. Many women have a sudden urge to speak out, to go deeper into their faith or spirituality, to organize others, or to take action. They seem to have the energy to get more involved in the world around them or their communities. It can often be the most productive time in women's life because they're no longer juggling both the daily circadian rhythm and the monthly infradian rhythm. While the loss of that monthly rhythm might initially throw off your energy, sleep, and mood, it also brings a new level of consistency. This is your time to harness that steadiness. Consistent sleep patterns, getting plenty of natural light, staying active, and eating mindfully will help keep your circadian rhythm in check and you feeling your best.

But why are humans one of only three species on the planet to undergo menopause? One intriguing evolutionary perspective is the grandmother hypothesis, which suggests that menopause evolved to allow women to shift their energy from reproduction to supporting their offspring and grandchildren. By doing so, they enhance the survival and success of their genes. Interestingly, this may also explain why women tend to live longer than men: Their presence continued to benefit their descendants even after their reproductive years ended. In contrast, men's evolutionary contributions were more focused on reproduction and physical survival during their prime years, which may not have created the same selection pressure for longevity. This unique human adaptation highlights the enduring power and influence of older women in shaping the future of their families and communities. Menopause isn't an end; it's a new beginning.

Understanding Male Hormonal Transitions

When we talk about men's hormonal changes, puberty often steals the spotlight. In truth, men undergo several key hormonal shifts throughout their lives. Each phase brings a new set of challenges and opportunities, influencing everything from mood and energy levels to physical health, sexual function, and vitality.

Preteen and teenager

During early childhood, boys, like girls, have low levels of sex hormones such as testosterone, androgens, and estrogen, with growth and development primarily regulated by other hormones.

Preteens: The hormonal surge

The calm of childhood eventually gives way to a powerful surge of hormonal activity in the preteen years — typically between ages 9 and 14. The brain starts to send signals to the testes via the hypothalamus and pituitary gland, which start releasing luteinizing hormone (LH) and follicle-stimulating hormone (FSH). These hormones travel to the testes, signaling them to ramp up the production of testosterone, the first step in initiating the physical changes that define male puberty.

Teenage years: Puberty hits

Once a boy enters his teenage years (traditionally around ages 12 to 15), the levels of testosterone and other reproductive hormones rise sharply, signaling the onset of puberty. This hormonal surge leads to the development of secondary sexual characteristics, such as increased muscle mass, the deepening of the voice, the development of an Adam's apple, and the growth of facial and body hair. It also triggers changes in the primary sexual characteristics — the reproductive organs themselves, including the testes, prostate, and penis, which mature during this phase. This is when sperm production, known as spermatogenesis, begins; before puberty, boys don't produce sperm capable of fertilizing a woman's egg.

Of course, these physical changes come with a side order of mood swings and behavioral changes. Boys might suddenly feel like they're ready to conquer the world — whether that means outcompeting their friends in everything or mastering the art of awkward flirting. Just as girls step into their Maiden phase with menarche, boys start to embrace their inner superhero, testing out their newfound powers and grappling with the responsibilities that come with them.

WARNING

Recent research indicates that boys, like girls, are beginning puberty slightly earlier than in previous decades, though this trend is less concerning for boys. However, differences exist among ethnic groups; for instance, studies reveal that Black boys often start puberty a bit earlier than their peers, which may influence their developmental timelines. It's important to note that the timing of puberty in boys can vary based on factors such as genetics, environment, and overall health. So for boys, significantly early puberty could signal more serious underlying medical conditions.

Reproductive years

As men move beyond their teenage years and into early adulthood, they enter a period characterized by stable levels of testosterone. During this phase, which typically spans from the late teens through the early 30s, testosterone plays a crucial role in maintaining muscle mass and bone density as well as reproductive health by supporting sperm production and sexual function.

TIP

Testosterone also influences mood, energy levels, and cognitive function, so men in this stage often experience high levels of motivation, confidence, and drive, which contributes to personal and professional growth. However, to make the most of your hormones, it's essential to maintain a healthy lifestyle because factors like stress, poor diet, and lack of exercise can negatively impact hormonal balance.

For more detailed information on how your sex and reproductive hormones function during this phase and how you can optimize them, visit Chapter 11.

Andropause

As men age, testosterone levels and growth hormone levels naturally decline. This gradual decrease, known as andropause, typically begins around the age of 30 and continues steadily throughout life. By the time men reach their 70s and 80s, testosterone levels are significantly lower, impacting muscle mass, energy, libido, sexual function, and overall vitality.

TIP

But andropause isn't the only hormonal shift men experience. As discussed in Chapter 12, men often see a decrease in testosterone and an increase in hormones like prolactin and oxytocin when entering a long-term partnership or after the birth of a child. These changes support bonding and caregiving behaviors, highlighting the complex and evolving nature of male hormonal health throughout life — an area that's gaining more and more understanding as research continues to emerge.

Interestingly, after a lifetime of hormonal and physical differences, men and women start to become more similar in this phase of life, which might explain why you often see older married couples adorably sporting matching outfits! As hormone levels shift and certain characteristics soften, the convergence of these changes can lead to a deeper emotional connection and shared experiences.

IN THIS CHAPTER

» **Understanding how your hormones interact with the other major systems in the body**

» **Accepting that every sight, sound, touch, taste, and smell you experience can set off a hormonal response**

» **Embracing exercise as a powerful tool to support your body's systems**

Chapter 5

Linking Hormone Health to Overall Health

If you're struggling to get your health where you want it to be, you're not alone. As I explore throughout this book, the way our modern lives are set up is certainly making it harder than ever before to be mentally, physically, and emotionally healthy. Although there are no quick fixes or shortcuts (trust me, I've looked for them!) understanding and harnessing the powerful role hormones play across your body is as close as you'll get.

In this chapter, you discover that hormones impact every tissue and cell in your body (unbelievable, right?). By exploring how hormones interact with and are influenced by your body's major systems, you'll gain insight into your body's remarkable ability to find balance and even heal itself.

I want to note that our understanding of how hormones interact with the body's systems — especially across the different stages of a woman's life — is still developing. For centuries, medical research overlooked women's unique physiology, defaulting to the assumption that women were just "small men" with less muscle mass. This led to critical gaps in knowledge of how hormones uniquely influence women's health from puberty to menopause. Thankfully, research is finally beginning to challenge these outdated assumptions, revealing how intricately hormones shape our bodies, minds, and health over time. As this knowledge evolves, so do the strategies we can use to support women's health in ways that are holistic, personalized, and in tune with these distinct physiological changes.

TIP

As you read through this chapter, consider doing an Internet search for images of the body's systems for a visual aid. Seeing the systems and how they're placed in the body can help you better understand how everything works together!

Nervous System

The nervous system, which is made up of a network of specialized cells called *neurons*, plays a crucial role in keeping you alive by helping your body respond to threats it perceives — whether they are real or imagined. You can think of neurons as electrical wires that communicate by transmitting signals across your body that assess your internal and external environments to answer the question, "Am I safe or unsafe?" The answer these neurons land on is important because your nervous system uses the answer to influence vital processes, such as hormone regulation, heart rate, digestion, and the body's stress responses, including fight, flight, freeze, or fawn.

TIP

Your nervous system and the endocrine system are two very important parts of your body's communication network, and they work together closely. In fact, 80 percent of your body's signals travel to your brain via the vagus nerve, which extends from your gut, through your heart and lungs, all the way up to your face and ear canal into your brain. It's a major power line and a key player in the nervous system. This is why nervous system work is an essential part of successful hormone balancing.

TECHNICAL STUFF

In Chapter 3, I mention the hypothalamus-pituitary-adrenal (HPA) axis. It's the feedback loop your nervous system uses to communicate with your endocrine system. Here's how it works: When you encounter a dangerous or triggering situation (Chapter 8 dives into the impact of trauma), the hypothalamus signals the pituitary gland to release hormones. These hormones then stimulate other endocrine glands, like the adrenal glands, to release cortisol and adrenaline — hormones that prepare your body to handle the stressor. Once the threat has passed, elevated cortisol levels signal the brain to reduce the production of these stress hormones, preventing prolonged overstimulation. This feedback loop ensures that your stress response is effective but temporary, protecting your body from staying in a heightened state of alert for too long.

REMEMBER

This relationship is also bidirectional: Just as the nervous system can trigger the release of hormones, hormones can also affect how the nervous system operates. For instance, cortisol levels that remain elevated due to chronic stress, low self-esteem, and unresolved emotions or trauma can impair memory, reduce concentration, and heighten anxiety — all of which have direct effects on the nervous system. In other words, hormonal imbalances can lead to various neurological and psychological conditions. Then, when your body is in a state of relaxation and safety, different hormones take the lead. For example, oxytocin can promote feelings of trust and bonding, helping to calm the nervous system, and serotonin helps regulate your mood, appetite, and sleep, which are essential for overall vitality and well-being.

TIP

Understanding the intricate relationship between the nervous and endocrine systems is the essential first step toward being able to recognize your current nervous system state at any given moment. This skill — known as *autonomic awareness* and is covered in Chapter 8 — empowers you to manage stress effectively and find calm when needed, helping you avoid the detrimental effects of living in a constant "survival mode."

I've only just scratched the surface of the nervous system here because it's an incredibly vast and intricate network, encompassing the central nervous system (CNS), peripheral nervous system (PNS), and autonomic nervous system (ANS). Other chapters in this book explore in greater depth the effects of both major (big *T*) and minor (little *t*) traumas, unprocessed emotions, and the influence of self-talk. This journey, particularly in Chapter 8, highlights the profound connection between mind and body, showing that they are indeed two sides of the same coin.

Digestive System

Often referred to as the "second brain," your digestive system plays a crucial role in both producing and regulating hormones. This connection is part of the *gut-brain axis*, a complex communication network that links your gastrointestinal tract directly to your brain and nervous system. Within this system, your gut microbiome — a diverse community of trillions of microorganisms, which Chapter 9 explores further — has a significant impact on both digestion and hormone regulation, influencing everything from mood to immune function.

TIP

Your gut even produces hormones. Ninety percent of serotonin, one of the "happy hormones" mentioned in Chapter 2, is produced in your gut. That's why taking care of your gut health is as much of a win for your mental health as it is your physical health. Ghrelin is another digestive hormone — the hunger hormone — that gives your brain the nudge when it's time to eat.

Your gut also plays a key role in regulating insulin — the hormone that manages blood sugar levels and metabolism — through other hormones like GLP-1 and GIP. GLP-1, which you might recognize from medications like Ozempic, is crucial for controlling insulin release after you eat, helping to keep your metabolism running smoothly.

WARNING

Now, I want to introduce one of the gut's most fascinating players — the estrobolome. This is a unique collection of microorganisms specifically involved in estrogen metabolism. When your estrobolome is functioning well, it helps maintain balanced estrogen levels, which is crucial for everything from reproductive health to bone density and mood regulation. However, if the estrobolome becomes imbalanced, it can lead to an excess or deficiency of estrogen. This imbalance can contribute to symptoms such as heavy or painful periods and increase the risk of conditions like breast cancer, endometriosis, osteoporosis, and cardiovascular issues.

REMEMBER

It's important to understand that the relationship between your gut and hormones is a two-way street, heavily influenced by the enteric nervous system (ENS) which is closely connected to your ANS (which I mention in the preceding section). The ENS is a vast network of neurons embedded in the walls of your gastrointestinal tract. It's responsible for controlling digestion and communicating with both your brain and endocrine system. When your body's fight-or-flight response is repeatedly activated and cortisol levels remain elevated, your ENS can become disrupted, leading to digestive issues such as acid reflux, bloating, and irritable bowel syndrome (IBS), and it can affect more serious conditions like Crohn's disease.

Additionally, high cortisol levels can contribute to a condition known as leaky gut, where toxins and partially digested food particles leak into your bloodstream. This breach triggers your immune system, sparking systemic inflammation — a response that affects your entire body and can contribute to various health issues, including autoimmune diseases, heart disease, and metabolic disorders. Not fun at all!

Hormones also play a significant role in controlling how quickly or slowly food moves through your digestive system, a process known as *gut motility*. For instance, during certain phases of the menstrual cycle or pregnancy, increased levels of progesterone can slow down gut motility, often leading to constipation. This is because progesterone relaxes smooth muscle tissue, including that of the gastrointestinal tract.

Similarly, fluctuations in estrogen can impact gut motility and the diversity of the gut microbiome. During menopause, when estrogen levels decline, some women may experience changes in digestion, including slower transit times or a shift in microbiome composition. These changes can influence everything from nutrient absorption to the way your body regulates hunger and satiety hormones, which is why understanding how your hormones interact with your digestive system can help you anticipate and manage these changes more effectively. For information on what impacts your gut health and the steps you can take to restore it, check out Chapter 9.

Immune System

You can think of your immune system as your body's personal defense squad that works around the clock to keep you safe from invaders like bacteria, viruses, and other harmful substances. This intricate network includes white blood cells, antibodies, the lymphatic system, and various organs, including the spleen and thymus. However, it's not a standalone force. It's deeply intertwined with your hormones to constantly communicate and coordinate and keep you healthy and resilient.

TIP

Take cortisol, for example. In small doses, this stress hormone is like a helpful firefighter, regulating inflammation and keeping your immune response in check. Healthy inflammation is your body's short-term way of handling injury or infection, boosting blood flow and immune activity to protect and heal. When stress sticks around and cortisol levels stay high, that helpful firefighter can turn into a troublemaker, suppressing your immune system and ramping up inflammation. If you've ever caught a cold right before a big exam or during a stressful work project, it's because stress has suppressed your immune system. So, managing stress isn't just a win for your mental health; it's also key to keeping your immune system strong and ready to fight off whatever comes your way.

REMEMBER

Estrogen also gives the immune system a boost, which is why women generally have stronger immune responses than men. There's a catch, though. While a strong immune system is fantastic for fighting off infections, it can sometimes go overboard, increasing the risk of developing autoimmune diseases, which means the immune system accidentally targets the body's own tissues. This is one reason why 80 percent of people with autoimmune diseases are women.

Conversely, testosterone acts as an immunosuppressant. This means it can weaken the body's immune response, which is one reason why men are less likely to develop autoimmune diseases. However, it also means that men might have a weaker initial immune response to infections, making them more susceptible to certain illnesses. (It turns out that "man-flu" may be real after all.)

Insulin, the tier 1 hormone responsible for regulating blood sugar levels, also interacts with the immune system in complex ways. Chronic insulin resistance, often caused by a lack of sleep, poor diet, skipping meals, lack of exercise or sufficient exercise recovery, low levels of muscle, exposure to endocrine-disrupting chemicals (found in plastics or processed foods), or chronic inflammation, can impair immune function and lead to systemic inflammation. This inflammation affects more than just your blood sugar levels; it also increases the risk of developing chronic diseases such as type 2 diabetes, cardiovascular disease, and even certain cancers. Additionally, insulin resistance can exacerbate conditions such as polycystic ovary syndrome (PCOS), which has its own set of immune-related challenges. Read more about PCOS and ways to treat its four different types in Chapter 6.

TIP

When your immune system is balanced and inflammation is under control, your metabolism works more efficiently, helping you maintain a healthy weight. So, by supporting your immune system, you're also giving your body a better chance at reaching and maintaining your weight-loss goals.

REMEMBER

Lastly, your thyroid hormones, such as T3 and T4, also play a crucial role in regulating both metabolism and immune function. When your thyroid is functioning properly, it helps regulate the production and activity of immune cells, ensuring that your body can effectively respond to infections without overreacting. However, when thyroid hormone levels are imbalanced — whether due to hypothyroidism (low thyroid function) or hyperthyroidism (high thyroid function) — your immune system can suffer. Conditions such as Hashimoto's disease and Graves' disease are examples of autoimmune disorders directly linked to thyroid dysfunction, highlighting the critical connection between the thyroid and immune health.

Lymphatic System

Lymphatic drainage massages and dry brushing aren't just trendy wellness fads. If done properly, they can help support the complex network of lymph vessels, nodes, and organs that work together to detoxify the body. This system plays a vital role in removing waste, toxins, and excess fluids from your tissues so they don't recirculate in the bloodstream.

TIP

When your lymphatic system is in top shape, it lightens the load on your liver which is crucial for processing and metabolizing hormones. (To learn more about the liver, refer to Chapter 3.) When lymph (a fluid containing white blood cells) flow is optimized, estrogen and other hormones are cleared from the body more effectively, preventing them from building up to levels that could trigger hormone-related conditions — such as PMS, fibroids, or endometriosis — and supporting the health of your immune system.

Estrogen isn't just along for the ride, though; it also has a say in how your lymphatic system works. Higher levels of estrogen, such as the levels a person has during the menstrual cycle, pregnancy, or hormone replacement therapy (HRT), can make the lymphatic vessels more permeable. This can lead to fluid retention and swelling, which is why some people feel bloated and puffy or notice swollen lymph nodes at certain times of the month.

Chronic stress and high cortisol levels can also put a damper on the lymphatic system, making your body more vulnerable to infections and reducing its detox power. (I hope you're noticing just how nosey cortisol is as you make your way through this chapter.) This stress-induced sluggishness can also mess with hormone metabolism, leading to imbalances that further strain your lymphatic system.

Thyroid hormones also play a significant role in influencing the lymphatic system, albeit indirectly. Low thyroid function, or hypothyroidism, can slow down metabolism, which may impact lymphatic flow and lead to symptoms such as mild swelling or reduced immune efficiency. Conversely, an overactive thyroid, such as in autoimmune Graves' disease, can increase immune activity, placing additional demands on the lymphatic system. This added immune load can worsen inflammation, making it harder for the lymphatic system to manage effectively.

REMEMBER

Importantly, the lymphatic system plays a major role in transporting and distributing hormones such as thyroid hormones (T3 and T4) throughout your body. This close partnership ensures that key hormones get where they need to go, but it also means that any disruption in lymphatic function can impact hormone distribution and overall balance.

TIP

Given how closely the lymphatic system and hormones are connected, taking care of this system is crucial. Incorporating the diet and lifestyle tips from Chapters 3 and 17 are a brilliant place to start, but stress management will always be essential. It's also important to stay hydrated, get regular exercise, and practice deep breathing or yoga. Because your lymphatic system doesn't have a central pump to move fluid around, it relies on your movement — so keep things flowing with regular activity!

Reproductive System

Your reproductive system is a network of organs and glands that governs sexual development, fertility, and reproduction. This system includes the ovaries, fallopian tubes, uterus, and vagina in women, and the testes, vas deferens (a tube that transports sperm from the testes to the urethra in preparation for ejaculation), prostate, and penis in men.

Hormones are the driving force behind the proper functioning of your reproductive system — something I talk about in more detail in Chapters 4 and 12 — and they influence everything from puberty to pregnancy and overall reproductive health. But the ovaries and testes do more than produce eggs and sperm; they're also responsible for releasing reproductive and sex hormones covered in Chapter 2 that significantly impact your mood, energy levels, bone density, and much more.

REMEMBER

The relationship between your reproductive system and hormones doesn't end there, though. Several other hormones play crucial roles in this complex system, influencing everything from fertility to overall health:

- **Cortisol:** Elevated cortisol levels can disrupt the balance of reproductive hormones. In women, this can interfere with ovulation, libido, pregnancy and menstrual cycles. In men, elevated cortisol can lower testosterone levels, affecting sperm production, sexual function, and libido.
- **Thyroid hormones (T3 and T4):** Hypothyroidism, or low thyroid function, can lead to irregular menstrual cycles and infertility in women. In men, it can reduce testosterone production and impair sexual function. Conversely, hyperthyroidism (excessive thyroid activity) can overstimulate the reproductive system, leading to issues such as absent menstrual cycles, ovarian cysts in women and reduced sperm quality, libido changes, or erectile dysfunction in men. I cover both conditions in more detail in Chapter 6.
- **Insulin:** Insulin resistance is a key factor in conditions like PCOS, where high insulin levels lead to increased androgen production, causing irregular periods and ovulatory issues. In men, insulin resistance can affect testosterone levels and sperm quality.
- **Prolactin:** Although primarily associated with lactation (the process of producing and releasing milk for newborns), elevated prolactin levels can actually inhibit ovulation in women, leading to menstrual irregularities. In men, it can reduce testosterone levels, leading to decreased libido and erectile dysfunction.
- **Human growth hormone (HGH):** In women, HGH influences ovarian function and follicle development. In men, it plays a role in sperm production and quality. As growth hormone levels decline with age, this can contribute to reduced reproductive capacity in both sexes.
- **Melatonin:** The sleep hormone helps protect reproductive tissues from oxidative damage. Additionally, melatonin influences the timing of key reproductive events, such as ovulation. When sleep patterns are poor or irregular, melatonin levels can become disrupted, which may negatively affect fertility by interfering with these important processes.

TIP

I know, getting on top of your hormone health can feel like trying to solve a complex puzzle with too many pieces. That's why when you're tackling hormone imbalances, it's essential to think of it like building a house: You need a strong foundation. By addressing the foundational hormones at the base of the hierarchy, you create stability, helping all your other hormones fit into place like the walls and roof of a well-built home. I discuss this approach in much more detail in Part 4 of this book.

Skeletal System

Bones aren't just hanging around inside your body waiting to be broken; they're active participants in managing your body's hormonal balance! The 206 bones in the adult skeleton work together to store essential minerals, produce blood cells, and even contribute to hormone regulation.

REMEMBER

Surprised? It's true! For instance, osteoblasts — the cells that build bone — also produce a hormone called *osteocalcin*. This multitasking hormone helps regulate insulin, improve insulin sensitivity, and manage fat storage, keeping your blood sugar in check and your energy levels balanced. Plus, your bones are crucial for maintaining the right balance of calcium and phosphorus in your body, which is vital for many bodily functions.

When it comes to the influence of your hormones on your skeletal system, during your growing years, hormones are the architects behind your bones' development. HGH, which is released by the pituitary gland, acts like the supervisor on a construction site, overseeing the production of insulin-like growth factor 1 (IGF-1), which directly stimulates bone growth. This duo ensures that your skeleton grows strong and sturdy as you move through childhood and adolescence. Thyroid hormones also play a supporting role, making sure that bone growth and maturation occur on schedule, so your skeletal framework develops as it should.

However, the work doesn't stop once you've reached your full height. Hormones continue to be crucial for maintaining bone density and strength throughout your life. For women, estrogen acts as a guardian of bone mass, slowing down the natural process of bone breakdown. However, after menopause, when estrogen levels drop, this protective effect weakens, leading to an increased risk of osteoporosis due to accelerated bone loss. Men, on the other hand, rely on testosterone to help maintain their bone density. Testosterone is a key player in keeping men's skeletons robust as they age.

WARNING

Another hormone that plays a pivotal role in bone health is vitamin D. Don't let the name fool you; it really is a hormone! The "sunshine vitamin" makes sure that calcium gets deposited into your bones where it's needed most. Without adequate vitamin D, bones can become weak and brittle, leading to conditions like rickets in children and osteomalacia in adults, where bones soften and become prone to fractures.

REMEMBER

Finally, your bones are constantly undergoing a process called *remodeling*, where old bone tissue is broken down and replaced with new tissue. This process is orchestrated by a delicate balance of cells — osteoclasts, which break down bone, and osteoblasts, which build it up again. Hormones like parathyroid hormone (PTH), calcitonin, and cortisol are the conductors of this complex process, so if cortisol levels become elevated, the balance can tip in favor of bone breakdown, which increases the risk of osteoporosis as bone density decreases.

TIP

Exercise plays a crucial role in maintaining this balance because physical activity stimulates the production of bone-building hormones and increases the activity of osteoblasts. Weight-bearing and resistance exercises are especially important for building and strengthening bones.

Cardiovascular System

Your cardiovascular system is the incredible highway network that keeps your body alive. It's made up of your heart, blood vessels, and blood, working together to transport oxygen, nutrients, hormones, and waste products to and from your body's cells. This system is essential for maintaining life, delivering the key elements your organs need to function, and carrying away what they don't.

REMEMBER

Your cardiovascular system doesn't just run on its own though; it's closely regulated by hormones, which play crucial roles in maintaining heart health, blood pressure, and overall function. For example, while your heart is the muscular engine of your cardiovascular system, adrenaline and noradrenaline can increase your heart rate during times of stress and excitement to prepare your body for fight-or-flight situations. While this is useful in short bursts, chronic stress can keep these hormones elevated, putting extra strain on your heart and increasing the risk of cardiovascular disease.

WARNING

Cortisol also has significant effects on your cardiovascular system. In times of stress, cortisol helps to regulate blood pressure and blood sugar levels, ensuring your body has the energy it needs. However, chronic high levels of cortisol can contribute to high blood pressure, weight gain, and an increased risk of heart disease.

The other tier 1 hormone, insulin, also plays a role by helping your blood vessels relax and improving blood flow to get crucial glucose (blood sugar) across your body to fuel you to fight or flee in stressful situations. However, insulin resistance can lead to high blood sugar levels and damage to blood vessels, increasing the risk of hypertension, heart disease, and stroke.

For women, estrogen offers a protective effect on the cardiovascular system. It maintains healthy blood vessels, supports good cholesterol levels, and improves blood flow. This is why premenopausal women generally have a lower risk of heart disease and why the risk of cardiovascular issues increases after menopause, when estrogen levels drop.

REMEMBER

This relationship works both ways: Your cardiovascular system also plays a crucial role in hormone regulation. Good blood flow is essential for delivering hormones to their target organs, ensuring that everything from your thyroid to your adrenal glands functions properly. If your cardiovascular health is compromised — say, by clogged arteries or high blood pressure — hormone distribution can suffer, leading to imbalances that disrupt your body's systems.

Integumentary System (Skin)

Your integumentary system, better known as your skin, is actually your body's largest and most visible organ. Consisting of the skin, hair, nails, and various glands, this system doesn't just protect you from environmental hazards by providing a protective barrier, it also regulates your temperature, acts as a first line of defense against infections, and interacts closely with your hormones. This relationship is particularly noticeable during periods of hormonal change, such as puberty, pregnancy, and menopause.

Here are some of the ways your hormones and your skin interact:

REMEMBER

- **Sebum production:** Ever wonder why your skin suddenly becomes oily or breaks out? You can thank hormones like androgens (including testosterone) for that. These hormones kick your sebaceous glands into overdrive, producing sebum, an oily substance that keeps your skin moisturized. During puberty, these hormones can go into overdrive, leading to oily skin and hair and acne. The same thing can happen during menstruation, pregnancy, or menopause, making your skin a bit unpredictable.
- **Collagen and elasticity:** Estrogen is your skin's best friend when it comes to staying firm and elastic. It promotes collagen production, which keeps your skin thick, bouncy, and wrinkle-free. But as estrogen levels decline with age,

especially after menopause, collagen production slows down, leading to thinner, less elastic skin and — you guessed it — wrinkles.

REMEMBER

- **Healing and inflammation:** Stress out too much, and your skin lets you know you need to relax. Chronic high levels of cortisol, the stress hormone, can slow down wound healing and make skin conditions like eczema, psoriasis, and acne worse by ramping up inflammation.
- **Melanin production:** Hormones also play a role in how much melanin your skin produces. Melanin is the pigment that gives your skin its color. During pregnancy, elevated levels of estrogen and progesterone can lead to hyperpigmentation, causing dark patches known as *melasma*.
- **Microbiome protection:** Your skin isn't just a blank canvas; it's a busy ecosystem of tiny microorganisms known as the *skin microbiome*. This community of friendly bacteria acts like your skin's personal bodyguard, keeping harmful invaders at bay and maintaining your skin's overall health. In times of hormonal ups and downs, such as puberty or pregnancy, this delicate balance can get thrown off, leading to unwelcome guests like acne or making your skin more sensitive than usual.

TIP

- **Vitamin D:** Your skin has the power to create vitamin D when it soaks up sunshine! Vitamin D isn't just great for your bones; it also boosts your immune system and even helps lift your mood. Of course, although catching rays is important, too much sun can cause damage and increase the risk of skin cancer. So, strike a balance: Enjoy the sunshine, but make sure you protect your skin with sunscreen, hats, and shade when needed!

Now that you know how closely your skin and hormones are connected, it's time to talk about pesky endocrine-disrupting chemicals (EDCs). You see, your skin is not an impenetrable barrier. Studies have shown that it can take as little as 26 seconds for chemicals from skincare products, lotions, or other topical applications to be absorbed into the bloodstream, and this rapid absorption is why it's important to be really mindful of what you apply to your skin (or let touch your skin). If you're not cautious, harmful chemicals can quickly make their way into your system and start affecting your hormonal balance.

TIP

Even small amounts of EDCs found on paper receipts you receive when shopping, perfume, make-up, or furniture (particularly in materials used to make them more durable or flame-resistant) can add up over time. Additionally, frequent exposure to such products may compromise the skin barrier and alter its microbiome, which has been linked to rising public health trends, such as increased allergies. For a full list of EDCs to avoid, where they're usually found, and where to find natural alternatives, refer to this book's online appendix at `www.dummies.com/go/hormonebalancefd`.

The good news is your skin also helps to detoxify your body through sweating. Regular exercise, staying hydrated, and visiting a sauna can all enhance this natural detox process and support your skin and hormone health.

Respiratory System

Your respiratory system is the incredible network that keeps you breathing in oxygen and exhaling waste gases — a process that happens so naturally, you probably don't even think about it. This system is made up of your lungs, airways, and the muscles that power your breathing, all working together to supply your body with the oxygen it needs!

Let's take a look at how your respiratory system and hormones work together to keep you healthy:

REMEMBER

- **Stress and breathing:** Ever notice how your breathing changes when you're stressed? That's because stress hormones such as adrenaline and cortisol kick your respiratory system into high gear as part of the HPA axis feedback loop, making you breathe faster and shallower. The goal is to flood your muscles with oxygen so you're ready to react to any threats or danger. While this can be a lifesaver in short bursts, chronic stress can lead to unhealthy breathing patterns such as rapid, shallow breathing or hyperventilation, which can worsen existing respiratory issues such as asthma.
- **Breathing and hormones:** On the flip side, your breathing rate can also influence the levels of carbon dioxide (CO_2) in your blood, which in turn affects your body's pH balance. When CO_2 levels are high (acidosis), it can trigger the release of stress hormones like cortisol and adrenaline to help manage the imbalance. Conversely, when CO_2 levels are low (alkalosis), it can suppress the release of these hormones. This bidirectional relationship is part of the body's complex feedback loops that help maintain balance.

REMEMBER

- **Estrogen and lung health:** For women, estrogen plays a complex role in respiratory function. It's often protective but not always straightforward. It generally supports lung health by maintaining airway integrity and enhancing immune defenses against respiratory infections. However, for some women, fluctuations in estrogen can act as asthma triggers, potentially contributing to the higher asthma prevalence among women compared to men. Hormonal shifts — such as during menstruation, pregnancy, perimenopause, or when using HRT — can worsen or improve asthma symptoms, highlighting how nuanced this relationship is.

» **Thyroid hormones:** Your thyroid hormones are also key players in your respiratory system. They help regulate the rate at which you breathe by controlling your metabolism. So, if your thyroid is overactive (hyperthyroidism), you might find yourself breathing faster than usual, whereas an underactive thyroid (hypothyroidism) can slow your breathing down, making you feel more sluggish.

Urinary System

Your urinary system is a high-efficiency waste disposal unit — constantly filtering out toxins, excess fluids, and hormones (once they've finished their job) to keep your internal environment balanced.

REMEMBER

While hormones play a significant role in how well your urinary system functions, urinary issues can also impact your overall hormonal balance. For instance, during puberty, pregnancy, and menopause, hormonal fluctuations can lead to urinary problems such as incontinence, urinary tract infections (UTIs), or overactive bladder. In men, hormonal changes can lead to an enlarged prostate (benign prostatic hyperplasia or BPH), causing urinary retention and frequent nighttime urination.

Here's how your urinary system works:

1. **Kidneys, the master filters:** The kidneys, which are located just below your rib cage, are bean-shaped organs that filter 120 to 150 quarts of blood daily. Nephrons in the kidneys remove waste products and excess substances, converting them into one to two quarts of urine daily.
2. **Ureters, the transport tubes:** Urine travels from the kidneys to the bladder through thin tubes called ureters, which use smooth muscle contractions to ensure there's no backflow.
3. **Bladder, the storage tank:** This muscular sac in the lower abdomen stores urine until it's ready to be expelled. The bladder can hold about 16 to 24 ounces of urine. It signals your brain when it's time for you to empty it.
4. **Urethra, the exit door:** Urine leaves your body through the urethra, a tube controlled by sphincters to ensure release only when you're ready.

Your hormones and urinary system interact in important ways. Here are a few examples:

- **Antidiuretic hormone (ADH):** Ensures you stay hydrated by signaling your kidneys to conserve water when you're dehydrated
- **Erythropoietin (EPO):** Stimulates red blood cell production in response to low oxygen levels
- **Aldosterone:** Helps regulate blood pressure by signaling the kidneys to retain sodium and excrete potassium, maintaining fluid and electrolyte balance

REMEMBER

Unfortunately, hormones can also contribute to some pesky urinary issues. For women, fluctuating estrogen levels during menopause can thin the urinary tract tissues, leading to more frequent UTIs, an overactive bladder, or stress incontinence. In men, dihydrotestosterone (DHT) can cause the prostate to enlarge, leading to BPH, which makes urination challenging, especially at night.

REMEMBER

Other conditions such as diabetes and PCOS can further complicate things. With PCOS, insulin resistance is often linked to central obesity, which increases abdominal pressure. This added pressure can strain the pelvic floor muscles, making stress urinary incontinence more likely. Meanwhile, in diabetes, high blood sugar leads to osmotic diuresis (where excess glucose in the blood causes the kidneys to excrete more water), forcing the kidneys to work overtime, which results in more frequent urination.

TIP

The lesson here is that when your urinary system and hormones are in sync, your body's balance and health are at their best. Symptoms like frequent urination, pain or burning, a sudden or strong need to urinate, incontinence, blood in urine, or bladder pain are signs that something might be off. If you experience any of these symptoms, it's a good idea to check in with your healthcare provider. Your body is always talking to you via its symptoms!

Your Senses

REMEMBER

Your senses and hormones are in a constant feedback loop, each influencing the other in fascinating ways. For instance, hormonal changes can heighten or dull your senses, altering how you experience smells, tastes, sights, and sounds. In turn, what you see, hear, touch, taste, or smell can trigger hormonal responses that affect your mood, energy levels, and even stress. Pretty interesting stuff! Let's take a closer look at how it all works.

Smell

Ever wonder why everything suddenly smells stronger (or more terrible)? When this happens, you can most likely blame your hormones! During pregnancy, for example, estrogen and progesterone can make odors way more intense — sometimes to the point of making a person queasy. Hormonal ups and downs during the menstrual cycle can also make certain smells more or less pleasant.

REMEMBER

This isn't a one-way street, though. Your sense of smell can also boss around your hormones! A whiff of something familiar and comforting may trigger a release of oxytocin, making you feel all warm and fuzzy. And you may have heard of pheromones, your body's invisible love notes. They're special chemicals your body naturally releases that can send signals to others without you even knowing it. These sneaky little signals can influence how attracted we feel to someone or how connected we are.

Sight

If you've noticed your vision getting sharper when you're stressed, that's cortisol kicking in to make sure you're ready to dodge any danger (or tackle that looming deadline). On the flip side, hormonal changes during pregnancy or menopause can cause dry eyes or blurry vision — because who needs to see clearly when you're already juggling so much, right?

TIP

Conversely, what you see can also do a number on your hormones. When you turn off the light (or put your blue light blocking glasses on) in the evenings, your body starts cranking out melatonin, helping you wind down when it's time to hit the hay. If your eyes land on something beautiful or heartwarming, dopamine jumps in to lift your spirits and give you an energy boost.

Hearing

Estrogen helps keep your hearing sharp, but changes in its levels during your menstrual cycle or pregnancy might make your ears a bit more sensitive or cause them to tune out certain frequencies. When stress hits, cortisol can turn up the volume, making loud noises seem even more jarring.

TIP

But guess what? Your ears can give your hormones a nudge, too. Listening to your favorite soothing playlist can lower cortisol levels, helping you relax. On the flip side, sudden loud noises — whether it's a car horn or your alarm clock blaring in the morning — can pump up adrenaline, prepping your body to react quickly.

Taste

REMEMBER

Craving pickles and ice cream? That's hormones at work! Pregnancy can flip your sense of taste upside down, making you love — or loathe — certain foods. If your thyroid is acting up, you might find that everything tastes a little off or doesn't have much taste at all.

The foods you enjoy can influence your hormone levels. Indulge in something sweet, and insulin rushes in to manage your blood sugar. Savoring a turkey sandwich? The tryptophan in it might give you a serotonin boost, helping you feel calm and content.

Touch

A hug or a cuddle isn't just comforting; it's hormonal! Oxytocin surges when you're physically close to someone you care about, deepening bonds and trust as well as lowering cortisol levels. When stress kicks in, cortisol can make your skin more sensitive, sometimes making even a gentle touch feel like too much.

Touch also has its own way of playing with your hormones. A soothing massage or a warm embrace can lower cortisol and ramp up oxytocin, leaving you feeling connected and relaxed. Don't forget about endorphins — your body's natural mood lifters. They're ready to kick in after a therapeutic massage.

The Power of Exercise

Your body is clearly a magnificent collection of interconnected systems, and right now you might be wondering, "What can I do now to start supporting all of these different systems as well as my hormones?" Well, exercise will always be one of the most powerful tools you have. (See Part 4 for information about other strategies.)

While it's usually celebrated for its physical benefits, such as building muscle and boosting cardiovascular health, its impact goes much deeper. When you exercise, your body experiences a cascade of hormonal responses that benefit you in countless ways such as stimulating the release of endorphins.

REMEMBER

These "feel-good" hormones boost your mood and reduce feelings of stress, making you feel more fulfilled and resilient. It has been found that almost all types of physical activity, including dancing and exercise, are more effective in reducing symptoms of depression than commonly prescribed medications. Moreover, physical activity also regulates cortisol, helping to buffer against the harmful effects of chronic stress.

TIP

However, it's important to consider the type, duration, and intensity of exercise, as these factors can impact cortisol differently across individuals. For example, high-intensity or prolonged exercise sessions may elevate cortisol unhelpfully in certain groups, particularly for peri- and post-menopausal women. As we age, a shift toward moderate-intensity activities and incorporating resistance training for muscle and bone health becomes especially beneficial. But ultimately, choosing enjoyable, sustainable physical activities will always be more effective than no exercise at all!

Regular exercise and muscle building also helps regulate insulin, which is crucial in preventing a range of hormone imbalances (particularly in tier 2 or 3 hormones such as estrogen and testosterone). By enhancing insulin sensitivity, physical activity helps cells use glucose more effectively. This insulin support also indirectly benefits the entire endocrine system, creating a more stable hormonal environment overall and helping to reduce inflammation, boost energy levels, and promote healthier body composition.

REMEMBER

Other benefits include enhancing your digestive health, supporting your immune function, and maintaining bone density. Clearly, exercise is a comprehensive, easy-to-implement and accessible form of preventative medicine which, when paired with a balanced diet, will help your body maintain balance and resilience across all its systems.

In a nutshell, exercise is much more than just a way to stay fit or reach your authentic body shape. It's a key component of a holistic approach to health. And when you make it fun, whether by dancing, playing team sports, or simply moving in ways that make you smile, exercise becomes something you look forward to, not just another task on your to-do list!

2

Investigating the Rising Rates of Hormonal Issues

IN THIS PART . . .

Explore the rapid rise of reproductive hormone imbalances worldwide and the biopsychosocial factors you may never have thought of that are driving it.

Examine the interrelated metabolic, adrenal, and mental health crises affecting individuals worldwide being driven by a complex web of environmental, societal, and modern lifestyle factors.

Discover what makes your hormonal profile unique by understanding the influences that shape your hormones from before birth through early life.

Understand how chronic stress, trauma, and unprocessed emotions overload your nervous system and what strategies you can use to boost your resilience.

Dive into the pivotal role of the gut-brain-endocrine axis and learn how tweaking your diet, lifestyle, and environment can positively influence your gut health.

Uncover how modern lifestyle changes — social media addiction, lack of purpose, and disrupted work models — are impacting our ancient hormones and the new frontiers of Western medicine seeking solutions.

IN THIS CHAPTER

» Understanding why women's reproductive health issues are increasing

» Examining the various reproductive health challenges affecting men

Chapter 6
Examining Escalating Rates of Global Reproductive Challenges

Rachel Carson, the American marine biologist and conservationist, warned in the 1960s that our Western way of living — with genetically modified foods, herbicides, pesticides, and exposure to chemicals and air pollution — posed a grave threat to our existence. She couldn't have foreseen just how prophetic her words would be or how we would introduce even more profound challenges to our health that amplify these dangers: the constant barrage of information from a 24/7 news cycle and social media, diet culture, the normalization of unrealistic body standards, sedentary lifestyles, increasing reliance on processed and fast foods, and overconsumption of sugar. Additionally, misinformation about health and wellness is pervasive and often makes these issues worse.

The evidence of the threat is everywhere. Rates of PCOS, endometriosis, and "unexplained" infertility are rapidly rising (though improved diagnostics have certainly helped detect more cases). Only 12 percent of Americans are metabolically healthy. British women spend 21 years of their life dieting. The global fertility rate has dropped 50 percent in the last 70 years (although in many ways this is a success story due to available contraceptives). And sperm concentration has dropped 51 percent since the 1970s. What was once a warning has now become a reality that demands our immediate attention.

Advances in interpersonal neurobiology have revealed that our individual health is profoundly influenced by our environment. Unfortunately, environmental influences aren't often discussed as part of traditional medical approaches. The truth is, our biology, psychological functioning, and social relationships are inextricably intertwined, meaning that the broader cultural, political, and economic forces in the world around us are as influential in shaping our health as our diet, lifestyle, and genetic predispositions.

This chapter explores the most pressing reproductive challenges currently facing populations, while Chapter 7 continues the discussion by looking at the metabolic, adrenal, and mental health challenges rising across the globe. In both, I examine how environmental, societal, and lifestyle factors are contributing to the rise in these imbalances to offer you a comprehensive understanding of why these health crises are so prevalent today.

TIP

This chapter and Chapter 7 lay the foundation for understanding the root causes of these complex conditions. Chapter 11 builds on this groundwork by taking a closer look at how modern lifestyle shifts are further undermining hormonal health. Actionable strategies for reclaiming control of your health and navigating the challenges of the rapidly evolving world are woven throughout all three chapters, providing you with the tools you need to begin addressing the underlying imbalances or stressors that are most relevant or prevalent for you.

Rising Reproductive Health Issues for Women

REMEMBER

If you've struggled with your reproductive or menstrual health and been told "it's just part of being a woman" or "there's nothing you can do" then welcome to the club. Symptoms such as severe premenstrual syndrome (PMS) or debilitating period pain have now become so common, they're thought of as "normal" when they're actually anything but. This normalization of women's discomfort is not acceptable, and it's caused us to lose touch with the profound power that lies within women's reproductive and menstrual system. Our bodies know how to work (they even produce natural pain-relieving chemicals during menstruation!).

REMEMBER

In many Indigenous cultures, menstruation is considered a sacred and powerful time rather than an inconvenience to be tolerated. Yet, somewhere along the way, we shifted from honoring women's cycles as a vital sign of their well-being to dismissing symptoms as an inconvenience. Here's the good news: You have the power to change this narrative and transform symptoms into opportunities for healing.

Period (menstruation) concerns

Chapter 4 discusses how a healthy menstrual cycle relies on a delicate and intricate balance of hormones. Insulin and cortisol, which are tier 1 hormones, influence on the entire hormonal landscape, affecting other key reproductive hormones such as estrogen and progesterone. Estrogen and insulin share a special relationship because estrogen helps regulate insulin sensitivity, and insulin resistance can disrupt estrogen balance. Similarly, progesterone and cortisol are closely linked; high cortisol levels from chronic stress can lower progesterone, further disrupting the menstrual cycle.

REMEMBER

Because insulin and cortisol have such significant influence, they also affect other critical cycle hormones such as follicle-stimulating hormone (FSH), testosterone, and luteinizing hormone (LH). Having adequate amounts of these hormones at the right time is essential for maintaining a healthy cycle, as is ensuring they are properly broken down and disposed of after they finish their jobs.

Before we take a closer look at what's causing the two most common period concerns, I want to explore some broader factors influencing menstrual health.

The sneaky saboteurs of your menstrual cycle

According to the CDC, a whopping 33 percent of U.S. adults admit they're not getting enough sleep, while 70 percent of high school students report getting insufficient sleep on school nights (averaging less than eight hours). With our modern lifestyles, we've developed a perfect recipe for sleepless nights. Over time, this disrupts not only melatonin and cortisol but may also lead to insulin resistance by disrupting the body's ability to regulate glucose, further aggravating hormonal issues such as irregular periods and severe PMS. Sleep really is your best friend!

REMEMBER

In addition, environmental pollution, particularly air pollution in urban areas, has been shown to significantly disrupt endocrine function. Studies indicate that exposure to pollutants, such as particulate matter (PM2.5), nitrogen dioxide (NO_2), and other airborne toxins, can interfere with hormone production, metabolism, and regulation, increasing your risk of imbalances such as insulin resistance and thyroid dysfunction that impact your cycle.

Unfortunately climate change is only going to make this issue worse by increasing global temperatures and worsening air quality to trigger something called *heat stress*. Heat stress has been associated with elevated cortisol levels and impaired reproductive hormone function, placing additional strain on the endocrine system.

REMEMBER

Then there's broader societal factors we often forget to consider — for example, economic upheaval, political unrest, and cultural pressures. For instance, economic hardship can lead to food insecurity and nutritional deficiencies, which interfere with ovulation. Political and social instability can trigger stress responses that put reproductive health on hold (because the body will always prioritize survival over reproduction). The result can be issues like spotting, irregular periods, or painful cycles. Essentially, menstrual issues can often be your body's way of saying, "We'll get back to reproducing when things calm down. . . whenever that is!" Even the pressure to meet certain beauty standards or achieve success in both family and career life can add to emotional stress and disrupt your hormonal balance.

Painful periods

Period pain (dysmenorrhea) is one of the most common and frustrating menstrual symptoms. In fact, a Japanese study showed that 80 percent of women experience period pain at some point in their lives. Another study of U.S. college students reported that 25 percent had moderate or severe pain before menstruation, and 60 percent had moderate or severe pain during menstruation.

WARNING

If your pain is so severe that you rely on medication to get through it, please don't brush it off. Often this is a signal that there's an underlying imbalance in the body. For instance, research has linked conditions associated with severe period pain, such as endometriosis, to an increased risk of ovarian cancer due to chronic inflammation and elevated estrogen levels, and much more research needs to happen to better understand these links. Additionally, relying on nonsteroidal anti-inflammatory drugs (NSAIDs) such as ibuprofen every month can harm your gut health, which in turn worsens hormone imbalances and period pain.

TIP

One major culprit behind period pain is exposure to endocrine-disrupting chemicals (EDCs) — those sneaky toxins hiding in everyday products. (Check out the online appendix at `www.dummies.com/go/hormonebalancefd` for a list of main offenders.) According to the Environmental Working Group, the average American woman is exposed to about 168 chemicals each day through different products, many of which mimic estrogen, causing the uterine lining to thicken more than it should. The result? Intense cramping as your body works overtime to shed that excess tissue during menstruation.

Another contributor that doesn't get enough attention is diet culture. The obsession with low-fat and low-carb diets has deprived many women of essential nutrients needed for proper hormonal function. Without the right building blocks to form different hormones (healthy fats or complex carbs; read more in Chapter 2), your body can't produce what it needs. Additionally, severe carb restrictions and lack of protein wreak havoc on your blood sugar, causing insulin spikes that over time lead to insulin resistance. This, in turn, increases androgens, which can result in heavier, more painful periods.

TIP

Nutritional deficiencies, especially in magnesium and omega-3 fatty acids (which are key for muscle relaxation and reducing inflammation), can also make period pain worse. To help ease the pain, try incorporating whole, nutrient-rich foods like leafy greens, nuts, seeds, and fatty fish in your diet.

A sedentary lifestyle doesn't help either. Many people spend long hours sitting at a desk, commuting, and enjoying the rise of convenience culture. (Yes, I'm also guilty of having groceries delivered instead of walking to the shops.) I talk more about the impact of a sedentary lifestyle in Chapter 11.

TIP

While we're on the topic of exercise, I want to debunk the myth that strength training makes women "bulky." It builds lean muscle and improves metabolic flexibility. In other words, muscle helps your body regulate insulin levels effectively, supporting healthy estrogen balance, lowering inflammation, and easing period pain. So this is your green light to lift those weights!

REMEMBER

Another contributing factor to painful periods is chronic stress, which is a major disruptor of hormone balance. For women especially, there is a constant pressure to do it all and be everything for everyone all the time (and make it look flawless on Instagram), which initiates a stress response and the production of stress hormones. When cortisol sticks around too long your progesterone stores become depleted, leading to more intense contractions and painful cramps. Chapter 9 covers more about how to take care of stress and ease the strain on your body.

Poor gut health, a sluggish liver, and an overburdened lymphatic system can also make things worse. Your liver is responsible for metabolizing hormones, but when it's overworked — thanks to toxins, alcohol, and medications — it struggles to process estrogen properly, which can result in a buildup that worsens period pain. Given our modern lifestyle, liver strain is becoming more and more common. Think of your liver working double shifts, trying to clear out toxins while also handling hormone overload!

Similarly, a sluggish lymphatic system can lead to toxin buildup, increasing inflammation and discomfort. Sitting for long periods (whether at work or during commutes), wearing tight clothing for hours (athleisure, I'm looking at you), and lack of movement all slow down lymphatic flow. Consequently, your body's ability to clear out waste efficiently is hampered, leading to inflammation that can worsen period pain. Refer to Chapter 3 for tips on taking care of your lymphatic system.

Lastly, modern diets packed with processed foods, inflammatory ingredients, sugar, and unhealthy fats are doing your period no favors. These foods disrupt gut health, particularly the estrobolome — a group of gut bacteria responsible for metabolizing estrogen. Chapter 10 takes a deeper dive into the estrobolome, but here's the gist: When the estrobolome is out of balance, estrogen recycling struggles or becomes dysregulated, leading to estrogen excess. Add stress, low fiber intake, and too much sugar, and you have the perfect recipe for a hormonal imbalance, with period pain as a clear warning sign.

Missing or irregular periods

REMEMBER

When your body senses that it doesn't have enough resources — whether due to poor nutrition, excessive stress, or physical exhaustion — it shifts its focus away from reproductive functions because your survival is the higher priority. So, if you've noticed your period becoming irregular (a condition called oligomenorrhea) or missing altogether (amenorrhea), it's most likely a signal that your body is conserving energy and perceiving your current environment to be unsuitable for reproduction. In short, your body is saying, "We don't have the energy for a baby right now!"

Here, I list some of the most common underlying factors:

- **Energy imbalance:** One of the most common causes is an imbalance in energy intake and expenditure. For example, women who follow restrictive diets, suffer from eating disorders or engage in extreme exercise routines (such as running marathons or training to be an Olympic athlete) may lose their periods due to the fact that ovulation is a very resource-intensive process, and the body needs sufficient body fat and calories to keep it running smoothly.

  Figure 6-1 illustrates an anovulatory cycle — meaning a cycle in which ovulation doesn't occur. In a typical menstrual cycle (which I describe in Chapter 4), progesterone levels rise significantly after ovulation as the body prepares for a potential pregnancy. In contrast, progesterone remains flat throughout the entire cycle shown in Figure 6-1, which indicates that ovulation didn't occur because progesterone is only produced after an egg is released.

  Estrogen (specifically estradiol) shows a moderate rise and fall, indicating some hormonal activity is still occurring. However, without the corresponding spike in progesterone, the body can't proceed through a healthy, full menstrual cycle.

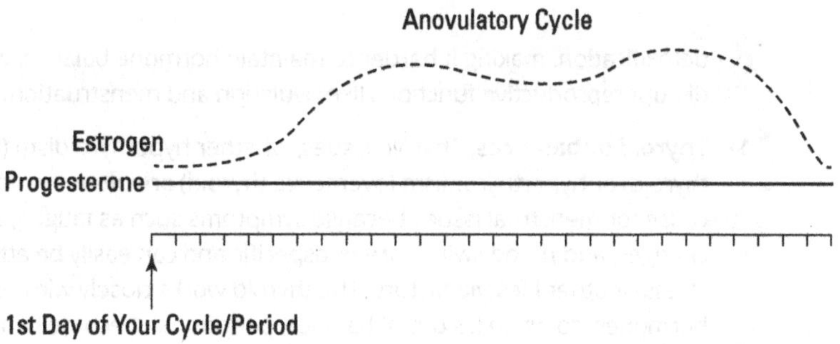

FIGURE 6-1: Anovulatory cycle.

REMEMBER

As a result, menstruation during an anovulatory cycle may be light, irregular, or completely absent. This cycle can also cause amenorrhea or oligomenorrhea as the hormonal balance is disrupted.

Additionally, without ovulation, it's common for the uterine lining to become unstable because it's not being regulated by the normal balance of estrogen and progesterone. This instability may lead to spotting or irregular bleeding, which isn't a true period because it lacks the structured hormonal shifts that come with ovulation.

REMEMBER

Most women will have a couple of anovulatory cycles each year, which can be considered normal, though what we consider "normal" may partly reflect what has become normalized due to modern lifestyle factors. However, persistent anovulation is abnormal and could signal underlying health issues that need attention.

- **Polycystic ovary syndrome (PCOS):** In women with this condition, the ovaries often produce excess androgens, which can interfere with ovulation and lead to irregular or absent periods. PCOS is also closely tied to insulin resistance, creating a cycle of imbalance that messes with the menstrual cycle. I talk about PCOS much more in the "Androgen excess" section later in this chapter.
- **Hypothalamic amenorrhea:** This form of amenorrhea happens when the hypothalamus — the brain's control center for regulating the menstrual cycle — stops sending signals to the ovaries to release eggs. It's usually triggered by high levels of stress, eating disorders, rapid weight loss, or excessive exercise, leading to prolonged stretches of time without a period.
- **Stress and emotions:** Stress, negative self-talk, low self-esteem, and unprocessed emotions also play a big role in menstrual irregularities by triggering cortisol production, signaling "danger" to the body. Essentially, your body is saying, "We've got bigger things to worry about than periods right now!"
- **Environmental toxins:** Just as the body may halt reproduction during times of stress or danger, it can respond similarly to toxin exposure, such as EDCs. Prolonged exposure to these toxins can shift the body's focus toward

detoxification, making it harder to maintain hormone balance, which may disrupt reproductive functions like ovulation and menstruation.

- **Thyroid imbalances:** Thyroid issues, whether hypothyroidism (underactive thyroid) or hyperthyroidism (overactive thyroid) are often overlooked as the cause for menstrual issues because symptoms such as fatigue, weight changes, and mood swings are nonspecific and can easily be attributed to stress or other lifestyle factors. The thyroid works closely with reproductive hormones, so when it's out of balance, periods can become heavy, prolonged, or irregular or stop all together due to the intricate relationship between thyroid function and reproductive health.

WARNING

- **Menopause and other medical conditions:** Irregular periods leading up to menopause can start as early as a woman's 30s, signaling that hormone levels are fluctuating. Other medical conditions, such as uterine fibroids, endometriosis, or even certain medications can also contribute to irregular periods or amenorrhea. If you experience persistent menstrual irregularities, please consult your healthcare provider to rule out these conditions.

Infertility

Infertility affects nearly 186 million people worldwide, with both genders contributing pretty equally to the underlying issues. Modern lifestyles are making natural conception more challenging than ever, particularly if you're unaware of the factors working against you. As one of my clients aptly put it, it's like "trying to plant a garden during a hurricane!"

With rising rates of obesity, insulin resistance, poor gut health, chronic stress, reproductive hormone imbalances, plus exposure to environmental toxins and all sorts of other stressors discussed throughout this chapter, our bodies are getting pretty overwhelmed. Add in the daily mental and emotional juggling act of modern life, and it's easy to see why our bodies might say, "We're in survival mode right now — reproduction needs to wait!" What's very comforting to know though is that once you understand these underlying factors, you can take control and make targeted, effective adjustments to the way you're living your life.

TIP

One often overlooked factor is the power of your subconscious beliefs, which you'll learn more about in the following chapters. In a nutshell, the subconscious mind is like a vast storage system, holding onto beliefs, memories, and patterns of behavior that influence how you think, feel, and react — even when you aren't fully aware of it. For example, if your only idea of childbirth comes from TV shows or stories of difficult births, your subconscious may hold onto these dramatized, traumatic, or negative portrayals, which can be one factor that affects your body's ability to relax and create optimal conditions for conception. While fear of childbirth isn't the sole cause of fertility challenges, it illustrates how subconscious beliefs can play a role in influencing your body's response.

For both men and women, fears about being a good parent, anxieties about the future, or societal pressures can trigger a stress response in the body that impairs sperm quality and testosterone production or disturbs the hormonal balance needed to conceive and maintain a healthy pregnancy. These subconscious fears, if severe enough, can also disrupt the hypothalamic-pituitary-gonadal (HPG) axis — the communication line between the brain and reproductive organs in both sexes — and the immune system, leading to inflammation that further impacts reproductive health.

REMEMBER

The key takeaway here is that fertility today requires more than a one-size-fits-all approach. A holistic strategy — one that includes optimizing diet, improving lifestyle, and managing emotional and psychological stressors — is the recipe for success. With the right tools and conscious effort, you can enhance your fertility and pave the way for conception, whether naturally or with support.

THE ROLE OF EPIGENETICS AND PARENTAL HEALTH

It's also important to consider that your lifestyle affects more than your fertility; it can also influence the health of future generations. Research shows that both the mother's lifestyle during pregnancy and the father's health at conception can significantly influence the baby's hormone profile through epigenetic imprinting.

For instance, inadequate maternal nutrition, particularly a diet low in essential nutrients like folate, can affect the genes involved in hormone regulation. Additionally, research has shown that chronically stressed men or those who consume a diet high in processed foods and low in essential nutrients are more likely to produce sperm with DNA damage or epigenetic changes that can impact gene expression in the embryo and potentially affect the child's hormonal regulation and susceptibility to metabolic diseases, obesity, or even cognitive and emotional health issues later in life.

For more practical tips on preserving your fertility, check out Chapter 4. In Chapters 15 through 17, you'll find even more strategies to support your journey. Remember, though, that if natural conception isn't your path, it's perfectly okay. Balancing your hormones and preparing yourself physically and emotionally will ensure you're the most confident, energized, and healthy parent — no matter how your family grows.

Androgen excess

Polycystic ovary syndrome (PCOS), one of the most common endocrine disorders, affects an estimated 10 to 15 percent of women globally, although that number is likely much higher. Why? Because many women remain undiagnosed, thanks to the wide range of symptoms and a lack of awareness.

Indeed, studies suggest that up to 70 percent of women with PCOS may not even know they have it. They often mistake their symptoms for something else or are told their symptoms are "just part of being a woman." Early diagnosis is crucial for managing PCOS effectively and preventing long-term issues like diabetes and heart disease. Thankfully, improved diagnostic tools that offer hope for earlier detection and better management are on the horizon.

Although the name polycystic ovary syndrome sounds modern, PCOS has likely been around for thousands of years. In fact, symptoms such as irregular periods, infertility, and excessive hair growth were documented in ancient medical texts from as early as ancient Egypt.

So, while PCOS isn't a new problem, today's lifestyle factors are making it much more common. Fortunately, thanks to modern science, it's also now largely manageable and, in many cases (mine included) even reversible by following a holistic approach that includes diet tweaks, lifestyle changes, and deep healing work to cultivate safety in the body by addressing stress, trauma, and unprocessed emotions.

Reasons PCOS is on the rise

The mainstream discourse on PCOS largely centers around modern dietary habits, particularly the consumption of processed foods, refined carbohydrates, and sugars, which contribute to insulin resistance and chronic inflammation — two primary drivers of the condition. Other factors, including a sedentary lifestyle, reduced muscle mass, and the accumulation of belly fat caused by hormonal imbalances, create a cycle that intensifies PCOS symptoms. Sleep disturbances, another common issue in PCOS, further disrupt cortisol and insulin regulation, making it even more difficult to adopt and maintain healthy habits, while further amplifying hormonal chaos.

Enhanced athletic performance and PCOS

REMEMBER

If PCOS were solely the result of poor diet and lifestyle, we wouldn't see such a high prevalence of the condition among elite female athletes, including Olympic athletes, who dedicate their lives to maintaining peak physical condition. Research shows that mild hyperandrogenism, a common feature of PCOS, is overrepresented among these athletes and contributes to greater muscle mass and increased bone density, which (according to some data) can provide an advantage in physical performance.

Clearly, PCOS is not just about poor diet and lack of exercise. Factors such as genetics, hormonal sensitivity, high levels of exercise, exposure to environmental toxins, and even unprocessed trauma can all significantly influence the development of PCOS. When you dig deeper, it becomes clear that this is a multifaceted condition that requires a much more comprehensive understanding than the conventional conversation and approach is offering.

The four types of PCOS

PCOS can manifest in different ways depending on its underlying causes, and research has identified four distinct types:

TIP

- **Insulin-resistant PCOS:** This is the most common form and is linked to — you guessed it — insulin resistance and blood sugar dysregulation. It's often associated with weight gain, particularly in the abdominal area, and symptoms such as fatigue and cravings for sugary foods. Managing insulin-resistant PCOS typically involves strategies to stabilize blood sugar levels, which can include dietary adjustments, muscle building, and sometimes medication.

TIP

- **Post-pill PCOS-like symptoms:** These symptoms can occur after discontinuing birth control pills, and it's typically a temporary condition. It happens because your body needs time to adjust and begin producing its own hormones after being regulated by the pill for years. In many cases, symptoms subside as your hormonal balance stabilizes, but you can proactively prevent or mitigate symptoms and support a smooth transition by addressing factors such as diet, exercise, and stress levels before you stop taking the pill.
- **Inflammatory PCOS:** In this type, your body produces extra androgens in response to systemic inflammation, which could be caused by stress, food sensitivities, or exposure to environmental toxins.
- **Adrenal PCOS:** This less common form occurs when the adrenal glands, rather than the ovaries, overproduce androgens, typically in response to stress, unresolved trauma or less common adrenal diseases. Women with adrenal PCOS often have normal insulin levels but elevated DHEA-S, a hormone from the adrenal glands. Stress management and healing trauma are key for this specific type of PCOS, along with a supportive diet and lifestyle.

Trauma and PCOS

The four PCOS categories in the preceding section show just how nuanced PCOS is and why managing it requires a holistic approach that acknowledges the intricate connections between your mind, body, and environment. Unresolved trauma and chronic stress — whether emotional, physical, or psychological — often play a profound role in how PCOS develops, so the following list explores how these factors come together:

- **Hormonal dysregulation:** Chronic stress — whether from unresolved trauma, emotional burdens, or the relentless pressures of modern life — throws off the balance between androgens (male hormones) and female reproductive hormones.
- **Insulin resistance:** Research indicates that both physical and emotional trauma can elevate the risk of developing insulin resistance. Elevated cortisol levels from chronic stress signal your body to release glucose into your bloodstream, energizing your cells for a fight-or-flight response. Then stress-related behaviors can worsen blood sugar imbalances and harm metabolic health. Over time, this creates a vicious cycle of insulin resistance, weight gain, and hormonal imbalance, all of which are common in PCOS.
- **Inflammation:** Chronic inflammation is deeply connected to stress and trauma because it activates your stress response and the HPA axis. It also fuels insulin resistance and disrupts ovarian function, worsening PCOS symptoms. Poor diet, lack of sleep, and inactivity can further exacerbate inflammation, making it even harder to manage the condition.

REMEMBER

- **Lifestyle factors:** When someone experiences trauma — whether physical, emotional, or psychological — the body often remains in a heightened state of stress, even long after the event. As a coping mechanism, many individuals unconsciously adopt habits, such as emotional eating to soothe stress, that intensify hormonal imbalances. Lack of exercise or irregular sleep patterns are also common responses to trauma because the nervous system is stuck in a state of hypervigilance that makes rest or physical activity difficult. The reliance on these habits can further disrupt cortisol regulation, insulin sensitivity, and reproductive hormones, creating a vicious cycle that worsens PCOS symptoms.
- **Neuroendocrine disruption:** Recent research also highlights how stress and trauma affect the neuroendocrine system. Changes in neurotransmitters and neuropeptides (the chemicals your brain uses to send messages between nerve cells) due to chronic stress can impair ovarian function and hormonal regulation, contributing to the hormonal imbalances seen in PCOS. This disruption of the body's natural hormone feedback loops can perpetuate the cycle of androgen excess, insulin resistance, and irregular menstrual cycles.

ADVERSE CHILDHOOD EXPERIENCES AND PCOS: STUDY OVERVIEW

In 2020, researchers from Monash University in Australia conducted a fascinating investigation into the connection between adverse childhood experiences (ACEs) and PCOS. The study examined more than 1,000 women and found a significant link between PCOS and a history of childhood trauma. Women with PCOS were far more likely to have experienced adverse events during their early years, such as emotional, physical, or sexual abuse, neglect, or household dysfunction. The study also revealed that these women had a higher prevalence of psychiatric conditions such as anxiety, depression, and other mood disorders, further suggesting that ACEs may be an important risk factor for developing PCOS. This study underscores the critical importance of considering mental health and past trauma when diagnosing and treating PCOS.

Endometriosis

Endometriosis (commonly shortened to *endo*) is a challenging condition that occurs when tissue similar to the lining of the uterus (the endometrium) grows outside the uterine cavity, commonly on the ovaries, fallopian tubes, and pelvic lining. In rare cases, it even ventures beyond the pelvis. Think of it weeds in a garden that not only sprout in the flower beds but also spread to the lawn and driveway — uninvited and hard to manage. These rogue cells thicken, break down, and bleed with the menstrual cycle, but they get trapped because they have nowhere to go. The result is inflammation, scar tissue, and adhesions that cause organs to stick together like they're in a dysfunctional group hug.

The true rates of endo are hard to estimate. According to a 2024 review from the University of York, endo takes about 6.6 years to diagnose and affects about 1 in 10 women. Due to widespread misunderstanding and frequent misdiagnosis, the actual prevalence is likely much, much higher.

REMEMBER

The hallmark symptom is severe pelvic pain, especially during menstruation, although women with endometriosis can experience delights such as heavy bleeding, irregular periods, pain during sex, and infertility. Sadly, many women spend years getting misdiagnosed, which leaves them to suffer with chronic pain that seriously impacts their quality of life and can often lead to anxiety, depression, and chronic fatigue. Additionally, endo can cause urinary, gastrointestinal, and musculoskeletal symptoms due to endometrial-like tissue deposits in more distant areas of the body, further complicating the condition.

Prevalence of endo

Since the late 1940s, there has been a stereotype in medical research and discourse portraying the "typical" endo patient as a white, middle-class, highly educated woman who is perceived as delaying childbirth. (A gross stereotype, I know.) This narrow view has led to significant gaps in our understanding, particularly concerning the experiences of women from diverse backgrounds.

REMEMBER

For example, endo wasn't even recognized as affecting Black women until the 1970s. Some of this bias stemmed from assumptions about racial differences in pain tolerance or misdiagnoses of pelvic pain as related to other conditions, such as pelvic inflammatory disease or sexually transmitted infections. It wasn't until 2012 that a team in Detroit found that Black women often experience more severe endometrial growths at different locations in their bodies compared to white women.

TIP

Clearly, there is a desperate need for more inclusive and comprehensive research to address these disparities and improve treatment outcomes. So, if you're struggling to get answers or a diagnosis, don't give up. Be persistent, advocate for yourself, and keep pushing for the care and answers you deserve.

Rising Rates of endo and further study

The increase in endo cases mirrors that of other hormone-related conditions such as PCOS, making it clear that modern lifestyles are playing a role. So far, EDCs, chronic stress, systemic inflammation, and poor gut health have all been linked to its development. But research into its causes and effective treatments remains insufficient. For this reason managing endo can seem like a daunting challenge, but by addressing the factors we are aware of holistically along with seeking medical support, you can turn endo's complexity into a vehicle for empowered self-care.

REMEMBER

Endometriosis, like many other chronic conditions, is not just a physical ailment but a message that something deeper needs addressing. It's deeply intertwined with the emotional and societal pressures women face and requires you to take a step back and assess the way you're living your life and any cultural/religious/family/workplace expectations on your shoulders. As world-renowned physician and trauma expert Dr. Gabor Maté points out, women often act as society's connective tissue or emotional glue, holding everything together, which he argues contributes to their higher prevalence of autoimmune and connective tissue diseases, such as lupus (90 percent of sufferers in the U.S. are women) and inflammatory arthritis (70 percent of global sufferers are women).

DOUBLE WHAMMY: PCOS AND ENDOMETRIOSIS

Interestingly, it's not uncommon for women to have both PCOS and endometriosis at the same time. Studies suggest that up to 10 percent of women with PCOS also have endometriosis. Why? Well, the shared hormonal imbalances, especially high estrogen and low progesterone, can create a perfect storm for both conditions to coexist. This overlap highlights the importance of a comprehensive, holistic treatment approach that addresses both the physical and emotional aspects of these complex conditions.

Endometriosis, although not classified as a connective tissue disease, shares similarities in its chronic inflammatory nature and systemic impact. What Dr. Maté's perspective invites us to do is explore the deeper emotional and psychological factors that may contribute to the physical manifestations of these diseases. Chapter 11 introduces you to two exciting fields tackling this question: psychoneuroimmunology and psychoneuroendocrinology.

Adenomyosis Versus endometriosis

It's also important to differentiate between endometriosis and adenomyosis, two conditions that are often confused. Endometriosis involves the growth of endometrial-like tissue *outside* the uterus, but *adenomyosis* occurs when endometrial tissue grows *into* the muscular wall of the uterus itself, which tends to lead to an enlarged, tender uterus. Both conditions cause similar symptoms, such as heavy bleeding and pelvic pain, but they require different treatment approaches.

Treatment options

TIP

I want to reassure you that yes, it is possible for some women to manage and even halt the progression of endo, although it requires dedication to a holistic treatment plan. As I've worked with women all over the world, I've found that by taking the best of what Western medicine has to offer and coupling it with diet and lifestyle changes, trauma resolution, and stress reduction, women can create a much more favorable environment for managing endometriosis. By helping the body return to its parasympathetic nervous system state — promoting relaxation and recovery — resources are redirected from stress responses toward healing and repair. This shift improves immune function, reduces systemic inflammation, and supports better management of endometriosis symptoms.

TIP

Drinking fresh ginger tea is an excellent example of a holistic daily habit you can implement right away because ginger contains powerful bioactive compounds, such as gingerol, which have strong anti-inflammatory and antioxidant effects. Studies show that ginger can help reduce inflammation, alleviate pain, and improve digestion, making it particularly beneficial for women with endo. Additionally, ginger has been shown to lower pro-inflammatory cytokines, which can help reduce the systemic inflammation associated with endometriosis. Plus, it's delicious with lemon. What's not to love?

When it comes to whether it's possible to heal endometriosis completely, the current evidence on the breakdown and reabsorption of misplaced endometrial tissue is limited, mainly due to the scarcity of research on the condition. However, managing inflammation and addressing the mind, body, and emotions always contribute to better long-term outcomes and symptom management.

Sometimes, surgery to remove endometrial lesions may be necessary to provide immediate relief, and that's completely understandable. However, it's important to approach surgery with care because repeated procedures can sometimes lead to scar tissue formation and other complications. If surgery is the best option for you, the goal is to make each intervention as effective and final as possible. By focusing on taking control of your health and slowing disease progression through holistic approaches, you can support your body in the long run and minimize the need for further surgeries.

TIP

You're the only expert in you, so if your symptoms persist or you feel something isn't right, trust your intuition and advocate for yourself. No one knows your body better than you do, and it's essential to push for answers and seek proper diagnosis if you're struggling.

Fibroids

Fibroids, also known as uterine leiomyomas, are like the uninvited guests at the uterine party. They're noncancerous, but they sure know how to make themselves known! They can grow within the uterine wall (intramural), causing heavy periods and pelvic pain, or under the uterine lining (submucosal), often leading to heavy bleeding and fertility challenges. Others like to form on the outer surface of the uterus (subserosal), pressing on nearby organs such as the bladder (necessitating frequent trips to the bathroom). Some even dangle from the outer or inner surface of the uterus (pedunculated), and can twist, causing sharp, sudden pain.

These muscular growths can range from tiny to "how is that even fitting in there?!" sizes, and in the U.S., around 70 to 80 percent of women will develop fibroids by the age of 50. One study showed an increase in diagnoses from

33 percent in 1980 to 40 percent in 2000. But don't worry; fibroids are generally considered "safe" when they're asymptomatic or cause mild symptoms that don't significantly impact daily life. They only become a concern when their size or location leads to complications like heavy bleeding, severe pelvic pain, or pressure on other organs, which can affect fertility and your overall quality of life.

High levels of estrogen and progesterone, influenced by factors such as obesity, poor diet and exposure to hormone-mimicking chemicals are understood to promote fibroid growth. Chronic stress, as always, gets in on the action, throwing hormonal balance out of whack by raising cortisol levels.

TIP

The real kicker is that our love for processed foods, sugar, and unhealthy fats fuels inflammation and insulin resistance, creating the perfect storm for fibroid growth. The good news is that tweaking your diet and lifestyle and following the steps outlined in later chapters can help you manage or reduce your fibroids.

Rising Reproductive Health Issues for Men

While issues such as declining testosterone levels, rising rates of erectile dysfunction, and the global sperm crisis are often dismissed as signs of aging or stress, they actually serve as crucial indicators of deeper imbalances in men's physical and mental well-being.

Historically, medical science and healthcare systems have paid far less attention to male reproductive health compared to women's, with limited research, narrow healthcare policies, and little social understanding or education on the subject. This neglect is partly fueled by the cultural stigma surrounding men's reproductive health; symptoms are often brushed off with embarrassment and shame. For example, have you ever heard of a men's infertility support group? They're hard to find because society has long associated male virility with strength, leaving men reluctant to admit to symptoms or issues, which in turn prevents them from seeking help unless there is a serious medical need. Even in cases of infertility, when men should undergo semen analysis and reproductive assessments, they won't happen 25 percent of the time.

To rectify this significant gap in knowledge and care, the global Male Reproductive Health Initiative (MRHI) was launched in 2018, marking a critical step forward in bringing attention to men's reproductive health and encouraging more comprehensive research and education on the topic.

Declining testosterone

A study published in the *Journal of Clinical Endocrinology and Metabolism* showed that men in the U.S. have 17 percent lower testosterone levels compared to men 20 years ago. U.K. statistics also mirror this trend as shown in a *British Medical Journal* report that shared that testosterone prescriptions have risen sharply in recent years, signaling more widespread deficiencies. So, what's happening? Is it simply due to an aging population? While it's true that testosterone naturally declines with age — around 1 percent per year starting at age 30 — there are many other factors at play that are disrupting men's testosterone levels, and those issues deserve urgent attention.

One of the biggest culprits is — you guessed it — EDCs. These sneaky chemicals (found in plastics and food packaging) and phthalates (found in personal care products, vinyl flooring, and many household items) can reduce testosterone and increase estrogenic activity, effectively throwing a wrench into your hormonal gears. Everyday exposure to these toxins, especially through diets filled with processed foods that strip the body of essential nutrients like zinc and magnesium (both crucial for testosterone production), makes it harder for men to maintain healthy testosterone levels.

WARNING

To further complicate things, traditionally male-dominated industries such as construction, manufacturing, and agriculture commonly expose workers to plastics and chemicals loaded with EDCs. For example, pesticides and herbicides used in agriculture contain chemicals that can disrupt hormone levels. In construction and manufacturing, workers frequently come into contact with solvents, heavy metals, and industrial lubricants. Additionally, materials such as PVC pipes and vinyl release phthalates and products like paint and insulation often contain toxic chemicals such as formaldehyde.

TIP

The level of exposure to these harmful substances varies greatly depending on the specific job, the duration of contact, and safety measures in place, but the good news is that while a career change may be off the table, there are still steps you can take to minimize exposure and protect your health — for example, wearing protective gear, reducing contact with harmful substances, and improving ventilation in work areas. Additionally, making healthy lifestyle choices can help mitigate some of the effects of these exposures.

The decline in traditional manual labor jobs over the past few decades has contributed to a more sedentary lifestyle with less daily physical activity. That decline combined with the increased consumption of processed foods — particularly among men, who are more likely to rely on fast food and ready-made meals — has fueled rising rates of obesity and metabolic dysfunction, such as insulin resistance. These factors are key contributors to reproductive struggles because excess body fat increases estrogen and lowers testosterone, creating a vicious cycle.

Beyond physical factors, changing gender roles and expectations also play a role, as men's lives are shaped by restrictive role expectations just as much as women's. Today, many men are expected to be both emotionally available caregivers and successful providers, a dual responsibility that previous generations may not have faced as intensely. This evolving landscape can be stressful for men in several ways. First, the pressure to excel as a financial provider in an increasingly competitive world can be overwhelming, especially as economic stability becomes more difficult to achieve for many people. At the same time, there is a growing expectation for men to be emotionally available and nurturing partners or fathers, a role that may conflict with the traditional, stoic view of masculinity that some men were raised with. This dual pressure can often leave men feeling like they are constantly falling short in one area or the other, fostering feelings of inadequacy and failure.

REMEMBER

Social isolation is another modern issue. Recent data shows that men are increasingly losing close friendships. A 2021 Survey Center on American Life poll found that 15 percent of men report having no close friends, a steep rise from just 3 percent in 1990. Only 27 percent of men say they have six or more close friends, a number that's halved over the past 30 years. When you combine stressors like financial burdens, work demands, loneliness, and the societal expectation to "be the provider," cortisol levels are likely to spike, driving testosterone levels down even more.

REMEMBER

Lack of sleep, irregular sleep patterns, poor gut health, too much screen time, and alcohol or drug use all play a role too. When life becomes overwhelming, men may turn to substances as a coping mechanism, further suppressing the endocrine system. In the U.S., 11.5 percent of men aged 12 and older have a substance use disorder, compared to 6.4 percent of women. Men are also more likely to binge drink, with 30.9 percent of men reporting binge drinking in the past month compared to 17.6 percent of women. The encouraging news is that the conversation around men's reproductive and mental health is finally shifting, and more men are stepping up to seek increasingly available support.

Decreasing sperm count

Between 1973 and 2018, the global average sperm count dropped by 51.6 percent, and its showed no signs of slowing down. That's an alarming trend regardless of whether you plan to have kids. Why? Well, much like a woman's menstrual cycle, sperm health can act like a report card for the entire body, especially a man's metabolic, hormonal, and cardiovascular health.

REMEMBER

The usual suspects are the culprits: EDCs; poor diet and nutrient deficiencies; obesity; sleep deprivation; sedentary lifestyles; chronic stress; overtraining or excessive endurance exercise; conditions such as type 2 diabetes, metabolic syndrome, and autoimmune diseases; smoking; excessive alcohol consumption; drug use; certain medications; and heat exposure (such as placing laptops directly on laps or wearing tight underwear).

Two less frequently discussed factors are air pollution and steroid misuse. Air pollution, particularly in urban and industrialized areas, is driven by vehicle emissions, industrial activity, and high population density. Steroid misuse is a growing concern often linked to body dysmorphia and societal pressure for men to achieve a muscular physique. These expectations are leading to alarmingly high rates of steroid abuse, which exacerbate hormone imbalances and pose significant health risks.

REMEMBER

One encouraging bit of news is that sperm count can improve within just 72 to 90 days — the time it takes for a fresh batch to regenerate. Simple diet and lifestyle changes outlined in Part 4 of this book can make a huge difference. And while there will always be factors beyond your control, such as air pollution in the city you live in, you can play a role in advocating for change. Let this be a reminder to focus on what you can control in your daily life, while also contributing to larger efforts for policy reform that improve the environment and public health for everyone.

Male sexual dysfunction

Male sexual dysfunction often gets swept under the rug of silence and shame. But here's what you should know: It's much more common than you realize, and there's nothing to be embarrassed about, it's essentially the body's way of waving a red flag and saying, "Hey, something's off, and I need your attention!" Symptoms are always communication from the body.

At its core, male sexual dysfunction encompasses any condition that prevents full sexual satisfaction, with the most common issues being erectile dysfunction (ED), Peyronie's disease (PD) — where fibrous scar tissue forms beneath the skin of the penis — and premature ejaculation (PE). The prevalence of male sexual dysfunction increases with age as you would perhaps expect, with more than 50 percent of men aged 40 to 70 reporting some degree of erectile dysfunction. The condition is a rapidly increasing concern for younger men too. For example, in 1995, more than 152 million men worldwide experienced ED, and projections for 2025 estimate this number will rise to approximately 322 million — an increase of nearly 170 million men.

WARNING

Ongoing research continues to explore modern factors contributing to this trend, such as excessive video gaming. Dr. Ashwin Sharma, a U.K.-based doctor, issued a public warning ahead of the release of EA Sports FC 25, citing studies such as one from 2016 that found that men who spent five hours or more using screens were almost three times more likely to report ED compared to those who limited their screen time to less than an hour. Sharma explained that the sedentary nature of gaming can negatively affect circulation and cardiovascular health, both of which are crucial for maintaining sexual function.

SLAY THE SHAME: A TOXIC SURVIVAL EMOTION

One of the most significant aspects of the conversation around male sexual dysfunction is shame, a particularly poisonous survival emotion. Survival emotions, like fear, anger, and disgust, evolved to help our ancestors react quickly to threats by triggering the fight-or-flight response. Shame is one of the most powerful of these emotions because it taps into our deep-rooted fear of social rejection. For our ancestors, being cast out of the tribe or community was a serious threat to their survival, so shame evolved as a way to keep us in line with social norms.

The challenge with shame is that it usually doesn't simply fade with time; instead, it lingers and festers, embedding itself deeply in the psyche. This unresolved shame often fuels chronic stress, keeping the body in a prolonged state of fight or flight. Over time, that interferes with critical physiological processes, particularly testosterone production and blood vessel function, two key components necessary for maintaining an erection and supporting overall sexual health. As shame persists, it creates a feedback loop, where emotional pain exacerbates physical dysfunction, and the resulting dysfunction further deepens feelings of inadequacy and shame.

How do you overcome shame? In many cultures, men are conditioned to hide vulnerability, leading to the suppression of emotions and avoidance — not just of intimacy, but also of seeking real solutions to sexual health concerns. To slay shame, you have to understand that it thrives in darkness; it only has power when kept hidden. The more openly men talk about their sexual health, the weaker shame's grip becomes. So whether through therapy, honest communication with a partner, or mindfulness practices, addressing your emotions is just as crucial as physical health when it comes to restoring hormonal balance and sexual function.

And while hormonal imbalances, poor health habits such as lack of sleep, and lifestyle habits such as smoking or drinking can all play a role, stress, anxiety, unresolved trauma, and relationship dynamics also significantly contribute to sexual dysfunction. Take chronic stress, for example: Whether the stress is from work, finances, family, or the societal expectation to "man up and provide," the associated elevated cortisol levels impair blood vessel function, making it more difficult to maintain an erection.

IN THIS CHAPTER

» **Examining the downward trend of metabolic health**

» **Analyzing the increasing prevalence of adrenal issues**

» **Unveiling what's behind our mental health decline**

Chapter 7
Unpacking Global Crises in Health

Building on the reproductive health crises explored in the previous chapter, here we broaden the lens to examine the interrelated metabolic, adrenal, and mental health crises affecting individuals worldwide. Though these crises may seem separate, they are intricately linked, driven by the same complex web of environmental, societal, and modern lifestyle factors.

Throughout this chapter, you'll uncover the forces driving the dramatic rise in metabolic disorders, explore the mounting pressure on our adrenal systems s, and dive into the roots of the global mental health decline. By understanding the connections between these crises and the hormones and systems in the body that they affect, you'll gain a deeper appreciation for the complexity of these issues and the power of addressing their root causes.

Understanding the Global Metabolic Health Crisis

The prevalence of serious illnesses and premature deaths linked to conditions such as high blood pressure and obesity has surged by 50 percent since 2000. This growing crisis in metabolic health places immense pressure on our already overstretched healthcare systems.

This shift marks a significant transition from a time when infectious diseases and maternal and child health were our primary health threats. Now, we're in an era where noncommunicable diseases, driven by metabolic risk factors like high blood sugar and elevated fat levels, are on the rise. Conditions such as heart disease, diabetes, and cancer are among the leading causes of ill health and premature death, a point emphasised in a report from the Institute for Health Metrics and Evaluation (IHME) at the University of Washington, which noted a 49.4 percent increase between 2000 and 2021 in the number of years lost to poor health and early death due to metabolic-related conditions. Distressingly, the impact is particularly severe in younger adults aged 15 to 49.

Future public health trends could be further complicated by rising obesity rates, pollution, climate change, and increasing substance use disorders, all of which contribute to worsening metabolic health and place additional strain on health-care systems. This is why I continually emphasize the connection between stress, emotions, and low self-esteem: Physical and emotional health are two sides of the same coin. Increasing rates of coping behaviors like substance abuse are a signal that deeper emotional issues are at play.

For example, a study from the YWCA in New Zealand found that 72 percent of young women experience negative feelings about their bodies at least once a day, with 25 percent feeling that way all day long. This leads to a significant amount of time avoiding sports, social gatherings, and fully participating in life. The situation in the U.S. is similarly concerning. IPSOS research shows that 79 percent of adults have experienced body dissatisfaction, and 66 percent of girls express a desire to lose weight. Even more alarming is that 46 percent of children aged 9 to 11 report engaging in dieting behaviors, often encouraged by their families.

REMEMBER

These statistics highlight a culture fixated on body image, where dissatisfaction starts young and continues to affect physical health, self-esteem, and social engagement. The pressure to meet unrealistic standards often leads to unhealthy behaviors, which adds fuel to the crisis in metabolic health. To effectively combat the global metabolic health crisis, we have to acknowledge the profound link between emotional well-being and physical health and start addressing the root causes, not just the symptoms.

The growing frustration with traditional weight-loss advice

REMEMBER

Many people find themselves stuck in the same cycle of dieting, restricting and bingeing, exercising intensely, or even considering more extreme measures like weight-loss medications, yet they often don't see sustainable results. There's a good explanation for that: A lot of what we've been told about weight loss is either outdated or incomplete. People are starting to realize that traditional weight-loss methods aren't working for a reason. The truth about our food — the hidden sugars, processed ingredients, and the way modern diets disrupt metabolism — has been downplayed for years. So while people are counting calories and hitting the gym, the real problem often lies in the quality of food and how it affects hormones, gut health, and energy levels.

Other key contributors to the crisis

Beyond the well-known factors driving the metabolic crisis, several additional contributors often work together, creating a perfect storm:

- **Sleep and circadian rhythms:** Lack of quality sleep throws off key hormones such as leptin (which tells you when you're full) and ghrelin (which triggers hunger) and can lead to overeating and weight gain. A study in the *Journal of Clinical Endocrinology & Metabolism* found that insufficient sleep even decreases insulin sensitivity by 30 percent, which means your body becomes less effective at processing glucose, leading to higher blood sugar levels.
- **The role of gut health:** The typical modern diet, rich in processed foods and low in fiber, can compromise your gut health, and that directly impacts your metabolism. Research shows that people with obesity tend to have less diverse gut bacteria, contributing to chronic inflammation and insulin resistance and making it harder to lose weight.
- **Sedentary lifestyles:** Sitting is the new smoking. More than ever, people are spending long hours being inactive at their desks, in front of the TV, while gaming, or while on their phones. Fewer than 25 percent of Americans meet the Centers for Disease Control and Prevention's (CDC's) recommended physical activity guidelines according, and this lack of movement slows metabolism, reduces insulin sensitivity, and promotes weight gain, even for those who diet or exercise occasionally.
- **Emotional eating and coping mechanisms:** Many people's eating habits change during times of stress or when dealing with negative emotions, leading to undereating, skipping meals, overeating, and further metabolic imbalance.

- **Socioeconomic barriers:** Access to healthy, affordable food is a significant barrier for many families. Processed, calorie-dense foods are often cheaper and more accessible than fresh, nutrient-dense options, particularly in low-income areas. Research published in the *American Journal of Public Health* shows a strong link between food insecurity and obesity, especially in children.

Type 2 diabetes and insulin resistance

In the U.S. alone, 10.5 percent of the population has diabetes, and a staggering 96 million Americans are living with prediabetes, where insulin resistance plays a central role. The U.K. faces a similar challenge, with around 4.9 million people diagnosed with diabetes — most of them type 2. However, this problem isn't limited to Western nations; countries like India and China are also experiencing alarming increases in diabetes, largely driven by the rapid adoption of processed foods and increasingly sedentary lifestyles.

The encouraging news is that type 2 diabetes and prediabetes are largely within your control to manage — and even reverse. If lifestyle choices contributed to the development of these conditions, whether knowingly or unknowingly, those same choices can be key to reversing them. Small, consistent changes can make a huge difference, and Part 4 of this book provides you with a comprehensive toolkit of strategies to help.

For now, I want to explain the difference between insulin resistance and its progression to type 2 diabetes:

- **Insulin resistance:** In this early phase depicted in Figure 7-1, your body's cells become less responsive to the effects of insulin. To compensate, your pancreas produces more insulin to keep blood sugar levels under control, which is why glucose levels stay relatively stable initially. However, there's also an impaired response to insulin stimulation in the target tissues — such as muscles, liver, and fat cells — which makes it harder for these tissues to effectively absorb glucose.
- **Type 2 diabetes:** Over time, the pancreas becomes overworked and can no longer keep up with the demand for insulin. This is where the insulin line drops; your pancreas simply can't produce enough insulin anymore. Meanwhile, glucose levels rise, indicating a loss of blood sugar control. At this stage, insulin resistance has progressed into type 2 diabetes, and your body can no longer manage blood sugar effectively without intervention through lifestyle changes or medication.

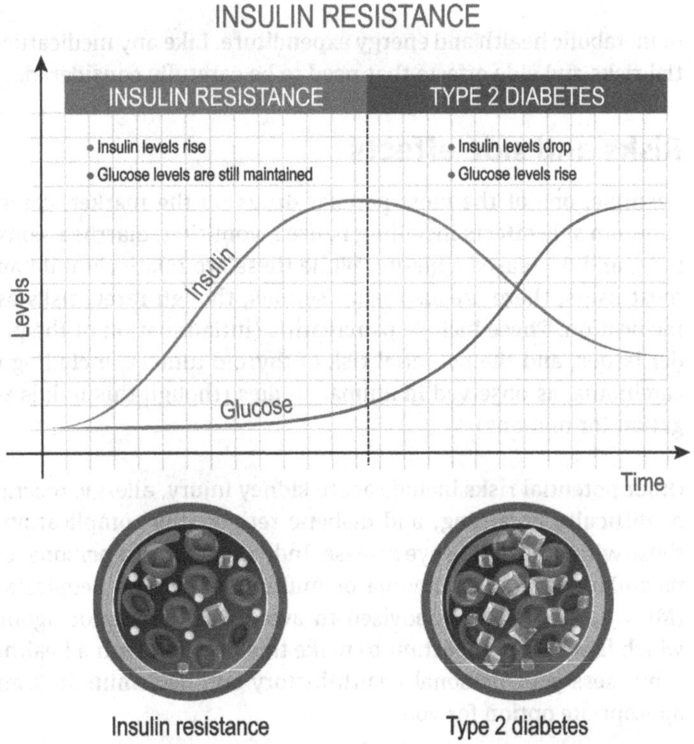

FIGURE 7-1: Insulin resistance.

designua/Adobe Stock Photos

The rise of weight-loss drugs

At the time of writing this book, Ozempic (semaglutide) has skyrocketed in popularity, making the pharmaceutical company behind them worth a staggering $500 billion. Ozempic, which was originally developed to manage type 2 diabetes, works by mimicking a hormone called GLP-1 (glucagon-like peptide-1), which helps regulate blood sugar, slow digestion, and reduce appetite. It often leads to significant weight loss, which, in a society fixated on narrow ideals when it comes body image, explains why the drug is increasingly being used off-label for weight management — even by individuals without diabetes.

REMEMBER

For many who have struggled with traditional diets and exercise, these new solutions can feel like a magic bullet, offering real hope for weight loss and metabolic health. For those with type 2 diabetes, it can be a vital part of managing their condition. However, it's important to remember that while these drugs can help you shed unwanted pounds, they're not a cure-all. They don't address the root causes behind metabolic dysfunction. Without addressing these underlying factors, the weight may return once the individual discontinues the medication. These drugs can also lead to significant muscle loss (especially when weight is lost rapidly), which will impact your metabolism because muscle is an essential driver of metabolic health and energy expenditure. Like any medication, there are potential risks and side effects that need to be carefully considered.

Risks and side effects

WARNING

Ozempic, one of the most popular drugs on the market, comes with a range of common side effects including nausea, vomiting, diarrhea, constipation, stomach pain, and decreased appetite. While these are relatively mild and manageable for most users, there are also more serious, though rarer, risks associated with the medication. These include pancreatitis (inflammation of the pancreas), gallbladder issues, and the potential risk of thyroid tumors, including medullary thyroid carcinoma, as observed in animal studies (though this link is still under investigation for humans).

Other potential risks include acute kidney injury, allergic reactions such as rashes or difficulty breathing, and diabetic retinopathy complications, particularly for those with preexisting eye disease. Individuals with a personal or family history of medullary thyroid carcinoma or multiple endocrine neoplasia syndrome type 2 (MEN 2) are generally advised to avoid GLP-1 receptor agonists like Ozempic, which is why it's important to make this decision with a healthcare provider who can assess your personal health history and determine if Ozempic is a safe and appropriate option for you.

Additionally, some women have reported unexpected pregnancies. While this may sound surprising, it actually aligns with the connection between metabolic and reproductive health, as described in Chapter 6.

REMEMBER

Side effects and adverse outcomes are possible with almost any drug and data on the long-term outcomes of these medications is still emerging. However, the severity of serious or unwanted effects may sometimes be overlooked in favor of speedy weight loss if the focus remains solely on immediate results rather than the broader impact on overall health and well-being.

Natural ways to boost GLP-1

TIP

If medication isn't the route you want or need to take, there are several natural methods to support GLP-1 production and enhance insulin sensitivity. A deeper dive into metabolic strategies is coming in Part 4, but here are a few tips to help you get started:

- **Eat GLP-1-boosting foods:** Incorporate more fermented foods (like kimchi), leafy greens, and healthy fats (such as olive oil), which can naturally help regulate GLP-1 levels.

- **Add GLP-1-boosting herbs and spices:** Cinnamon is well-known for stabilizing blood sugar and boosting GLP-1 secretion. Other options include turmeric, with its anti-inflammatory properties, and ginger, which improves insulin sensitivity and stimulates GLP-1. Fenugreek seeds, cayenne pepper, garlic, and bitter melon are other great additions to a diet aimed at improving GLP-1 function.
- **Eat more protein:** A study found that individuals following a diet with 30 percent protein, featuring meals like chicken, tuna salad, and meat with rice, experienced reduced hunger and a 50 percent increase in GLP-1, keeping you feeling satiated. For plant-based sources, options such as lentils, chickpeas, quinoa, tofu, tempeh, and edamame are excellent protein-rich alternatives. You can find a list of proteins sources in the online appendix at `www.dummies.com/go/hormonebalancefd`.
- **Drink apple cider vinegar (ACV) before meals:** Studies show that apple cider vinegar (ACV) can help reduce post-meal blood sugar spikes by improving insulin sensitivity and promoting a feeling of fullness. One approach is to drink 1 to 2 tablespoons of ACV diluted in water before meals. You can also incorporate it into your diet by using it as a salad dressing.
- **Walk after meals:** A 15 to 20 minute walk after meals has been shown to lower blood sugar and improve insulin sensitivity, which aligns with the traditional Indian philosophy of taking 100 steps after eating to aid digestion.

Hypo- and hyperthyroidism

As covered in Chapter 2, thyroid hormones play crucial roles such in regulating metabolism, thermogenesis (the body's heat production), food intake, and fat oxidation. Beyond that, they're vital for reproductive health in both men and women.

If left unchecked, thyroid issues can have far-reaching consequences. Research from the U.S. and Taiwan, published in the journal *Neurology*, found a link between an underactive thyroid later in life and an increased risk of developing dementia. Additionally, a study published in *Annals of Neurology* revealed that low levels of thyroid hormone during pregnancy increase the risk of autism-like symptoms in the child by four times.

REMEMBER

How prevalent are thyroid issues? In the U.S., the American Thyroid Association estimates that approximately 20 million Americans are affected by some form of thyroid disease, with up to 60 percent of those individuals unaware of their condition. However, once diagnosed, thyroid dysfunction is highly treatable, so the next two sections explore the most common thyroid hormone imbalances in more detail to help you better understand how you can manage and optimize your thyroid function.

Hypothyroidism

Hypothyroidism is when your thyroid gland just can't pull its weight in producing enough T3 and T4, so everything in your body slows down. (Think of it like switching from a sports car to a bicycle.) The pituitary gland then attempts to compensate by releasing more thyroid-stimulating hormone (TSH), signaling the thyroid to ramp up hormone production. However, in hypothyroidism, your thyroid can't keep up with these demands, leading to a cascade of symptoms that reflect the overall reduction in metabolic efficiency. Common symptoms include the following:

- Fatigue
- Weight gain
- Cold intolerance (always reaching for a sweater)
- Depression
- Constipation
- Thinning hair

Hyperthyroidism

Hyperthyroidism occurs when the thyroid goes into overdrive and produces too much T3 and T4. The leading cause of hyperthyroidism is Graves' disease, an autoimmune disorder that accounts for 70 to 80 percent of cases. Normally, the thyroid responds to signals from the pituitary gland to regulate hormone production, but in hyperthyroidism, it continues to produce excessive amounts, which sends your metabolism into overdrive as the body struggles to cope with the accelerated pace. Symptoms include

- Unexplained weight loss
- Increased heart rate
- Anxiety
- Heat intolerance (feeling uncomfortably warm)
- Insomnia
- Muscle weakness

Investigating the root causes

REMEMBER

Iodine deficiency remains a major cause of thyroid dysfunction worldwide, but too much iodine — often because of supplements or diet — can also disrupt thyroid function. In countries like Australia, the leading cause of thyroid problems is Hashimoto's disease, an autoimmune disease. To truly understand why are these conditions are becoming more common, we need to take a closer look at the toll that modern work demands, chronic stress, and lifestyle factors are taking on our thyroid health. A study by Dr. Young Ki Lee, a specialist at the National Cancer Center, found that people working more than 53 hours per week were significantly more likely to develop hypothyroidism compared to those working more manageable hours.

Although we still have much to learn about the complex interactions between stress, lifestyle, and thyroid health, here's what we do know about the key root-cause drivers:

- **EDCs:** As with other hormone-related conditions discussed in this chapter and the previous one, chemicals such as BPA, phthalates, and pesticides interfere with thyroid hormone production and signalling.
- **Chronic stress:** Family or cultural pressures, workplace stress, long hours, financial strain, and the juggling act of modern life all directly affect the hypothalamic-pituitary-thyroid (HPT) axis, the feedback loop that regulates thyroid hormone production. Unregulated stress can lead to adrenal fatigue and further complicate thyroid health.
- **Nutrient deficiencies:** Key nutrients such as iodine, selenium, and zinc are essential for healthy thyroid function. However, with the rising consumption of processed, nutrient-poor foods — partially driven by cultural shifts toward convenience — people are often missing out on these vital nutrients. For example, selenium, a critical nutrient for thyroid health, is easily found in Brazil nuts, with just one or two nuts providing the daily recommended intake. Yet, many diets lack even this small but essential source. Additionally, global food insecurity and reliance on low-quality, affordable food options further exacerbate these deficiencies, making it harder for people to maintain optimal thyroid function.

TIP

- **Autoimmune disorders:** Hashimoto's disease and Graves' disease occur when the immune system mistakenly attacks the thyroid gland, leading to chronic inflammation and dysfunction. Rising chronic inflammation, poor gut health, environmental toxins, chronic stress, and trauma also exacerbate these conditions.
- **Eating disorders and undereating:** Societal ideals around thinness, particularly for women, can lead to prolonged calorie restriction, which slows down

thyroid function as the body conserves energy. The result is symptoms like fatigue, cold intolerance, and weight gain.

- **Obesity and insulin resistance:** As I mention earlier in the chapter, obesity and insulin resistance are significant contributors to hormonal imbalances, including thyroid dysfunction. Excess body fat increases inflammation, which can disrupt the thyroid's ability to function properly. Studies also show a strong correlation between metabolic health issues like type 2 diabetes and hypothyroidism, creating a feedback loop where poor thyroid function worsens metabolic issues, and vice versa.
- **Sedentary lifestyles:** Movement and exercise support metabolic health, and a sedentary lifestyle can slow down the entire endocrine system, including the thyroid. Without regular movement, the body may struggle to maintain optimal thyroid function.

The impact on women

Thyroid disorders disproportionately affect women, who are 8 to 10 times more likely than men to develop hypothyroidism. This gender disparity is largely due to the complex interactions between thyroid hormones and female sex hormones, particularly estrogen and progesterone, especially during key life stages such as pregnancy, postpartum, and menopause. During these transitions, fluctuations in hormone levels can disrupt normal thyroid function.

Adding to this, women have a significantly higher incidence of autoimmune diseases such as Hashimoto's and Graves' diseases, which further contribute to thyroid dysfunction. Unfortunately, the symptoms that arise are often mistakenly attributed to the natural changes of these life stages rather than recognized as potential signs of a thyroid disorder.

To determine whether these symptoms are "normal" or indicative of a thyroid issue, it's important to seek thorough testing. Refer to Chapter 14 for guidance on testing.

Accurate thyroid testing

TIP

If you're looking to thoroughly assess your thyroid health, it's recommended to request a comprehensive thyroid panel that includes tests for T3, T4, reverse T3, and thyroid antibodies. This provides a more complete picture of thyroid function because standard tests by primary care physicians often measure only TSH, which is useful, but it may not detect underlying issues such as autoimmune conditions or imbalances in the active thyroid hormones. A more detailed panel can help identify key markers that could otherwise be missed in a basic TSH test.

Unfortunately, in many healthcare systems, such as the U.K. and U.S., testing for T3 and reverse T3 is not part of the standard thyroid function tests offered, nor is it typically included in monitoring or assessing response to treatment. To ensure you get the testing you need, consider advocating for a full panel with your physician. Be prepared to explain your symptoms and the potential benefits of comprehensive testing. If insurance or healthcare protocols remain a barrier, seeking guidance from a functional medicine practitioner or metabolic specialist can be another option, though this may also involve additional private costs. For more on combining Western medicine with functional approaches, refer to Chapter 14.

Assessing Adrenal Dysfunction

Adrenal dysfunction occurs when the adrenal glands, which regulate cortisol levels and help the body respond to stress, become overworked and unable to keep up with the body's constant demands. Modern phenomena such as "information overload" and "digital fatigue" have been shown to significantly contribute to adrenal strain.

You see, when the body is continuously bombarded with stressors such as work deadlines, nonstop news, or endless social media scrolling and comparing oneself to others, the adrenal glands can start struggling to effectively produce the necessary hormones, resulting in chronic exhaustion, difficulty handling stress, and a range of other physical and emotional symptoms.

REMEMBER

To put modern pressure on our adrenals into perspective, according to British television producer and author John Lloyd, a single edition of the *New York Times* now contains more information than someone from Shakespeare's era would have encountered in their entire lifetime. Back then, life moved at a slower pace. News was local, and change happened gradually. Today, we're exposed to global events, cultural shifts, and political debates in real time every single day. This relentless flood of information can overwhelm our brains and adrenal glands, leaving our cortisol levels in a constant state of overdrive.

Our "normal" isn't normal

We've come to accept a constant state of stress as a normal part of daily life, but in reality, it's anything but normal. Studies show that 75 percent of adults report feeling moderate to high levels of stress on a regular basis. For many people, that stress is nearly unrelenting. What's more, many people carry unresolved emotional trauma from childhood, past relationships, or recent life events, which adds even more weight to an already heavy burden. (Read Chapter 8 for more on this.)

Social media has also turned many of us into "comparison junkies" as we continually measure our self-worth against the polished and often unrealistic images of others' lives. The pressure to maintain a perfect appearance, succeed in every area, and keep up with societal expectations fuels negative self-talk and low self-esteem that puts our adrenal glands on constant high alert.

WARNING

Political polarization and the relentless stream of bad news also contribute to our collective angst to create an environment where everything feels like a battleground. Combined with the capitalist treadmill of productivity and achievement, we find ourselves constantly striving toward unattainable goals, convinced that we must do more, achieve more, and be more.

However, it's equally important to recognize the freedoms and opportunities many of us enjoy in the West — access to education, healthcare, and the autonomy to make personal choices — privileges not universally available. While these advantages equip us with a strong foundation for a better quality of life, they can also be eroded by the consumer-driven pressures that fuel this relentless cycle.

Living this way shouldn't be the baseline, and it doesn't have to be. Each of us can consciously create a lifestyle that acknowledges the need for rest, boundaries, reflection, and real human connection.

High and low cortisol: What it means for your body

Cortisol is not a villain. You need it to help appropriately respond to stress and regulate your energy, metabolism, sexual arousal, and immune responses. But when it remains elevated for too long, you begin experiencing symptoms such as

- Anxiety, irritability, and restlessness
- Weight gain, especially around the abdomen
- High blood pressure and blood sugar spikes
- Sleep disturbances, like difficulty falling or staying asleep

On the flip side, when the adrenal glands become overworked, cortisol production eventually drops to protect the body, which leaves you feeling

- Fatigued, no matter how much sleep you get
- Mentally foggy and struggling to concentrate

- Weak, with low stamina and motivation
- Emotionally depleted, leading to feelings of depression or apathy

Low cortisol levels are essentially your body's way of signalling that it can no longer keep up with the constant demands placed upon it. Essentially, the body has shifted into survival mode, and energy is conserved by shutting down nonessential functions, leaving you exhausted and burnt out. If this sounds like you, don't worry! You'll learn how to take back control of your cortisol levels step by step in Chapter 9 as well as Part 4 of this book.

Declining Mental Health

In 2023, the White House acknowledged that the nation faced "a mental health crisis," with 40 percent of U.S. adults experiencing depression or anxiety in 2021. Gallup estimated that 22 percent of Americans had symptoms severe enough to disrupt their daily lives for two weeks or longer. One-third of U.S. teens had anxiety disorders, and nearly one in five faced a major depressive episode in 2023. This concerning trend isn't limited to the U.S. Globally, the World Health Organization reports that nearly 1 billion people are now living with a mental health disorder, with depression and anxiety leading the way.

Anxiety and depression

REMEMBER

The hormonal shifts we've discussed in this chapter — particularly in cortisol, dopamine, estrogen, and thyroid function — are tightly linked to mental health conditions such as anxiety and depression. In many ways, the mental health crisis is another dimension of the larger global hormone health crisis, showing how deeply interconnected our emotional and physical well-being truly are.

Recognizing these connections is a powerful reminder that addressing the mind, body, and emotions holistically is essential for navigating the complexities of hormone health. Later chapters will continue to explore mental health, but understanding that broader societal factors such as cultural expectations and long work weeks are contributing to mental illness can be incredibly empowering. By acknowledging these external influences, you can begin to recognize your agency, reclaim control and create a life that lights you up.

Cognitive function

The global hormone health crisis is not only impacting mood and emotions but is also contributing to a widespread decline in cognitive function, where the ability to think critically, focus, and innovate is weakened. Hormones such as cortisol, insulin, and thyroid hormones are crucial for brain health, memory, and concentration, so when these hormones become imbalanced, cognitive processes suffer.

Chronic stress, elevated cortisol levels, and inflammation, for instance, can impair memory, decrease focus, and lead to the all-too-common experience of "brain fog." Taking the steps toward hormone balance outlined in Part 4 of this book will help you to think much more clearly, focus for longer, and tap into your full cognitive potential. Imagine what you could get done as this version of yourself?

IN THIS CHAPTER

» **Uncovering the hidden influences before your birth**

» **Exploring how early life shapes your hormones**

» **Demystifying the real impact of genetics**

Chapter 8
Understanding Your Unique Hormonal Profile

This chapter explores the key factors that shape your unique hormonal profile, beginning before you were born (or even thought about!). I explain how your parents' and grandparents' health and lifestyle choices, through the lens of epigenetics, generational trauma, and exposure to endocrine-disrupting chemicals (EDCs), can have lasting impacts on your hormonal system.

You also find out how early life experiences and genetic factors contribute to your hormonal balance. Research continues to evolve in this fascinating area, but this chapter provides you with valuable insights into how these influences work together to shape your hormonal well-being and how you can take proactive steps to optimize your health no matter where you're starting from or what your early life looked like. And if you're planning to have children, the information in this chapter can help you create the best possible foundation for their hormonal health.

Investigating Influences before Birth

Your hormonal journey begins long before you're born — even before you're conceived! Emerging research in the field of epigenetics is shedding light on just how far back these influences can reach. For now, what we do know is that it's not only your parents' health and lifestyle that matter but also the health and environment of your grandparents and even earlier generations.

REMEMBER

Epigenetics refers to changes in gene expression that don't alter the DNA sequence itself but instead act like a set of instructions that tell your genes how to behave. These instructions can be modified by factors such as environment, diet, stress levels, and even chemical exposures your ancestors faced. This means that the conditions in which you were conceived and grew in the womb can have lasting effects on how your body responds to hormones throughout your life, potentially shaping your health in ways we are only beginning to understand.

REMEMBER

Here's an example of how far these influences can reach: When a woman is pregnant with her daughter, the developing fetus already contains the eggs that may one day become the woman's grandchildren. Therefore, the environment and experiences of the woman — such as her exposure to stress, nutrition, exercise, trauma, and toxins — can influence not only the hormonal environment of her unborn daughter but also the developing eggs within that daughter. These eggs carry the genetic and epigenetic information that will later impact the grandchild's hormonal health.

This multigenerational connection highlights the profound and far-reaching influence of ancestral health and environmental exposures, underscoring the importance of taking care of your health not only for yourself but for future generations.

Parental preconception health

It takes two to tango, of course. The combined health of both parents before conception (the moment when a sperm cell from a male fertilizes an egg cell from a female) is a critical factor in shaping the environment in which an embryo develops and lays the foundation for the child's development.

That's quite a lot of responsibility, and it's easy to feel overwhelmed when you start considering all the factors that can influence your child's hormonal health before they're even born. Or perhaps you're reflecting on your own conception and upbringing, and you feel frustration or anger about the choices your parents made or the circumstances they were in and how those things have affected you. Another possible situation is that you don't have the privilege of knowing your biological background or the health and lifestyle choices of your parents, as is the case for many who are adopted or raised in circumstances separate from their biological parents.

REMEMBER

Here's the reassuring truth: The human body is incredibly resilient. Whether you're planning for the future or reflecting on the past, there's a lot you can do to support your health. If you're preparing to become a parent, making informed, proactive choices now can set the stage for a healthier future for your children. If you're looking back, understanding the factors that shaped your development can empower you to make positive changes in your own health. Efforts to improve your nutrition, manage stress, process trauma, reduce exposure to environmental toxins, or make other positive changes at any stage — before conception, during pregnancy, or afterward — can have profound benefits.

Maternal health and influence

A mother's health before and during pregnancy is understandably one of the most critical factors influencing fetal and endocrine development. The mother's womb is the child's first "home" or environment after all! Let's take a closer look at the key factors that shape this environment and ensure the best possible start for a child's hormonal health:

TIP

- **Nutrition and diet:** Getting the right nutrients before and during pregnancy is crucial for a baby's developing endocrine system. Folic acid is essential not just for preventing neural tube defects but also for supporting the healthy development of the fetal brain and hormone production. Iodine plays a key role in the development of the fetal thyroid gland, which regulates metabolism and growth. Omega-3 fatty acids are important for the development of the fetal brain and eyes, both of which rely on well-functioning hormonal pathways. Adequate protein, iron, calcium, and vitamin D are also critical because they support the growth of the fetal skeletal system and proper hormonal regulation.
- **Stress and mental health:** Chronic stress, unprocessed emotions, and unresolved trauma before and during pregnancy can lead to elevated maternal cortisol levels, which not only impact the mother's health but also directly affect the developing fetus. High cortisol levels, even before conception, can alter the hormonal environment, potentially influencing the early development of the fetal hypothalamic-pituitary-adrenal (HPA) axis — a crucial part of the endocrine system. During pregnancy, cortisol can cross the placenta (refer to Chapter 2 to learn more about how hormones move around the body), programming the baby's stress response and making them more susceptible to anxiety, depression, and hormonal imbalances later in life.

TIP

- **Physical health and exercise:** Regular, moderate exercise before and during pregnancy helps regulate blood sugar levels, reduces the risk of gestational diabetes, and healthy weight gain, all of which contribute to better hormonal supports balance. Maintaining a healthy weight and building muscle is absolutely crucial because both undernutrition and obesity are linked to adverse outcomes such as preterm birth and gestational diabetes.

- **Environmental exposures:** Exposure to environmental toxins, including endocrine disruptors like bisphenol A (BPA), phthalates, and pesticides, can have significant effects on fetal hormonal development. This issue is so critical that I'm dedicating an entire section later in this chapter, empowering you with the knowledge and tools to reduce your exposure and protect your health.

REMEMBER

- **Maternal age:** Advanced maternal age (typically 35 years or older) is associated with an increased risk of pregnancy complications, such as gestational diabetes, preeclampsia, and preterm birth, which can affect the hormonal environment of the fetus. Older maternal age is also linked to a higher likelihood of chromosomal abnormalities, such as Down syndrome, which can influence the child's development and endocrine function. Additionally, as women age, changes in their own hormonal balance, such as reduced levels of estrogen and progesterone, may impact the pregnancy and the developing fetus, potentially leading to challenges in brain development and overall hormonal regulation in the child. However, with advances in prenatal care and increased awareness of these risks, many women of advanced maternal age have healthy pregnancies and thriving children. With careful monitoring, a healthy lifestyle, and proactive medical support, older mothers can provide an excellent start for their babies!

Paternal health and influence

REMEMBER

While a mother provides the child's first "home," it is increasingly clear that the father's health and genetic contribution at the time of conception play an equally pivotal role in shaping the future health of the child. Sperm quality, which can be influenced by various factors such as diet, exercise, age, stress, trauma, and exposure to toxins, plays a significant role in the health of the child (refer to Chapter 6 for a deeper dive). Additionally, the placenta, which acts as the primary boundary between the mother and the developing fetus, is not only influenced by maternal factors but is also significantly shaped by paternal genes. These paternal genes can program the placenta's development and function, which in turn can have lasting effects on the child's health and susceptibility to diseases in adulthood. Therefore, the father's preconception health should be carefully considered to ensure the best possible start for the child:

TIP

- **Nutritional status and lifestyle:** A father's nutritional status before conception is key to producing healthy sperm that supports proper hormonal development in the fetus. Essential nutrients such as folate, zinc, and omega-3 fatty acids are critical. For instance, low folate levels in fathers have been linked to an increased risk of birth defects and developmental issues in their offspring. Additionally, unhealthy lifestyle conditions and choices such as obesity, smoking, and excessive alcohol consumption can lead to epigenetic changes in sperm, potentially increasing the child's risk of metabolic and hormonal disorders like type 2 diabetes and obesity.

REMEMBER

- **Stress and mental health:** Chronic stress, unprocessed emotions, and unresolved trauma in fathers can lead to hormonal imbalances, particularly elevated cortisol levels, which can negatively affect sperm quality. Stress can also cause epigenetic modifications in sperm, potentially predisposing children to stress-related disorders, anxiety, or depression later in life.
- **Environmental toxins and exposure:** Exposure to endocrine disruptors, heavy metals, and pesticides can damage sperm DNA and disrupt normal hormonal functions. You can refer to Chapter 6 for a closer look at how this works, and you'll also find more about endocrine disruptors and toxins later in this chapter.

REMEMBER

- **Paternal age and genetic factors:** The age of the father at the time of conception can significantly impact the child's health. Advanced paternal age (typically 40 years or older) has been associated with an increased risk of neurodevelopmental disorders in children, such as autism spectrum disorder (ASD). Older fathers are also more likely to pass on genetic mutations that can interfere with normal brain development and hormonal signaling pathways, potentially leading to conditions like attention-deficit/hyperactivity disorder (ADHD), schizophrenia, and bipolar disorder. However, with proper health management, informed decisions, and supportive medical care, older dads can contribute to a healthy future for their children.

Gestation

REMEMBER

During gestation, the approximately 40-week period when a fetus develops inside the mother's womb, every choice and external influence can have a lasting impact on the child's life, especially in shaping their hormonal development. Nutrition, stress management, physical activity, and avoiding environmental toxins are all significant, but it's important to recognize that these factors don't operate in isolation. They interact in complex ways, influencing not just the immediate health of the fetus, but also how the child's endocrine system will respond to the world after birth.

For example, the nutrients a mother consumes do more than contribute to physical growth; they help program the hormonal systems that will regulate everything from metabolism to stress responses later in life. Similarly, a mother's emotional state and stress levels create a hormonal environment that the developing fetus adapts to, potentially setting patterns that will affect their ability to manage stress, seek out safe relationships, and maintain emotional health as they grow. If the hormonal environment is marked by chronic stress, the child may be more prone to risk-taking behaviors or have difficulty forming healthy relationship attachments because their body is primed to operate in a heightened state of alertness or anxiety.

Additionally, the physical activity a mother engages in helps regulate her own hormones, creating a stable environment that supports the optimal development of the fetal endocrine system. This physical environment, along with protection from harmful environmental toxins, ensures that the fetus's hormonal development proceeds without unnecessary disruption, laying the groundwork for a healthy start.

REMEMBER

As I keep reminding you throughout this book, the body is remarkably adaptable and resilient because of *bioplasticity*, which is the body's continuous ability to regenerate and heal, with cells around the body renewing at varying rates throughout life. So, please take comfort in knowing that even if conditions during gestation weren't perfect, the body has a remarkable ability to self-repair, allowing the endocrine system to adapt.

Generational trauma

Generational trauma, also known as *intergenerational* or *transgenerational trauma*, refers to the transmission of trauma from one generation to the next. But what is trauma, exactly? Chapter 9 explores the topic in much more detail, but in simple terms, trauma is any experience or event that overwhelms your ability to cope and makes you feel unsafe emotionally, psychologically, or physically. It can take many forms, including something that happens *to* you, such as abuse or something that is *withheld* from you, like emotional support, love, belonging, or a sense of safety. Both deeply influence how you respond to stress and interact with the world around you.

REMEMBER

Trauma can be categorized into two types: Big *T* trauma and little *t* trauma. Big *T* trauma includes major, life-altering events such as abuse, natural disasters, or serious accidents. These are the kinds of experiences that most people easily recognize as traumatic. On the other hand, little *t* trauma refers to less obvious, yet still impactful, experiences such as ongoing stress, emotional neglect, or feelings of rejection. While these experiences might seem less significant on the surface, they can accumulate over time and have profound effects on a person's emotional, psychological, and hormonal health.

Intergenerational trauma occurs when the effects of these traumas are passed down from parents to children, often without conscious awareness. This transmission can happen through learned behaviors, coping mechanisms like binge eating or alcoholism, emotional patterns, and even biological changes.

REMEMBER

For example, when a person experiences trauma, their body responds by activating stress hormones, such as cortisol and adrenaline. This heightened state of stress can lead to changes in hormonal regulation and may also alter the expression of genes through epigenetics. These epigenetic changes, which do not modify the DNA sequence itself but influence how genes are turned on or off, may sometimes be passed from parents to their children if they occur in germ cells or due to environmental exposure around the time of conception. For instance, studies on Holocaust survivors have shown that their children and grandchildren exhibit altered stress hormone levels and increased vulnerability to anxiety and depression, suggesting a potential transgenerational impact of trauma.

Let's dive deeper into how the transmission of trauma across generations can impact your hormonal profile:

- **Chronic stress response:** Individuals who inherit generational trauma may have an overactive hypothalamic-pituitary-adrenal (HPA) axis, the system responsible for regulating the body's response to stress. This can lead to chronically elevated cortisol levels, making the individuals more susceptible to stress-related disorders, including anxiety, depression, and post-traumatic stress disorder (PTSD). Because cortisol is a tier 1 hormone, it can also disrupt other hormonal systems, such as reproductive hormones and thyroid function, leading to a range of health issues.
- **Altered stress hormone sensitivity:** People affected by generational trauma may have a heightened sensitivity to stress hormones, meaning they might experience stronger or more prolonged stress responses than others in similar situations. This hypersensitivity can aggravate mental health issues and increase the risk of developing conditions such as insulin resistance, type 2 diabetes, high blood pressure, and obesity.
- **Impaired immune function:** The interplay between stress hormones and immune function is complex, but it's well established that prolonged exposure to high cortisol levels can suppress immune responses, leading to a higher risk of illness or contribute to the development of autoimmune diseases.
- **Impact on reproductive health:** Generational trauma can also affect reproductive health by disrupting the balance of sex hormones and contributing to fertility issues, menstrual irregularities, and complications during pregnancy. Additionally, epigenetic changes resulting from trauma may influence the development of reproductive tissues, potentially leading to conditions like polycystic ovary syndrome (PCOS) or endometriosis in women and reduced sperm quality in men.

REMEMBER

Although the effects of generational trauma can be profound and certainly need further research, it's important to recognize that these patterns or effects are not set in stone. Recent research suggests that while epigenetic changes can be inherited, they are also potentially reversible. By adopting the strategies shared in this book, you can reverse some of the harmful epigenetic modifications you've inherited from previous generations to be a cycle breaker by reducing the likelihood that you'll pass the effects on to future generations.

Exposure to endocrine disruptors and toxins

WARNING

The fetal endocrine system, which is responsible for regulating hormones that control development and growth, is highly sensitive to disruptions. Research increasingly shows that fetal exposure to endocrine-disrupting chemicals (EDCs) found in food, plastic, personal care products, clothing, and furniture can have lasting impacts on the developing endocrine system.

Because EDCs (such as BPA, phthalates, and dioxins) can mimic or block natural hormones like estrogen and testosterone, they can interfere with normal tissue and organ development. The World Health Organization (WHO) has estimated that more than 800 chemicals are suspected to be EDCs, and a significant portion of these chemicals are found in consumer products that pregnant women and infants are exposed to daily. For instance, one study in the U.S. found that more than 95 percent of the population had detectable levels of phthalate metabolites in their urine, including pregnant women.

Despite widespread evidence of harm, EDCs continue to be prevalent because sufficient regulations are not yet in place to prevent their use. In the European Union, for instance, a study estimated that exposure to certain EDCs could result in over €150 billion in healthcare costs annually, largely due to health effects impacting fetal and child development.

One of the most concerning aspects of EDC exposure is its impact on the hypothalamic-pituitary-gonadal (HPG) axis, a key hormonal pathway that regulates reproductive development. EDCs can disrupt the HPG axis by altering the production, release, and function of gonadotropins and sex steroids, which are crucial for the normal development of reproductive organs. For example, prenatal exposure to phthalates has been linked to reduced levels of testosterone in male fetuses, leading to incomplete masculinization and potential reproductive issues later in life.

Another frightening discovery was that EDCs can cause changes in how a baby's genes are "tagged" during development in the womb, a process known as

DNA methylation. This tagging helps determine which genes are turned on or off. When EDCs interfere with this process, they can disrupt genes crucial for hormone regulation. What's even more concerning is that these changes can be passed down to future generations, potentially affecting not just the baby but also their children and grandchildren.

WARNING

For example, one study on BPA exposure (commonly found in plastic or food and beverage cans) in utero found that fetuses exposed to this chemical had altered DNA methylation patterns in genes related to endocrine regulation, and the changes persisted into adulthood. This suggests that prenatal exposure to EDCs not only disrupts fetal development but also increases the risk of endocrine disorders, such as thyroid dysfunction and metabolic syndrome, later in life.

Given that many EDCs are pervasive in the environment and found in everyday products, there is a growing need for stricter regulation and policies aimed at reducing exposure, particularly for pregnant women. Public awareness campaigns and further research into safer alternatives to these chemicals are crucial steps in protecting future generations from the harmful effects of EDCs.

TIP

In the meantime, we all need to take our health into our own hands and take proactive steps to reduce our exposure. In the online appendix at `www.dummies.com/go/hormonebalancefd`, I provide a list of common EDCs and where they're found so that you can assess the products in your environment and take steps toward reducing your exposure.

Considering Early Life Influences

While the foundation of your hormonal health is largely laid before you are even born, the journey doesn't stop there. The first years of life are a critical period when your environment continues to shape your hormonal profile. This is where nurture meets nature, and your experiences can significantly influence how your endocrine system functions for the rest of your life.

TIP

While a well-balanced diet made up of whole, nutrient-dense foods, consistent exercise, and strength training are all well-known foundations of a healthy lifestyle — and their significance can't be overstated — this section explores the deeper, often overlooked contributors that build upon the essential foundations.

Adverse childhood experiences

Adverse childhood experiences, or ACEs, are traumatic events that occur in childhood and can include both Big *T* traumas, such as physical or sexual abuse, and little *t* traumas, such as emotional neglect or conditional love. ACEs encompass a wide range of experiences, including growing up in a household affected by substance abuse, mental illness, emotional instability, domestic violence or a lack of financial security, emotional attunement, love, safety, or bonding.

REMEMBER

The stress associated with ACEs can cause chronic activation of the HPA axis. When activated repeatedly or over prolonged periods, the HPA axis can become dysregulated, leading to persistently high levels of cortisol, the body's primary stress hormone. This can interfere with the normal development of other hormonal systems, such as those regulating growth, metabolism, and reproduction.

WARNING

Studies have shown that children who experience multiple ACEs are at an increased risk of developing endocrine-related health issues later in life, such as obesity, type 2 diabetes, and cardiovascular disease. Additionally, there is growing evidence and research linking ACEs to conditions like PCOS and endometriosis. The long-term impact of ACEs on hormonal health underscores the importance of early intervention and support for at-risk children because addressing these issues early can mitigate some of the harmful effects on their endocrine systems.

Parental care and bonding

The early attachment between a child and their caregivers plays a critical role in shaping your emotional, psychological and physical health. Secure attachment, where a child feels safe and nurtured, promotes healthy development of the endocrine system, particularly the HPA axis. This secure bonding environment helps regulate stress responses, ensuring that cortisol levels remain within a healthy range. In contrast, insecure attachment or lack of consistent nurturing can lead to chronic stress and dysregulation of the HPA axis, which has far-reaching consequences for hormonal balance.

REMEMBER

Additionally, the quality of parental care can influence the development of oxytocin pathways in the brain. A nurturing environment promotes the release of oxytocin — a hormone crucial for bonding, social behaviors, and emotional regulation — which supports healthy development of the brain's stress-regulation systems and enhances the child's resilience to stress later in life.

Exposure to a toxic world

From the air we breathe to the food we eat, modern life exposes us to a host of chemicals and pollutants that can interfere with the delicate balance of our endocrine system.

Because of children's smaller stature, developing organs, and the higher rates at which they absorb substances relative to their body weight, they're particularly vulnerable to environmental toxins. For instance, exposure to heavy metals such as lead and mercury — which are often found in older homes, certain foods, and contaminated water — can disrupt neurological development and endocrine function, leading to long-term health issues. Additionally, heavy metals can be stored in bones for decades, potentially reentering the bloodstream during periods of bone remodeling, such as pregnancy or aging, further compounding their health impact.

REMEMBER

As investigated in Chapters 6 and 7, air pollution has also been linked to disruptions in hormonal balance, particularly in children living in urban areas. Studies have found that exposure to pollutants like particulate matter and polycyclic aromatic hydrocarbons (PAHs) can interfere with the endocrine system, potentially leading to developmental delays and increased susceptibility to chronic conditions such as asthma and diabetes. Even seemingly innocuous plastic toys or household items can be sources of EDCs, such as phthalates and BPA.

Given the pervasiveness of these toxins, it might seem overwhelming to try to protect yourself and your family. However, by becoming informed and making conscious choices — such as opting for cleaner, safer products, advocating for healthier environments, and supporting policies that reduce pollution — you can significantly reduce your exposure to these harmful substances. While you can't eliminate every toxin from your life, you can take meaningful steps to minimize their impact and trust your body's resilience to handle the rest. You can find resources and tips on how to live a 'low tox life' in the online appendix at `www.dummies.com/go/hormonebalancefd`.

Understanding Genetic Contributions

While our genes provide the blueprint for our biological functions, including the intricate workings of the endocrine system, it's crucial to recognize that your genetic makeup is just one part of the story.

Although your genes can influence your hormonal profile — shaping everything from your metabolism to your stress response — they do not necessarily determine your destiny. Environmental factors, lifestyle choices, and even your mindset can all interact with your genetic code, altering how your genes are expressed and how your endocrine system functions. In other words, while your genes set the stage, you have significant control over the script.

Individual variation in endocrine systems

REMEMBER

Every individual's endocrine system is unique and shaped by a complex interplay of genetic and environmental factors. This variation means that even if two people have the same levels of hormones in their bloodstream, they can experience entirely different effects in their bodies. For instance, two individuals might have identical levels of thyroid hormones, but one may feel energetic and balanced, whereas the other struggles with fatigue and mood swings.

REMEMBER

One key reason for this difference lies in hormone receptor sensitivity. Hormones exert their effects by binding to specific receptors on cells, much like a key fits into a lock. However, not all locks are the same; the sensitivity and responsiveness of these receptors can vary widely between individuals. This means that even with the same hormone levels, one person's receptors might respond more strongly or weakly compared to another person's, leading to different physiological and emotional experiences.

Genetic differences can influence how your body produces, processes, and responds to hormones, leading to differences in metabolism, stress responses, and reproductive health. For example, certain genetic variants can affect how your body metabolizes estrogen or insulin, potentially increasing your susceptibility to conditions like PCOS, thyroid disorders, or insulin resistance.

REMEMBER

It's not just genetics at play. This variability in receptor sensitivity can also be influenced by lifestyle choices. Chronic stress, diet, and exposure to environmental toxins can alter receptor sensitivity, further contributing to differences in how hormones are felt and utilized by the body. This is why understanding your unique hormonal profile requires more than just looking at hormone levels on a lab test; it involves considering how your body responds to these hormones at the receptor level and learning to listen to what your body is telling you. Your symptoms are often the most reliable guide, signaling how well your hormones are functioning and where adjustments might be needed.

Your genes don't define you

REMEMBER

While genetics certainly play a role in your endocrine system, they don't seal your fate. The field of epigenetics has shown us that gene expression can be influenced by external factors, meaning that the way your genes are "read" and "used" by your body can change based on your environment, experiences, and behaviors. For example, positive lifestyle changes such as improved nutrition, regular physical activity, and stress management can modify gene expression, leading to better hormonal balance and overall health.

This concept of genetic flexibility offers a powerful message: Your genes provide potential; they don't decide your destiny. By making informed and proactive choices, you can influence how your genes express themselves, promoting a healthier endocrine system and reducing the risk of hormone-related conditions.

So, whether you have a family history of endocrine disorders or are simply looking to optimize your health, understanding that you have control over how your genetic information is expressed can be a relief. It allows you to confidently take steps that can positively shape your health, regardless of the hand you were dealt at birth.

This perspective shifts the focus from what might seem like inevitable genetic outcomes to a more dynamic understanding of health — one where your actions and environment play a crucial role in determining your hormonal balance and overall well-being.

IN THIS CHAPTER

» Getting to know your nervous system and how it works

» Unearthing the truth about stress

» Unpacking the influence of unresolved trauma

» Examining the power of unprocessed emotions

» Exploring the wide range of treatment options

Chapter 9
Overloading the Nervous System

The nervous system has always drawn significant attention — and rightly so. It's the fundamental system that allows you to perceive, interact with, and adapt to the world around you. It governs your body's stress response, and its primary purpose is ensuring your survival by managing your reactions to internal or external threats.

Without the nervous system, survival wouldn't be only difficult; it would be impossible. In fact, its importance is evident from the very beginning of life because it's one of the first systems to develop as a person transitions from a fetus to a fully formed infant.

The truth is that the hormone health you seek is impossible without prioritizing the well-being of your nervous system. Unfortunately, in our hyperconnected, always-on modern world, our nervous systems are increasingly teetering on the edge of overload. Without a clear understanding of how this system operates and how to care for it, you risk missing its vital cues or early warning signs, allowing chronic stress, hormone imbalances, and other health issues to silently undermine your quality of life over time.

This chapter dives into the fascinating and emerging intricacies of the nervous system. You find out how to identify which of its two primary states — sympathetic or parasympathetic — you're in at any given moment. I also introduce polyvagal theory, a nuanced understanding of how your body responds to stress, danger, and even everyday situations like an awkward Zoom meeting. Additionally, I explain the powerful role that unresolved trauma and unprocessed emotions play in nervous system health, so by the end of this chapter, you'll be equipped with both traditional and cutting-edge tools to cultivate nervous system resilience and create a more balanced, harmonious internal environment that supports your overall health.

Meeting Your Nervous System

Although humans are considered the most advanced species on Earth, we still carry survival mechanisms that are inherited from our evolutionary ancestors. Research in evolutionary science shows that all mammals share fundamental survival strategies such as the fight-or-flight response and, in extreme cases, the freeze reaction. So although we've now developed more complex abilities such as problem-solving, abstract thinking, the use of tools and technology, and advanced communication, these ancient neural circuits remain deeply rooted in our biology.

REMEMBER

The nervous system was originally designed to help people survive the African savanna, where humans sometimes confronted life-threatening dangers like lions and hyenas. But clearly most modern people no longer navigate those same threats: We now face concrete jungles and the digital wilderness of social media and the internet. The threats we face are no longer occasional or short term; you may find yourself constantly bombarded by stressors every time your phone pings with a news alert, you accidentally like your ex's Instagram post, or your boss asks for a meeting without explaining why. You're using ancient survival biology to cope with a very different world, and it's no wonder your nervous system may be struggling to keep up.

To put the importance of your nervous system into perspective, it begins to develop very early in the fetal stage, even before the spine or brain are fully formed. It plays a crucial role in orchestrating the development of key organs and bodily functions, ensuring that everything is properly connected and communicating effectively. In fact, it acts as the scaffolding from which these critical body structures emerge, laying the foundation for your physical, emotional, and mental well-being long before birth.

Epigenetics and generational trauma

REMEMBER

The health and functioning of your nervous system aren't influenced only by your current environment. They can also be shaped by what you inherit from your parents and ancestors. Emerging research in epigenetics (the study of traits you inherit) shows that trauma, stress, and even certain behaviors can leave a biological imprint on your nervous system and can be passed down through generations. This means that your nervous system's health may not only be a product of your own life experiences, but also those of your parents, grandparents, and beyond.

For example, if your ancestors endured chronic stress or trauma such as slavery, abuse, the holocaust, forced migration, war, or famine, their nervous systems likely adapted to those survival demands, and those adaptations could be passed along to you. This is why certain responses, such as heightened anxiety or sensitivity to stress, may feel ingrained, even if you don't face the same challenges your ancestors did. Understanding this connection helps explain why you react differently from others when faced with the same situations. Reactions can involve untangling the past and working with the biology you've inherited to build a healthier future and embrace your role as a cycle breaker.

Your nervous system's "fingerprint"

REMEMBER

Each person's nervous system operates uniquely and is shaped by a complex interplay of individual experiences, genetics, and environment. These factors create a distinct set of emotional patterns, triggers, and stress responses in you, much like your fingerprint identifies you and no one else. For example, losing a job might be a deeply destabilizing event for someone living paycheck to paycheck, whereas an executive with financial security may feel less immediate concern in the same situation. However, even the executive may experience significant stress if their identity and self-worth are closely tied to professional achievement. In a similar vein, societal pressures can create emotional stress, which varies greatly from one individual to another.

TIP

Likewise, the ways you prefer to take care of your nervous system is highly individual, reflecting your personal needs and what brings you the most calm and balance. As you explore this chapter, please keep this in mind. Take what resonates with you and feels right for *your* body and mind. You don't need to apply every technique or suggestion. Focus on what feels right for *you*.

The silent navigator of your life

In Chapter 5, I explain that your nervous system's role is to make sure all parts of your body "talk" to each other efficiently, keeping everything running smoothly and adapting to the demands of your environment. The nervous system is made up of a network of specialized cells called *neurons* that constantly scan your internal and external environments to determine whether you're safe or unsafe. This question guides many of the nervous system's functions, including regulating hormone levels; supporting reproductive processes; controlling blood sugar levels, heart rate, and digestion; and activating the fight/flight/freeze/fawn responses when you encounter danger.

How do the nervous and endocrine systems work together?

As soon as your nervous system perceives something as threatening to your safety (even if it's not truly dangerous, just unfamiliar — but more on that shortly), it triggers a stress response that's been hardwired into humans over millions of years. Your nervous and endocrine systems work closely together here as part of your body's communication network. In fact, about 80 percent of the signals from your body travel to your brain via the vagus nerve — a major "power line" that plays a crucial role in regulating this communication. The vagus nerve stretches from your gut through your heart and lungs and all the way to your face and brain. Once your brain receives the signals, it then tells your endocrine system to release hormones that prepares your body for action and helps you respond to the perceived threat. In a nutshell, your nervous system is capable of influencing how every system in your body functions, and it even influences your choice in romantic partners.

Why does your nervous system seek the familiar?

REMEMBER

Your nervous system is most comfortable with things that are familiar, and it's largely shaped by your early experiences. The relationships you had with your caregivers when you were young play a huge role in determining what your nervous system interprets as "safe" as an adult. For example, if you experienced secure, loving, and supportive relationships with your parents or primary caregivers, your nervous system may be more likely to seek out similar traits in romantic partners and gravitate toward people who provide emotional safety and security. On the flip side, if you experienced inconsistent or even unsafe emotional environments growing up, your nervous system might interpret that type of relationship as "normal" or "familiar," making you more likely to be drawn to partners who reflect those dynamics, regardless of whether it's good for you.

How do relationships affect hormonal balance?

REMEMBER

This gravitation toward safety is important to understand in the context of hormone balancing because the people around you have a significant impact on your stress levels and overall health. When your nervous system feels emotionally safe in a relationship, stress hormones like cortisol decrease, while hormones that promote well-being, such as oxytocin, increase. Healthy relationships also support relaxation, encourage positive lifestyle choices, and enhance overall happiness.

In contrast, relationships that mirror unhealthy patterns from childhood can keep your nervous system on high alert, triggering chronic stress responses. This can disrupt hormonal balance, increase inflammation, and trigger coping behaviors like overeating, undereating, substance abuse, overworking, or emotional withdrawal, all of which can further compound hormonal imbalance.

What is the importance of connection?

The importance of human connection cannot be overstated. (I cover this more extensively in Chapter 11.) Social isolation is not just an emotional experience but a biological one because it triggers stress responses that can harm the body over time. Research continues to link loneliness and a lack of close relationships to increased inflammation, which, when chronic, is associated with a wide range of serious health issues.

Research consistently shows that partnered individuals tend to eat better, exercise more, and are less likely to engage in harmful behaviors such as smoking or excessive drinking, all contributing to a protective effect on overall health and longevity. Studies on long-term, cohabiting, and married couples indicate that they live longer than their single counterparts on average. Men in heterosexual partnerships generally experience more pronounced health benefits than women, often due to the additional emotional and caregiving responsibilities that can fall disproportionately on female partners.

REMEMBER

Now, while the research might make it sound like long-term partnership is the magic bullet, remember that it's not about whether you're single or partnered; it's about the quality of the connections you have. Whether you're spending time with a close friend, family member, or even a beloved pet, moments of genuine connection are nourishing for your nervous system, which doesn't care about your relationship status. Your nervous system just wants you to feel safe and supported, like you belong, and are surrounded by love, in whatever form that comes.

What about your brain?

REMEMBER

You might be asking, "But isn't my brain the 'command center' of my body?" Well, this belief is actually a bit of an oversimplification. Recent research suggests that the brain is more of a coordination hub, challenging the long-held view that the mind and body are two distinct units that interact with each other. Since human bodies existed long before the evolution of the modern mind, it's clear that the two are deeply interconnected. You can't have a body without the mind, nor a mind without the body. A more fitting description is the *BodyMind*, a concept introduced by pioneering researcher Candace Pert and long embraced by Eastern medicine.

You can think of yourself as a computer, with your mind as the software and your nervous system as the hardware. The hardware (your brain and nervous system) processes information, while the software (your thoughts, beliefs, and emotions) shapes your actions and decisions. This is why mind-body work is essential for balancing hormones; it helps create safety and resilience in both.

Operation of the nervous system

Your nervous system's reliance on a simple "safe" or "unsafe" response is like having a light switch with only on and off settings. It works for basic survival needs, but it's not always suited to the complexity and fast pace of modern life.

To start getting your nervous system to work *for* you, rather than *against* you, imagine its different components as parts of a car, each playing a crucial role in how smoothly or erratically your body navigates the world:

- **Autonomic nervous system (ANS):** The ANS is your car's automatic transmission. It runs in the background, handling essential functions such as heartbeat, digestion, and breathing without you thinking about it. It also regulates your response to stress, helping you shift between high gear (fight or flight) and low gear (rest and digest). The ANS consists of two main branches or "gears" the SNS and PNS:
  - **Sympathetic nervous system (SNS):** Think of the SNS as your car's accelerator. When you encounter stress, your SNS is pressed, speeding up your heart rate, raising blood pressure, and flooding your body with adrenaline to prepare for flight-or-flight action.
  - **Parasympathetic nervous system (PNS):** The PNS is your brake pedal. After the stress passes, the PNS slows everything down, lowering your heart rate, reducing blood pressure, and allowing your body to recover and restore itself. It governs rest, digestion, and relaxation as well as the more extreme "freeze" response, a survival mechanism that can occur during intense stress or perceived danger. (Read more on this shortly.)
- **Enteric nervous system (ENS):** The ENS is your car's onboard computer, which is specifically responsible for managing your gut. It communicates directly with both the sympathetic and parasympathetic systems, adjusting digestion based on whether you're relaxed or stressed. This explains why stress can upset your stomach, a sensation reflected in sayings like *gut-wrenching* or *butterflies in your stomach*.

» **Extrinsic sensory neurons:** These neurons are like your car's sensors. They specifically connect your gut to your central nervous system (brain and spinal cord), transmitting sensory data such as pain, stretch, or chemical changes, ensuring your body responds appropriately to what's happening internally.

The sympathetic nervous system

REMEMBER

To survive, you need to react quickly in the face of a threat, which is why you can find yourself feeling anxious or tense without understanding why. Then, after the initial reaction, you can engage in logical human thinking. The SNS plays a crucial role in accelerating your body's response, which isn't always a bad thing. Sometimes you need to push through to make a work deadline! The key is not letting your SNS stay active too long. It's great for short bursts but not for running the show all day.

PHYSICAL SIGNS THE SNS IS ACTIVE

An increased heart rate is the most obvious physical sign that the SNS is active. Your body pumps more blood to your muscles and initiates rapid, shallow breathing so you take in more oxygen. You may experience elevated blood pressure as blood vessels constrict to direct blood flow to vital organs and muscles. Muscle tension, especially in the shoulders, neck, and jaw, is also common as your body gets ready to respond physically to a threat.

REMEMBER

Other noticeable symptoms include dilated pupils to improve vision, digestive issues like bloating or constipation as digestion slows, and cold hands or feet due to blood being redirected to core organs. Sweating often occurs as your body tries to cool down, whereas hypervigilance makes you more alert, although it can make focusing on nonimmediate tasks difficult. You may have trouble sleeping due to elevated cortisol levels, and cravings for sugary or salty foods may increase as your body seeks quick energy. Irritability, anxiety, and a sense of being "on edge" are common emotional responses, often accompanied by dry mouth or frequent urination.

BEHAVIORAL SIGNS THE SNS IS ACTIVE

TIP

If you feel disconnected from your body or have been in a state of stress for so long that it's hard to recognize what's normal, your behavior can offer important clues. When the SNS is activated, it often triggers coping behaviors that may provide temporary relief but ultimately perpetuate stress.

REMEMBER

You may notice emotional eating, particularly with cravings for sugary or salty foods. Some people turn to substances like alcohol or nicotine to numb anxiety. Procrastination or avoidance of stressful tasks is common, as is overworking or staying constantly busy to maintain a sense of control. Over a longer period, this activity can often lead to burnout. Compulsive behaviors like mindless scrolling, online shopping, overexercising are also ways people cope with stress, and they may experience irritability, aggression, or social withdrawal. Some may overconsume caffeine or stimulants to keep up with energy demands.

TRIGGERS FOR THE SNS

The triggers that prompt the SNS are highly individual and can range from emotional triggers to physical stressors, many of which are part of daily life. Here are some examples:

- **Environmental overstimulation:** Constant notifications, social media, long work hours, or chaotic surroundings can overstimulate your SNS, keeping your body in a low-level state of stress.
- **Physical stress:** Factors like lack of sleep, poor diet, blood sugar fluctuations, toxin exposure, irregular sleep patterns, or dehydration can all make the body more susceptible to triggering the SNS, preventing proper recovery and regulation.
- **Unresolved trauma:** Past traumatic experiences, or the negative thought patterns they create, can keep you in a state of hypervigilance. Read more about this in the "Exploring the Influence of Unresolved Trauma" section later in this chapter.
- **Unprocessed emotions:** When emotions such as sadness, anger, or fear are suppressed rather than acknowledged and expressed healthily, your body may interpret them as unresolved stress, keeping the SNS activated. I cover how to process these emotions for better regulation later in this chapter in the "Revealing the Influence of Unprocessed Emotions" section.

REMEMBER

To shift out of SNS overdrive, it's essential to understand that you can't will your mind and body to relax. Instead, you must actively engage your body through the methods it inherently understands: movement and breath. The good news is that your ANS is not static in how it responds to stress. With the right tools and techniques (covered later in this chapter as well as in Chapter 17), you can retrain it to react more calmly and efficiently.

The parasympathetic nervous system

The PNS helps your body "catch its breath," to lower inflammation, repair tissues, regenerate of cells, and restore hormonal balance. This is often why so many of people lose weight, get pregnant, or feel like a whole new person when they're relaxed and regulated on holiday!

PHYSICAL SIGNS THE PNS IS ACTIVE

One of the most noticeable physical signs the PNS is active is a slower heart rate because your body no longer feels the need to prepare for action. Your breathing becomes deep and steady, allowing for better oxygen exchange and signaling relaxation throughout the body. Additionally, digestion improves; you have increased saliva production and enhanced gut motility, which make it easier for your body to process food and absorb nutrients. You may also experience lower blood pressure as your blood vessels widen and circulation improves. Muscle tension decreases, especially in typically tight areas like the neck, shoulders, and jaw, leaving you feeling physically relaxed. Warm hands and feet are also common, as blood flow returns to the extremities. This state of relaxation often brings a sense of calm or drowsiness. Your body is prepared for rest.

BEHAVIORAL SIGNS THE PNS IS ACTIVE

When the PNS is active, you may find yourself more open to social interaction and feel emotionally present and relaxed around others. It also supports a deeper sense of connection because your nervous system feels safe and ready to engage with those around you.

REMEMBER

Your behavior may also become more mindful and grounded. You'll be able to focus on the present moment without the diversions of stress or anxiety. In this state, you're more likely to engage in calming activities like reading, meditating, or spending time in nature because your body naturally gravitates towards restorative behaviors. Overall, you feel relaxed, unhurried, and more at peace with your surroundings — so much so that even minor annoyances (like a driver cutting you off) won't trigger an intense reaction.

TRIGGERS FOR THE PNS

You can only communicate with your nervous system via movement and breath because it evolved long before humans' rational brains developed. Practices such as deep breathing, singing, humming, massage, exercise, somatic (body-based) techniques, and meditation work well because they bypass the busy cognitive mind and speak directly to the nervous system, sending the messages "Hey, I'm safe" and "I've got this."

TIP

One of my favorite simple but powerful somatic techniques is rocking (I list more in Chapter 17). It taps into the primal comfort we associate with being rocked as babies, making it a deeply nurturing and effective way to activate the PNS. Whether you're sitting in a rocking chair, swaying side to side, or gently rocking on the floor, this technique promotes a deep sense of calm and safety.

TIP

Social connection and positive interactions, like laughing with a friend, hugging a pet, or sharing a meal with loved ones, can also activate the PNS. Other simple practices such as progressive muscle relaxation or splashing cold water on your face can stimulate the vagus nerve. Ultimately, anything that promotes breathing, movement, and a sense of safety will help, so find what works for you!

Polyvagal theory

Polyvagal theory, which was developed by Dr. Stephen Porges, explains how the ANS regulates your body's responses to safety, stress, and social connection.

Figure 9-1 shows a visual representation of this theory and the roles of the two branches of the ANS: the SNS and PNS. The figure provides a breakdown of how each branch of the ANS functions in real time and illustrates the nuances of the body's complex responses to different environmental and social stimuli, from states of calm to states of heightened stress:

- **Dorsal vagal (PNS):** Triggered by extreme stress or trauma, this pathway puts your body into a freeze or immobilization state, leading to numbness, dissociation, or withdrawal. It's a protective response when things feel overwhelming, but staying in this state too long can make it difficult to reconnect with life and is strongly linked to depression.
- **Sympathetic (SNS):** The SNS triggers the fight-or-flight response, which is great when you need a quick boost of energy (like swerving to avoid a car in traffic), but it's not where you want to stay 24/7.
- **Ventral vagal (PNS):** This represents the "safe and social" state — basically, your body's happy place. This is where you want to be for everyday life.

Polyvagal theory helps us understand that our bodies are constantly shifting between the different nervous system states throughout the day, depending on whether we perceive safety or danger. The goal isn't to completely avoid the sympathetic fight-or-flight or parasympathetic freeze responses all together. These reactions are natural and part of how we navigate life's challenges. Instead, the focus should be on expanding your window of tolerance, so you can handle stress more effectively and recover faster with greater ease.

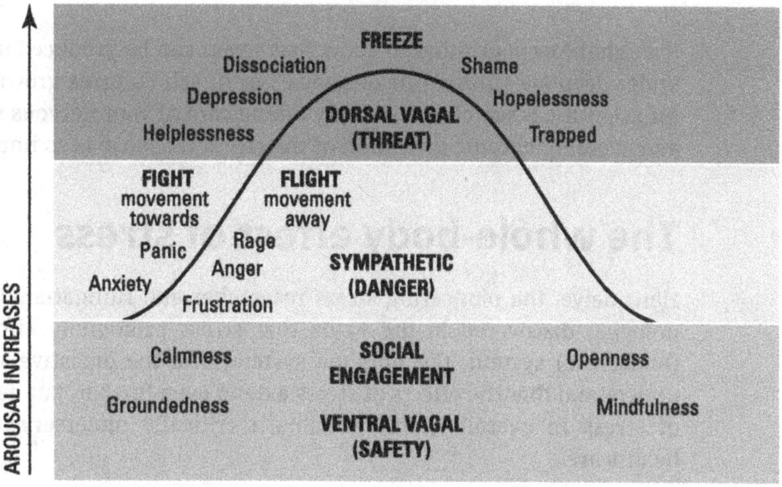

FIGURE 9-1: States of arousal according to the polyvagal theory.

REMEMBER

This means that when you're triggered, whether by a stressful email or an unexpected confrontation, your fight/flight/freeze reaction might initially kick in, but you can shift back into a relaxed state more quickly. Over time, this is how you rewire your nervous system, training it to respond differently to triggers. I dive deeper into rewiring in the "Examining Treatment Options" section later in the chapter.

Defining Stress

The hypothalamus-pituitary-adrenal (HPA) axis, which I talk about in Chapter 3, is closely intertwined with the nervous system. When the nervous system detects a perceived threat or something unfamiliar, it signals the hypothalamus to activate the HPA axis. This triggers a cascade of hormonal responses, including the release of cortisol and adrenaline, which prepare the body to respond to the challenge by heightening alertness, increasing heart rate, and mobilizing energy — ultimately helping to ensure your safety.

Stress isn't what you think it is

If I ask you to give me a definition of stress, you will likely explain that it's a sense of nervous agitation or anxiety. But these sensations don't actually define stress. In fact, you can be stressed with no awareness of its presence. You see, stress is not about feelings; it's a measurable set of objective physiological events in your body that involves your brain, hormones, immune system, and various organs.

It might blow your mind to know that stress can be produced in patients who are under deep anesthesia (unconscious!) or in cell cultures grown outside the body for scientific research. This is why taking care of your nervous system proactively and avoiding chronic activation of the stress response is so important.

The whole-body effect of stress

Hans Selye, the pioneering stress researcher and Hungarian-Canadian endocrinologist, discovered in the 1930s that stress profoundly affects the hormonal (endocrine) system, the immune system, and the digestive system. Today, we understand that the effects of stress extend even further, but despite this, the role of stress in overall health remains a critically underserved area in modern healthcare.

Stress first impacts the hormonal system, causing visible changes in the adrenal glands — your body's stress hormone factories. Then it weakens the immune system and wreaks havoc on the digestive system, damaging the intestinal lining and disrupting gut health.

Over time, the continuous flood of cortisol begins to affect every tissue in your body. The overstimulation of your adrenal glands leads to exhaustion and adrenal fatigue, disrupting the production of essential hormones like estrogen, testosterone, and progesterone, which results in menstrual irregularities, infertility, sexual dysfunction, and a decreased libido. The constant release of cortisol also dampens your immune system, leaving you more susceptible to illness, and weakens your digestive system, contributing to issues like leaky gut and irritable bowel syndrome (IBS).

REMEMBER

Chronic stress further disrupts your body's natural balance (homeostasis) by slowing metabolism, altering thyroid function, and increasing the risk of metabolic disorders such as insulin resistance and type 2 diabetes. Mental health also takes a hit, creating a vicious cycle where stress and hormonal imbalances feed off each other, damaging both mind and body.

Exploring the Influence of Unresolved Trauma

Your nervous system is deeply shaped by your early experiences, especially trauma — whether it's big *T* or little *t* trauma. (I cover the difference in a moment.) As Gabor Maté wrote in *The Myth of Normal: Trauma, Illness, and Healing in a Toxic*

Culture (Avery, 2022), "The earliest established components of an infant's psychobiological makeup are those most formative of his lifelong outlook." Our early experiences lay the groundwork for patterns of behavior that persist into adulthood unless we actively work to rewire them.

REMEMBER

Here are some words of wisdom: Don't mistake ropes for snakes. Imagine you're walking through a forest and suddenly spot a coiled rope on the path. In a split second, you mistake it for a snake and your nervous system immediately kicks into gear, triggering a stress response as if the danger is real. Even after you realize it's just a rope, your body remains in fight-or-flight mode for a while, as if still bracing for the threat. This is similar to what happens with unresolved trauma. Your nervous system remains on high alert, reacting to perceived dangers that aren't actually present. In modern life, you may feel anxious over a harmless email from your boss. Your nervous system, conditioned by past experiences of criticism or rejection, interprets the message as a serious threat, even though it may be completely innocuous to someone else without a similar past.

Defining trauma

Trauma is defined as any experience in which you don't feel safe physically, psychologically, or emotionally, and your ability to cope is overwhelmed. It's important not to convince or gaslight yourself into thinking your experiences don't "count" as trauma just because they don't fit a stereotypical definition or now seem less significant than they did when they occurred.

REMEMBER

Trauma is highly personal. What overwhelms one person may not affect another in the same way. What truly matters is how you were made to feel in that moment — not how you judge the experience now.

At the core of trauma responses lies your fundamental human need for love, connection, safety, and belonging. From birth, your nervous system seeks safety through attachment to others and guides behaviors that aim to secure love and avoid rejection. When this need is disrupted, whether through trauma, neglect, or adverse circumstances, your nervous system adapts in ways that may have helped you survive at the time but can manifest later in life as avoidance, repression, or emotional shutdown. While these responses once served a purpose, over time, they can contribute to burnout, illness, and hormone dysregulation.

TIP

Although you can't undo past trauma, you can rewire its effects on your nervous system by calibrating it to a new sense of safety and resilience.

Understanding the trauma scale

Trauma can be categorized two ways: big *T* Trauma and little *t* trauma:

REMEMBER

- **Big *T* trauma** refers to major, life-altering events that overwhelm the nervous system, triggering strong survival responses such as hypervigilance, perfectionism, or an intense need for control. This is often seen in individuals who have faced events like severe accidents, abuse, or sudden loss, leaving their nervous system in a prolonged state of high alert.
- **Little *t* trauma** involves smaller, more repetitive experiences such as ongoing criticism, neglect, or bullying. Although these experiences are often less dramatic, they can accumulate over time, leading to similar coping mechanisms as Big *T* trauma. For example, someone raised with emotional neglect might develop people-pleasing behaviors, leaving their nervous system in a constant state of low-level tension, even in objectively safe situations.

REMEMBER

However, trauma isn't only about what happened to you; it's also encompasses what you didn't receive: your unmet needs. *The biology of loss* is a concept that focuses on how the absence of emotional connection or nurturing during early childhood can profoundly shape brain development. When a child doesn't receive the emotional support, safety, or security they need, it leaves a lasting imprint on their nervous system, shaping how they navigate stress, relationships, and their own sense of resilience as adults.

Understanding how trauma shows up in your life

REMEMBER

To understand how trauma shows up in your life and heal from it, you first have to understanding the relationship between your conscious and subconscious mind. Your conscious mind is the part you're aware of — your thoughts, decisions, and actions in the present. However, much of what drives your nervous system's reactions, especially to stress or trauma, lies in the subconscious mind, which stores memories, emotions, and patterns that influence your nervous system's responses without you even realizing it.

Unresolved traumatic experiences are stored in your subconscious as physical and emotional memories. This is why you might find yourself reacting to a situation with anxiety or fear even when you "know" logically that there's no real danger.

REMEMBER

Your subconscious mind, working with your nervous system, holds onto beliefs the trauma created such as "I'm not good enough" or "I'm not deserving of success." These narratives were created to shield you from perceived danger in the future but often keep your nervous system in a heightened state of stress so you play small (holding back, avoiding risks, and staying within your comfort zone), and live according to narratives that limit your growth and evolution.

TIP

By becoming aware of the stories looping in your subconscious, you can begin to identify the root causes of your reactions and emotional patterns. Techniques that allow you to access the Theta brainwave state — such as mindfulness, EMDR, meditation, and breathwork — are particularly powerful as they bridge the gap between the conscious and subconscious mind, allowing you to rewire these narratives to ones based in high-self-worth such as, "I am good enough just the way I am." I cover solutions in more detail at the end of this chapter in the "Examining Treatment Options" section.

Revealing the Influence of Unprocessed Emotions

REMEMBER

Emotions are not just physical sensations, They're the result of complex hormonal and chemical secretions in the body. For example, when you feel joy, your brain releases dopamine and serotonin, which contribute to a sense of happiness and calm, helping the nervous system shift into a state of safety and allowing the body to rest, digest, and repair. On the other hand, emotions such as anger or fear trigger the release of stress hormones like cortisol and adrenaline, preparing your body for a fight-or-flight response. In this way, emotions are deeply tied to your body's chemistry and directly affect how your nervous system and hormones function.

Understanding emotions

The late neuroscientist Candace Pert was a trailblazer in understanding the biochemical nature of emotions. Her work has shown that emotions communicate with every single cell to influence vital systems like your immune and endocrine functions.

REMEMBER

Survival emotions — fear, shame, anger, and sadness — are what you need to pay attention to because they're your body's way of signaling danger or unmet needs. When they surface, your brain activates your nervous system to release hormones that gear your body up for action. If you suppress these emotions — whether by pushing down anger, burying grief, avoiding confrontation, or internalizing shame — they don't just disappear. Instead, they can get stuck in your body (as I describe in the next section), which can cause various physical and psychological problems.

Feeling and processing emotions properly allows your body to return to a balanced state. Think of it like emotional digestion: If you don't process what's happening, it's going to cause discomfort and imbalance over time.

Retaining emotions: How emotions get stored in the body

When you suppress emotions, they get "stuck" in the body. Here's a brief overview of how that happens:

REMEMBER

- **Stress hormones:** At the chemical level, emotions trigger the release of hormones such as cortisol and neuropeptides that can keep the body in a heightened state of alert. Although the body metabolizes the hormones over time, repeated activation of the stress response can lead to ongoing tension, inflammation, and disruptions in your body's ability to return to hormonal balance.
- **The vagus nerve:** The vagus nerve (read more in the "Meeting Your Nervous System" section earlier in this chapter) helps the body recover from stress, so when emotions are unprocessed or stress is prolonged, vagal tone can be reduced, meaning your body's ability to relax is compromised. This can lead to prolonged physical symptoms like muscle tension or digestive issues.
- **Fascia and muscle tension:** The idea that emotional stress is "stored" in the muscles and fascia is still being explored, but there's growing evidence that emotional trauma and chronic stress can contribute to physical tension and discomfort, which therapies like somatics and body-based practices (covered in the "Examining Treatment Options" section of this chapter) aim to address.

Exploring the Relationship between Anger and Disease

Research as early as the 1950s and 1960s highlighted the connection between emotional stress and conditions like multiple sclerosis (MS). In many cases, patients reported significant life stressors prior to the onset of their symptoms and had difficulty acknowledging or expressing their anger. These results suggested for the first time that unresolved emotional tension plays a role in the progression of disease.

We now understand that when anger remains unprocessed, it keeps the stress response active, leading to elevated cortisol levels and holding the nervous system in a prolonged state of fight or flight. Over time, this impairs the body's ability to return to rest and repair, heightening the risk of disease and disrupting the hormone balance required for optimal health.

Ways to express and metabolize anger in a healthy way

TIP

Learning how to channel anger constructively while honoring your emotional experience is the aim of the game. Here are some effective techniques:

- **Communication:** Speak up clearly and calmly. Instead of letting anger fester, verbalize your emotions. Say what you need in the moment — whether it's asking for more space, respect, or acknowledgment. Clear communication lets you release anger before it builds into resentment.
- **Movement:** Get physical. If your body's calling for a bigger release than communication can provide, try screaming into a pillow or throwing it on the bed repeatedly. Sometimes your body needs this kind of outlet. (Children do this intuitively.) You can also walk, run, or dance to let the anger move through your body.
- **Breath:** Try deep belly breaths or box breathing to ground yourself.
- **Boundaries:** Anger often arises when boundaries are crossed. Setting clear limits on your time, space, and energy prevents you from overextending yourself, building up resentment or feeling frustrated.

Signs you're holding on to emotions

You might not consciously realize you're holding on to emotions, but your mind and body can send you signals. You can experience effects triggered by hormone imbalances, such as irregular menstrual cycles, low libido, metabolic struggles, or persistent fatigue, but there are other common signs:

TIP

- **Physical tension and pain:** You can experience pain, particularly in the shoulders, neck, back, and hips, which tense up in times of stress to provide support and protection. Over time, persistent stress can lead to chronic muscle tension, resulting in pain and discomfort.

» **Digestive issues:** If you're holding onto emotions such as anxiety, shame, sadness, or anger, you may notice digestive problems like bloating, constipation, or IBS flare-ups. Stress and emotions directly affect your health via the gut-brain connection, which is the topic of Chapter 10.

» **Emotional reactivity:** Overreacting to small incidents (for example, you snap at someone over a minor inconvenience) could be a sign that you're carrying emotional baggage.

» **Frequent illness:** A weakened immune system, manifesting as frequent colds or infections, can be a sign of ongoing emotional strain.

» **Avoidance or numbing behaviors:** If you find yourself turning to distractions or numbing activities, you could be trying to avoid dealing with emotions. These habits are often coping mechanisms to suppress what you don't want to feel.

» **Sleep disruptions:** Difficulty falling asleep or waking up frequently during the night can also be a sign of emotional and stress hormone overload. When your nervous system is stuck in a heightened state of alert due to unresolved emotions, it can interfere with your body's ability to relax and enter restful sleep.

» **Frequent mood swings:** Do you find yourself feeling inexplicably sad, angry, or anxious without understanding why? This emotional unpredictability can be a sign that there are deeper, unresolved emotions beneath the surface, driving these sudden shifts in mood.

Examining Treatment Options

Since each individual's BodyMind connection (read about BodyMind in the "What about your brain?" section earlier in this chapter) is unique, there is no one-size-fits-all solution. This section explores various traditional and emerging methods to help reset and rewire your subconscious mind and nervous system. You may want to experiment with several so you can choose what's best based on your needs and preferences.

Traditional methods

Traditional methods are therapeutic approaches that have been widely studied, practiced, and integrated into mainstream healthcare and mental health practices over time. Here are some of the most commonly used techniques and their potential benefits:

- **Cognitive Behavioral Therapy (CBT):** CBT, one of the most well-researched and widely used therapies, offers a practical approach to recognizing and reframing unhelpful thought patterns that contribute to stress and anxiety. It can be very effective in helping individuals manage their stress by focusing on the conscious mind. However, it's worth considering that CBT primarily addresses *conscious* thought processes and may not fully delve into subconscious patterns.
- **Mindfulness and meditation:** Mindfulness and meditation, which are rooted in ancient practices, are now well-supported by modern science. By regularly focusing your attention on the present moment, you can activate the PNS, lower cortisol levels, improve mood, and enhance overall nervous system regulation to promote rest, relaxation, and healing.
- **Deep breathing exercises:** Breathing techniques, such as diaphragmatic breathing or the box breathing method, are simple yet powerful ways to engage the PNS. By slowing down the breath, you signal to your nervous system that you are safe, reduce the fight-or-flight response, and calm the body. Deep breathing also improves oxygen flow, which supports hormonal regulation.
- **Progressive muscle relaxation (PMR):** This technique involves tensing and relaxing different muscle groups to help reduce overall physical tension. Becoming aware of where you're holding stress helps you release it more effectively. PMR is often recommended for those with high levels of anxiety or chronic muscle tension due to stress.
- **Yoga, tai chi, qigong, and other ancient practices:** These ancient practices are not only physical exercises but also the original forms of somatic healing. These practices emphasize the connection between mind, body, and breath, helping individuals to become more attuned to where they hold tension and stress. By focusing on intentional movement and breathwork, they activate the PNS and promote emotional regulation.

New and emerging methods

REMEMBER

Research increasingly highlights the brain's incredible adaptability, or *neuroplasticity*, which is its ability to reorganize and form new connections, particularly in response to trauma, stress, or learning. This means that even long-standing patterns tied to trauma and stress can be reshaped. So while traditional methods such as talk therapy remain valuable, emerging techniques such as the following are showing great promise in reaching deeper layers of mind, body, and nervous system healing:

TIP

- **Eye movement desensitization and reprocessing (EMDR):** This powerful technique is designed to help individuals process traumatic memories by using guided eye movements (or other bilateral stimulation) to help the brain integrate distressing experiences and reduce the emotional charge associated with them. It offers a direct path to reprogramming the brain's stress response and supporting nervous system regulation and has proven particularly effective for treating trauma, post-traumatic stress disorder (PTSD), and anxiety.
- **Somatic therapy:** Somatic therapy recognizes that trauma and stress are often stored in the body as physical sensations. Through techniques like body awareness, movement, and safe, gentle touch, it helps release stored tension and unprocessed emotions and encourages new, healthier patterns of brain-body interaction.
- **EFT (emotional freedom techniques) tapping:** This method combines cognitive reframing with physical stimulation of acupressure points by tapping on specific areas of the body, which helps release energy blockages caused by stress, anxiety, or trauma. A groundbreaking study involving veterans with PTSD found that EFT reduced symptoms in 90 percent of participants, who showed significant improvements after just six sessions. These results suggest that EFT not only helps alleviate emotional distress but also promotes neuroplasticity by allowing the brain to rewire its response to stress.
- **Hypnosis:** By inducing a relaxed, focused state, hypnosis allows for the reprogramming of adaptive beliefs that live in the subconscious mind, such as "I'm unlovable," along with our emotional responses and behaviors. Research shows that hypnosis can effectively reduce stress and anxiety by tapping into the brain's neuroplastic potential, making it an invaluable tool for trauma recovery and stress management.
- **Neurofeedback:** Neurofeedback is a noninvasive method that trains your brain to regulate its own activity. By monitoring brainwaves in real time and providing visual or auditory feedback, individuals learn to shift brainwaves into healthier patterns. Hypnosis improves focus, relaxation, and emotional control. It's especially useful for conditions like anxiety, ADHD, and sleep problems, and it helps the brain naturally respond better to stress without medication.
- **Vagus nerve stimulation (VNS):** VNS can be achieved through practices like controlled breathwork, humming, singing, cold exposure, and other targeted techniques that directly activate the vagus nerve. (Read about the vagus nerve earlier in this chapter in the "Meeting Your Nervous System" section.) This stimulation helps transition your body from a state of stress to relaxation

and enhances the parasympathetic response. As a result, VNS promotes recovery, supports hormonal balance, and optimizes the body's natural ability to heal.

- **Theta brainwave therapy:** Theta brainwave therapy works by guiding individuals into a deeply meditative state, where theta brainwaves — which are associated with deep relaxation, creativity, and healing — are dominant. By calming the nervous system and reducing stress, theta therapy lowers cortisol levels and promotes the release of hormones that support relaxation and recovery. Additionally, accessing the subconscious mind in this state allows for more effective rewiring of emotional patterns, helping to restore long-lasting emotional stability and fostering an overall sense of balance in the body and mind.
- **Non-Sleep Deep Rest (NSDR):** NSDR uses guided relaxation techniques to help the body mimic the restorative effects of sleep, promoting nervous system regulation, reducing stress, and enhancing focus. Unlike theta brainwave therapy, NSDR doesn't specifically target the subconscious but provides a quick way to deeply rest, regulate, and restore energy.

IN THIS CHAPTER

» Exploring the powerful connection between the gut, brain, and hormones

» Identifying key factors that impact your gut health

» Taking steps to rebuild and nurture your gut

Chapter 10
Endangering the Gut and Its Microbiome

Welcome to the fascinating world of the gastrointestinal system, also known as your gut. It's an intricate and multifaceted network responsible for important processes such as digesting food, influencing hormone regulation, absorbing nutrients, and eliminating waste. Although gut health is now recognized as one of our most critical public health challenges, with up to two-thirds of the U.S. population experiencing recurrent digestive disturbances (such as bloating, gas, and abdominal discomfort), for many there are still questions about what gut health actually means.

Indeed, a 2023 study found that a surprising majority of Americans remained unfamiliar with the gut microbiome, a vast ecosystem comprising trillions of microorganisms that reside in the digestive tract. The same survey found that many of them weren't aware of the importance of their gut health and ways to enhance it, with more than half of respondents expressing confusion due to the overwhelming amount of information available about diet and nutrition. Additionally, 85 percent failed a quiz assessing basic gut health knowledge, with only one-third aware that antibiotics can destroy both beneficial and harmful bacteria within the gut. So, if you find yourself feeling confused or overwhelmed by the subject of gut health and the all-important microbiome, you're certainly not alone, and it's not your fault.

One major reason for all this confusion is the fact that researchers have yet to identify a universal definition of a "healthy" microbiome because it varies significantly from person to person. While emerging studies suggest that our dietary choices either support beneficial bacteria or contribute to less favorable strains (read more in the "Understanding What Influences Gut Health" section later in this chapter), much more research is needed to determine exactly which foods and products produce optimal results in different individuals. This uncertainty has opened the door for companies to capitalize on the trend by promoting products such as supplements, powders, and snacks marketed as being friendly to the microbiome or gut. At the time of writing, in the U.S., the Food and Drug Administration (FDA) does not approve or verify claims made by supplement manufacturers before their products enter the market, leaving consumers largely responsible for educating themselves and holding these companies accountable.

To successfully navigate the flood of mainstream information (and often, misinformation) around gut health and make effective decisions, you need to empower yourself with knowledge. This chapter not only covers the gut health basics but explains its influence on hormone balance, affecting everything from cortisol to serotonin, and how this delicate interplay can directly impact your energy levels, mood, and metabolism.

Getting to Know The Gut-Brain-Endocrine Axis

REMEMBER

The gut is often referred to as our "second brain" because of the intricate communication network known as the gut-brain axis (see Figure 10-1), which facilitates continuous interaction between the digestive system and the brain. This interaction is largely mediated by the enteric nervous system (ENS) — a complex web of neurons embedded in the gut — and the vagus nerve, which acts as a direct conduit between the brain and digestive system.

The ENS functions both independently and in conjunction with the sympathetic and parasympathetic nervous systems to respond to your internal and external environments by regulating essential digestive processes such as muscle contractions, enzyme secretion, and nutrient absorption. (Read more about the ENS in Chapter 9.) This complex system is also where the concept of "gut instinct" comes from because the gut-brain connection allows emotional and intuitive signals from the body to influence decision-making and emotional responses, often before the conscious mind even registers them.

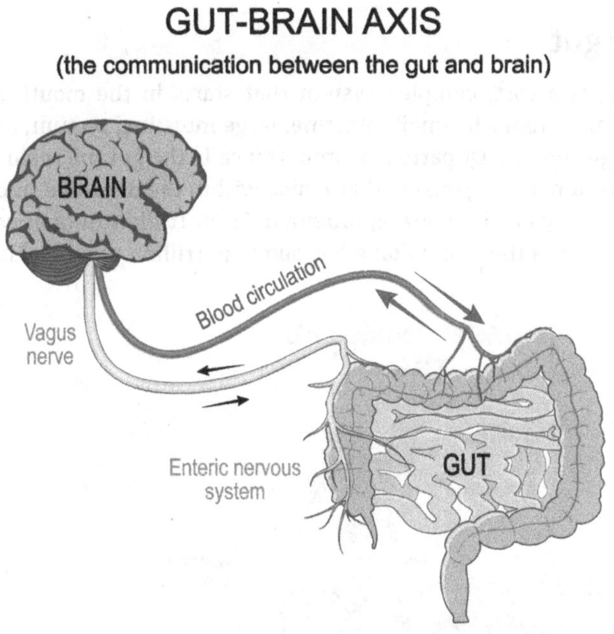

FIGURE 10-1: The gut-brain axis.

designua/Adobe Stock Photos

However, this system of communication goes beyond just the physical connections between the brain and gut. It also includes pathways such as hormonal signals, chemical messengers in the blood, metabolic processes, and immune responses. This chapter takes a deeper dive into the gut-brain-endocrine axis, which looks at the essential role of hormones such as cortisol, insulin, and serotonin in maintaining balance between these systems. Much like a high-functioning communication network, this axis depends on uninterrupted signalling to maintain homeostasis (balance), just as we rely on a strong Wi-Fi connection to ensure that all our devices are syncing and communicating properly. When the signal is strong and stable, everything runs smoothly, allowing for seamless coordination between devices. But when the connection falters, it potentially triggers symptoms such as fatigue, painful periods, mood swings, and even more serious conditions such as insulin resistance, thyroid disorders, or autoimmune diseases.

Investigating the gut, brain and endocrine relationship

The following sections explore the intricate connection between your gut, brain, and endocrine system, revealing how they work together to influence nearly every aspect of your health.

Your gut

The gut is a vast, complex system that starts in the mouth and includes your esophagus, stomach, small intestine, large intestine, rectum, and lastly, the anus (see Figure 10-2). Of particular importance is the gut microbiome, a collection of trillions of microorganisms that reside within the digestive tract. To put this into context for you, there are approximately 30 trillion human cells in the human body, whereas the microbiome has about 39 trillion microbial cells.

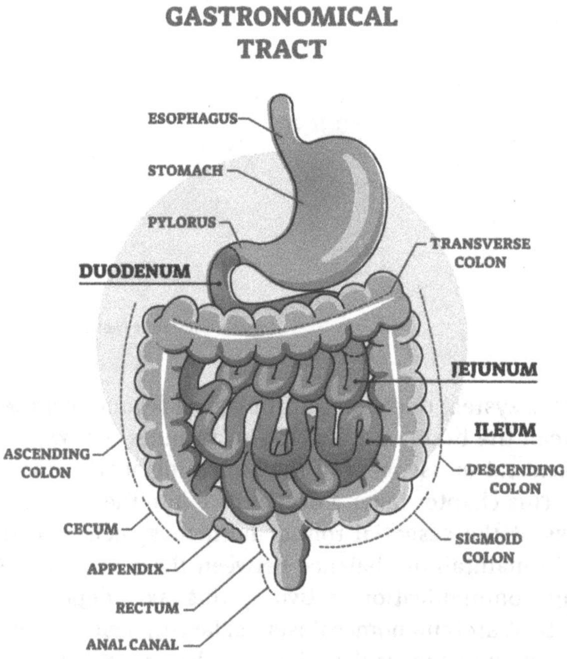

FIGURE 10-2: GI tract.

REMEMBER

These microscopic organisms are famously known for breaking down food, absorbing nutrients, and synthesizing essential vitamins, but their role extends into hormone regulation as well. For example, 90 percent of your serotonin, one of your "happy hormones" which contributes to mood stabilization and helps regulate appetite, is produced in the gut, and the gut microbiome also significantly influences the regulation of cortisol, thyroid hormones, and insulin. The estrobolome — a specific subset of gut bacteria — also plays a key role in metabolizing and regulating estrogen levels.

Your gut bacteria influence the availability of nutrients and signal the release of biologically active peptides, such as galanin and ghrelin, from enteroendocrine cells (specialized gut cells that release hormones in response to what's happening in the digestive system). Galanin is believed to play a role in stimulating the stress response by influencing cortisol and adrenocorticotropic hormone release (ACTH signals the adrenal glands to release cortisol). It also contributes to metabolic regulation, though much of this evidence currently comes from animal models. Similarly, ghrelin is well-documented for its role in modulating both stress and nutritional balance through its on cortisol release.

REMEMBER

In fact, the gut-brain-endocrine connection is so strong that stress alone can shift the composition of your microbiome, leading to a cycle where stress affects gut health, and gut health, in turn, influences emotional well-being. In studies involving germ-free rodents, researchers found that gut microbiota abnormalities could even trigger symptoms of major depressive disorder.

What makes the gut microbiome so captivating is its uniqueness in every individual. While it's shaped by what we consume and when we consume it, it is equally influenced by factors such as sleep, exercise, social interactions, genetics, and the surrounding environment. Even slight shifts in these areas can disrupt or enhance the delicate balance of microbes, potentially leading to significant effects on digestive, hormone, and overall health.

It's also important to note that your microbiome is not important just during your lifetime but also across generations. Research from University of Helsinki showed that the gut health of mothers can influence the development of their babies' immune systems and nervous systems while they're a fetus, which points to a growing understanding that a balanced gut microbiome is essential for long-term health stability across generations. Refer to Chapter 8 to learn more about transgenerational impacts.

Your brain

REMEMBER

Stress is a major disruptor of the gut-brain-endocrine axis, but your emotions play a significant role in this process too. Negative or survival emotions such as fear, anger, or sadness activate your body's fight-or-flight response, flooding your system with stress hormones that alter the balance of your gut's microbiome.

The gut bacteria that help regulate digestion and keep inflammation in check become less effective under chronic stress, leading to slowed digestion, a weakened immune system, and more inflammation. This chronic inflammation then disrupts hormonal balance, as inflammatory signals interfere with hormone production and regulation, particularly cortisol, insulin, and estrogen. Over time, this creates a vicious cycle between the brain and gut, with stress weakening the gut's ability to function properly, and a poorly functioning gut contributing to further emotional and physical stress. It's no wonder gut issues are often accompanied by anxiety, depression, or brain fog.

REMEMBER

On the flip side, positive emotions can help restore balance. Regulating your nervous system using the techniques and therapies detailed in Chapter 9 can lower the production of stress hormones and increase feel-good neurotransmitters such as serotonin, which is primarily produced in your gut. Joy, love, and feelings of gratitude can have a powerful and positive impact, as do developing high self-esteem and maintaining strong social bonds.

The brain also has a significant influence over the gut's key functions, such as the movement of food (gut motility), the production of digestive substances like acid and mucus, and the way fluids are handled in the intestines. These processes are essential for maintaining a protective mucus layer in the gut, which provides a habitat for various groups of bacteria to grow and thrive. When the gut-brain-endocrine communication is disrupted, it can lead to changes in this protective layer and potentially trigger digestive issues or other gut-related problems.

In addition, there's strong evidence that the microbes in your gut can influence brain function by affecting brain chemicals and interacting with the systems that control stress, anxiety, and memory. Interestingly, these effects are specific to certain strains of bacteria, meaning that specific probiotics may have potential as a supportive therapy for neurological conditions such as anxiety and stress-related disorders.

Your endocrine system

We are still in the early stages of uncovering the full complexity of the endocrine system — a system that turns out to be far more intricate than previously imagined. It's not governed only by the traditional hormones we've long studied; it's also influenced by chemicals secreted by newly identified microbes in the gut that far exceed the output of the nervous system in terms of both volume and variety. Due to the complexity of these systems, the scientific community is still piecing together how these chemical signals contribute to overall health, metabolism, and disease, but now experts acknowledge that gut bacteria are a dynamic endocrine organ in its own right.

What's especially intriguing is that the gut microbiome can act as both primary and secondary messengers in the body's biochemical pathways. As primary messengers, the chemicals secreted by microbes directly influence bodily functions, such as altering insulin sensitivity or modulating cortisol levels in response to stress. As secondary messengers, microbial chemicals can influence the release of other hormones or activate processes such as inflammation, which then trigger further hormonal cascades.

REMEMBER

This emerging picture underscores the gut microbiome's significant role in endocrine regulation — one that is reshaping our understanding of the body's hormonal systems and its profound influence on both health and disease. The implications for medicine, nutrition, and overall wellness are exciting.

The ripple effect across the body

Evidently, the health of your gut-brain-endocrine axis profoundly affects the state of your body's other systems. For example, chronic stress and gut imbalances elevate cortisol levels, which in turn can lead to increased blood pressure, irregular heart rhythms, and a heightened risk of cardiovascular diseases such as heart attacks and strokes.

REMEMBER

Equally critical is the role of the gut in immune regulation. Approximately 70 percent of immune cells are located in the gut — often the body's first point of contact with many external substances, including food, pathogens, and chemicals. The trillions of microorganisms that form the gut microbiome play a vital role in training the immune system to identify and respond to harmful invaders and potential threats, which is essential in preventing harmful pathogens from entering the bloodstream and causing infection or inflammation.

WARNING

New studies have also shown that exposure to harmful chemicals, such as those found in food contact materials (FCMs), can disrupt the balance of the gut microbiome. Researchers have identified 189 potential carcinogens in food packaging that can leach into food, exposing individuals to chemicals that may promote diseases like breast cancer. Essentially, when your gut microbiome is balanced and healthy, it helps to protect you from the impact of these chemicals by preventing chronic inflammation and related conditions such as autoimmune disorders, allergies, and persistent infections. However, researchers have identified a connection between the brain and gut that weakens immune defences during periods of psychological stress.

TECHNICAL STUFF

Research published in *Cell* involving over 1,000 male mice has zeroed in on a little-known structure in the digestive system called Brunner's glands, which are located in the small intestine. These glands might not sound exciting, but they play a critical role in gut health by producing mucus that protects the lining of the intestine and encourages the growth of good bacteria. Here's where it gets interesting: When the central amygdala, a part of the brain involved in emotional processing, was suppressed — either by stress or through experimental techniques — Brunner's glands went quiet. The result? Less mucus production and a perfect environment for harmful bacteria to thrive. On the flip side, when the amygdala was activated, it sent signals through the vagus nerve to stimulate the glands, increasing mucus and promoting the growth of beneficial bacteria.

Probiotic treatments helped to partially reverse the negative effects of amygdala suppression, showing the power of gut health interventions.

REMEMBER

This research indicates that mental states like stress aren't just emotional — they have real, physical impacts on gut health and, by extension, the immune system. Stress hormones such as cortisol and the health of the vagus nerve play a central role in this interaction, highlighting how deeply interconnected our mental health, nervous system, and hormonal balance are. Taking care of the nervous system, especially through practices that support vagus nerve function, is going to be key to maintaining overall health and the resilience of your gut. (Refer to Chapter 9 for tips on supporting your nervous system.)

Because a balanced gut microbiome plays such pivotal role in hormone regulation, it therefore directly influences the health of your skin. Elevated cortisol levels often triggered by gut imbalances, for instance, can lead to increased oil production, resulting in breakouts and inflammation. Hormonal disruptions involving estrogen and androgens may similarly manifest as skin issues, such as dryness, sensitivity, or unwanted hair growth. Ultimately, healthy skin is a reflection of your internal health, and maintaining a well-functioning gut microbiome is key ingredient.

Understanding What Influences Gut Health

Our understanding of what constitutes a "healthy microbiome" continues to evolve, but generally, it's characterized by a balance of beneficial bacteria such as *Lactobacillus* and *Bifidobacterium*, which play essential roles in digestion, immune regulation, and even mood stabilization. To get even more granular, we're also discovering that gut health is also about the specific subspecies and strains of those bacteria. For example, different subspecies within the *Lactobacillus* genus can have vastly different effects on health. For example, *Lactobacillus crispatus* is typically considered beneficial, supporting vaginal health and immune function, whereas certain strains of *Lactobacillus reuteri* have been implicated in inflammation and may contribute to gastrointestinal disorders in some cases. This means that it's not only about maintaining a balance of "good" bacteria but also about which specific strains are present and active in the gut.

REMEMBER

Dysbiosis on the other hand, which is the term used for an imbalance in the microbiome, occurs when harmful bacteria such as *Clostridium difficile* or *E. coli* outcompete the beneficial strains. However, it's important to note that dysbiosis takes many forms, and its impact varies from person to person, which makes it difficult to diagnose based on a standard definition. Moreover, the concept of dysbiosis is context dependent: The uniqueness of each individual's gut microbiome means that factors affecting one person's gut health might not have the same effect on another's. As you continue through this chapter, pay close attention to the challenges and strategies that align with your own experiences and circumstances, considering how they can be thoughtfully applied to your personal journey.

Diet

WARNING

Navigating the modern diet landscape often feels like walking through a maze of confusing labels and empty promises thanks to food companies that know exactly how to sell us on their products (using nutritionists with social media followings to do it for them, as exposed by the *Wall Street Journal*). They spend massive amounts on advertising to position their ultra-processed foods as "healthy" or "natural," using buzzwords such as *low-fat*, *whole grain*, *high-protein*, or *gut friendly* to make their products seem nutritious and distract you from the fact that many of them (although of course not all) are filled with unhealthy additives, thickeners, sweeteners, emulsifiers, sugars, and preservatives. Although the FDA has reviewed and approved these ingredients as "generally regarded as safe," some studies have highlighted potential concerns that need further research to fully understand their long-term effects. To make things even trickier, food companies self-fund research to promote their products, ensuring that it's difficult for the untrained eye to identify biased and unbiased nutritional information.

In this section, I want to equip you with the knowledge you need to make informed decisions.

Ultra-processed foods

Seventy-three percent of the food on the grocery store shelves in U.S. is ultra-processed, and it's currently the top-ranked country for ultra-processed food (UPF) consumption in the world, followed by the U.K. Although some products may seem obviously processed — such as ready-made meals, chips, and sodas — many that seem healthy can often be UPFs in disguise. Examples include protein bars, flavored yogurts, and even whole grain breads

REMEMBER

These foods are not just processed. Most have been industrially engineered to be hyperpalatable, hitting what scientists call the "bliss point" — a perfect combination of sugar, fat, and salt that makes them incredibly appealing to our taste buds. This design keeps us wanting more because these foods stimulate the brain's dopamine reward system, much like addictive substances do. While these foods may be delicious, they lack real nutrition and leave us unsatisfied, leading us to eat more without ever feeling full. This overconsumption not only contributes to obesity, cardiovascular disease, and diabetes but also triggers inflammation in the body, exacerbating issues like insulin resistance, mood swings, and even reproductive health problems.

REMEMBER

UPFs often have long ingredient lists of things you've never heard of and can't pronounce and that haven't been properly researched for their long-term effects. These added ingredients strip away the natural nutrients and fiber found in whole foods. Without fiber, the beneficial bacteria in your gut starve, leading to a less diverse and less healthy microbiome, slowed digestion, and a sense of being unsatisfied, which can lead to overeating. Additionally, artificial sweeteners, emulsifiers, and preservatives used in UPFs have been found to damage the gut lining, increase intestinal permeability (often referred to as "leaky gut," which is illustrated in Figure 10-3), and interfere with neurotransmitter production in the brain. This can have cascading effects on both gut and brain health, disrupting the gut-brain-endocrine axis and leading to cognitive impairment and psychological issues. In fact, for every 10 percent increase in calories consumed as UPFs per day, adults experience an 11 percent higher risk of depression.

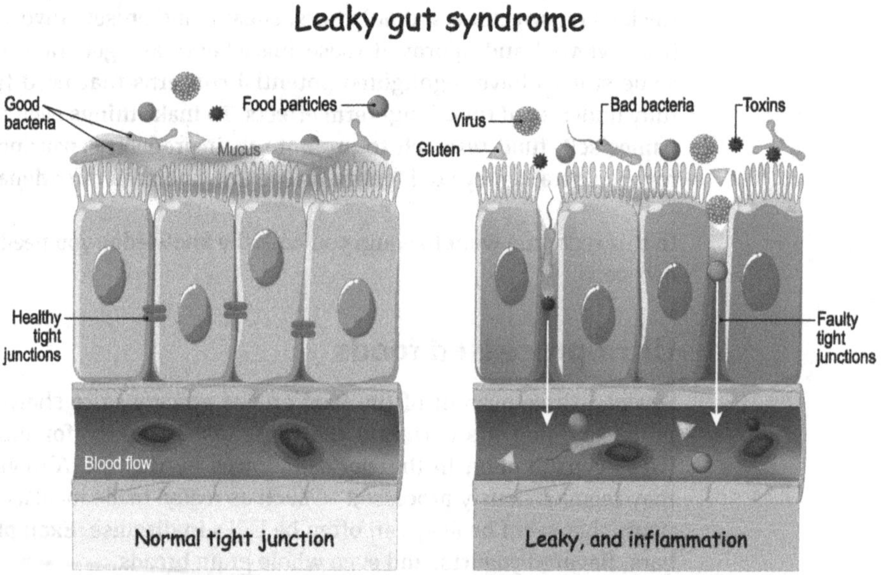

FIGURE 10-3: The mechanics of leaky gut syndrome.

designua/Adobe Stock Photos

So, while UPFs may be convenient, they are far from your gut or hormones' best friend. Much more research is still needed to determine which UPFs cause the most harm and exactly how they do so, but this should be the responsibility of food companies and government regulatory bodies. At the same time, we can all educate ourselves to make informed choices. As a simple guideline: If an ingredient list is long and includes items you wouldn't find in your kitchen, it's probably not something that should go in your mouth!

Lack of diet diversity

TIP

If you've been eating the same meals on repeat, it's time to switch it up. Your gut's likely craving a bit more excitement! According to Dr. Megan Rossi (The Gut Health Doctor), eating at least 30 different plant-based foods per week is key to supporting a diverse range of beneficial bacteria in your gut. Different fibers and nutrients feed various strains of bacteria in your microbiome, so without diversity, some of those helpful bacteria can start packing their bags. I walk through how you can introduce a larger range of foods later in this chapter in the "Applying diet interventions" section. I promise it's not as difficult as it sounds.

Exposure to endocrine-disrupting or "forever" chemicals

REMEMBER

Research published in *Environmental Health Perspectives* showed that early exposure to "forever chemicals" (per- and polyfluoroalkyl substances, or PFAS) commonly found in products such as nonstick cookware, water-repellent clothing, food packaging, and even contaminated drinking water, can lead to lasting disruptions in the gut microbiome of mice that predisposed them to metabolic disorders later in life, such as obesity and insulin resistance. Although this study was conducted on animal models, the findings raise important concerns about human health, suggesting that early-life exposure to these environmental contaminants could be contributing to the rising rates of metabolic diseases, including obesity and type 2 diabetes, in adults.

Genetic or epigenetic influences

REMEMBER

Certain individuals may indeed have a genetic predisposition to gut-related issues, but what's particularly promising is the role of epigenetics. This field of study explores how lifestyle factors — such as diet, exercise, and environmental exposures — influence gene expression without altering the underlying DNA sequence. In other words, although you may have inherited certain genetic tendencies, you have significant power to modify how those genes express themselves through conscious lifestyle choices.

Antibiotics and other medications

The interaction between your gut and medications is more of a dynamic balance than a one-sided conversation. While your gut microbiome can affect how medications are metabolized and absorbed, medications in turn can influence the composition and health of your gut. Understanding these interactions allows you to make more informed decisions about supporting your gut while using any necessary treatments:

- **Digestive medications:** Well-established treatments, such as laxatives for constipation or anti-diarrheals for IBS, can often improve gut function. However, these medications may not be suitable for everyone, so please work with a healthcare provider to determine the safest and most effective option for your specific needs.
- **Antibiotics:** Although they're often crucial for clearing harmful infections, antibiotics don't differentiate between beneficial and harmful bacteria, which means both can be depleted and result in digestive discomfort. Repeated or prolonged use may also contribute to antibiotic resistance, reducing their long-term effectiveness. So, to help restore gut health and prevent further imbalance, follow the steps outlined at the end of this chapter.
- **Metformin:** This common medication for type 2 diabetes can cause some digestive issues (diarrhea or bloating) but research suggests it may also help foster beneficial bacteria in the gut over time. If you're experiencing discomfort, talk to your doctor about adjustments or additional support for your gut.
- **Chemotherapy and radiation:** These therapies can cause significant damage to the gut lining and disrupt the balance of good bacteria, often leading to issues such as inflammation, diarrhea, or nausea. Although the side effects can't be fully avoided, it's possible to nurture your gut health during and after treatment with supportive foods, probiotics, and lifestyle changes (under the guidance of your healthcare team).
- **Nonsteroidal anti-inflammatory drugs (NSAIDs):** Pain medications such as ibuprofen and aspirin but can irritate your gut lining. Long-term use may increase gut permeability (leaky gut) and raise inflammation levels.
- **Proton pump inhibitors (PPIs):** PPIs, which are prescribed for acid reflux, reduce stomach acid production, which can help alleviate discomfort but may also allow harmful bacteria to thrive and lead to small intestinal bacterial overgrowth (SIBO) over time.

REMEMBER

Just because these medications can affect your gut doesn't mean you should avoid them. If a qualified healthcare professional prescribes any of these drugs, it's because the benefits outweigh the risks. However, if you're concerned about potential gut side effects, be sure to communicate your concerns with your healthcare team. There are plenty of ways to support your microbiome while continuing necessary treatment.

Our modern lifestyle

REMEMBER

People living in rural areas where there's more exposure to natural microbes due to their direct contact with the environment tend to have more diverse microbiomes and therefore, stronger immune systems. But here's something interesting: Research on people who move from regions with low asthma rates to highly urbanized areas where asthma and allergies run rampant showed that their microbiomes shifted, leaving them more susceptible to these conditions.

It's not just city living that impacts our microbiome. Over-sanitization plays a big role too. The hygiene hypothesis suggests that in our quest to stay ultra-clean — scrubbing away dirt and germs with hand sanitizers, antibacterial wipes, and harsh cleaning products — we're also wiping out the good bacteria that help strengthen our immune system. In fact, studies show that a little exposure to everyday germs can help train your immune system. This is why oversanitation has been proposed as a contributing factor to the rise in childhood and adult allergies and atopic disorders such as asthma and eczema.

That being said, it's important to note that the data supporting the hygiene hypothesis shows correlations rather than definitive causes, and other environmental factors likely play a role too. Still, the concept serves as a useful lens to understand how modern habits might impact our immune health.

Illness

Just as your gut health can influence your immune response, illness can significantly impact your gut-immune function. When you're fighting off an illness — whether it's a mild cold or a more severe infection — your body triggers an inflammatory response that can compromise the gut lining's ability to function optimally. This inflammation can disrupt nutrient absorption, cause bloating, and alter bowel habits.

Interestingly, many women report experiencing more severe premenstrual syndrome symptoms following a period of illness. This can be linked to immune system strain and the gut's central role in regulating inflammation and hormone balance.

Exercise

A sedentary lifestyle doesn't do the gut any favors either. Regular physical activity boosts the diversity of beneficial bacteria in your microbiome, helping everything move along in your digestive system more smoothly and reducing issues such as bloating or constipation. It also lowers inflammation and supports a stronger gut barrier, keeping everything in balance.

Environment

Elements in the physical environment can affect your gut lining. For example, pollution, toxin exposure, and even household products can directly harm your gut microbiome. Certain dishwasher tablets, for example, were recently shown to contain chemicals that damage the gut lining, creating tiny holes that allow toxins to enter the bloodstream — worsening inflammation and gut imbalances.

REMEMBER

However, it's not only the physical environment that affects the gut. You've likely heard the saying, "You are the company you keep," and this wisdom extends to your gut health. The emotional and social environment you cultivate can have a profound impact on your digestive system. Just as chronic emotional stress can lead to disruptions in your gut's balance — resulting in inflammation, digestive discomfort, and mood disturbances — positive and supportive relationships can help ease stress and promote gut health. A supportive circle not only strengthens your emotional resilience but also contributes to a balanced and healthy gut.

Restoring Gut Health

WARNING

Despite mainstream media and commercial momentum, critical gaps in our scientific understanding of gut health remain. Many insights into the relationship between the microbiota and human health stem from animal studies, and further rigorous human trials are necessary before we can confidently translate these findings into concrete dietary recommendations.

The gut microbiome's remarkable adaptability, or plasticity, is what makes it an extremely appealing target for health interventions. We know that short-term dietary changes can induce notable shifts in gut microbial populations. However, it's the long-term dietary habits that tend to result in more stable and resilient microbial communities. Interestingly, the microbes most responsive to dietary changes often represent a small fraction of the overall microbiome. This raises the question of whether altering these minor populations is sufficient to drive significant physiological changes in the body.

REMEMBER

Given the current limitations in research, it's important to make decisions based on what we do know. Getting back to the foundational habits listed covered in the following sections remains the most reliable way to support your gut health and hormone balance.

Employing lifestyle interventions

While the gut-brain-endocrine connection may seem complex, nurturing it involves simple, accessible steps that will add up to make a big difference over time:

WARNING

- **Taking probiotics/prebiotics:** While probiotic (beneficial bacteria found in fermented foods) and prebiotic (fiber) supplements are often marketed as quick miracle fixes for gut health, many fall short of their promises. These supplements are not strictly regulated, so they may not always contain the strains or quantities listed on their labels. Factors such as encapsulation, storage conditions, and resistance to stomach acid and bile can also affect whether the probiotics reach the colon alive in sufficient numbers to provide benefits.

  So while probiotics do show promise, more research is needed to identify targeted strains for specific conditions, and current evidence doesn't support using probiotics for prevention. Choosing products tested by third parties for quality and potency is essential if you want to maximize the potential benefits. However, a diverse, nutrient-rich diet often proves just as effective — if not more — at supporting your gut. As always, food is medicine!
- **Managing stress and taking care of your nervous system:** Incorporating practices such as meditation, yoga, and breathwork into your daily routine can significantly lower cortisol levels and reduce gut inflammation by activating the vagus nerve and regulating the ENS. Even daily choices to spend time outdoors, engage in enjoyable hobbies, or foster meaningful connections can help regulate your nervous system. Moreover, addressing unresolved trauma, learning to process emotions effectively, and building a supportive, positive community are critical steps in nurturing both your mental and gut health.
- **Moving your body regularly:** Regular, moderate physical activity such as walking, swimming, or cycling will help you maintain a well-functioning and resilient gut-brain-endocrine axis.
- **Being mindful of medications:** While medications are often necessary, it's important to be mindful of their impact on your gut health. If you're taking antibiotics, prioritize eating prebiotic-rich foods and a diverse array of plant foods to help replenish beneficial bacteria.

TIP

- **Reducing exposure to environmental toxins:** Prioritizing organic produce, filtering your drinking water, and selecting natural cleaning products are key strategies to reduce toxin exposure. If you live in an urban area, it's also essential to carve out time for fresh air in natural environments to counterbalance the impact of pollutants. These small changes can significantly reduce your body's toxic load, supporting both hormonal and gut health. For a more detailed exploration of toxins and actionable steps to mitigate their impact, I encourage you to refer to Part 4 and the online appendix at `www.dummies.com/go/hormonebalancefd`.

Applying diet interventions

TIP

Research shows over and over again that a varied, whole-foods, nutrient-rich diet is key to fostering optimal gut health. This doesn't mean you have to embark on a strict or complicated eating plan. In fact, it's as easy as mixing in a variety of colorful fruits, veggies, and grains throughout the week, or trying out new ingredients such as fermented foods and fiber-rich legumes. Here are some recommendations:

- **Eat prebiotic and probiotic foods:** Incorporating probiotics, the friendly bacteria found in fermented foods like yogurt, kefir, and sauerkraut, can support your gut. For optimal results, pair these with prebiotic-rich foods, like garlic, onions, and asparagus, which feed these beneficial bacteria. Think of probiotics like planting seeds, and prebiotics as the fertilizer that helps them grow!
- **Aim for 30 plant-based foods a week:** This might sound daunting at first, but it's easier than you think. Include a mix of fruits, vegetables, grains, nuts, seeds, and legumes in your meals. A simple salad with a handful of mixed greens, a few roasted veggies, and a sprinkle of seeds checks off several boxes. And don't forget to season your protein (chicken, tofu, lentils, lamb, and so on) with herbs and spices!
- **Focus on whole, nutrient-dense foods:** Skip ultra-processed options and choose whole grains, nuts, seeds, and fresh fruits and vegetables. These foods are packed with fiber, which is fuel for your gut bacteria and helps them produce beneficial short-chain fatty acids that reduce inflammation.
- **Consume polyphenols for the win:** Dark chocolate, berries, and green tea are great for your gut because they're rich in polyphenols, which are antioxidants that support the growth of beneficial gut bacteria.
- **Watch your sugar and processed food intake:** Opt for fiber-rich alternatives that promote a healthy microbiome and keep your blood sugar levels stable. Fresh fruits, like berries and apples, provide natural sweetness along with

essential vitamins and antioxidants. Nuts and seeds, such as almonds or chia seeds, offer a satisfying crunch, healthy fats, and fiber to support sustained energy. Whole-grain crackers or vegetable sticks paired with hummus can be a great savory alternative, providing both fiber and nutrients without the blood sugar spikes.

- **Reduce alcohol and substance use:** Reducing alcohol consumption can lead to substantial improvements in gut health, as excessive alcohol consumption disrupts the gut microbiome and contributes to inflammation. Additionally, recovery from substance abuse will often necessitate targeted dietary interventions to rebalance the gut bacteria as substances such as opioids, and stimulants, can damage the gut lining, alter microbial populations, and promote inflammation.

IN THIS CHAPTER

» Investigating how contemporary lifestyle changes are disrupting our hormonal balance

» Discovering the impact of a lack of purpose and fulfillment

» Speculating about the reasons for more prevalent hormone imbalances

Chapter 11

Unpacking Modern Life's Impact on Our Ancient Hormones

Dr. Barry Sears, the American biochemist and creator of the Zone Diet, once said, "To control your hormones is to control your life." While I agree, I would take it a step further and say this: Reclaiming your life from the pressures of modernity is key to achieving hormonal balance and taking control of your life.

This book departs from the traditional, mainstream, fragmented view of hormone balance, where the body is often reduced to a set of hormones or hormone-producing organs to be "managed" like a machine. This reductionist approach, sometimes referred to as the "technological fragmentation of the body," treats hormones as isolated elements in a system to be optimized — often with consumer-driven solutions — while neglecting the deeper, interconnected layers of our physical, emotional, and mental health. Instead, throughout this book, I've presented a more holistic perspective that embraces the complexity of modern life itself, not just the mechanics of the endocrine system.

Whereas Chapters 6 and 7 explore the global increase in the most common hormone-related health issues, this chapter builds on that foundation by diving into how to cultivate a more intentional, aligned way of living — one that harmonizes purpose, physical movement, emotional connection, and mindful use of technology to help counteract hormonal imbalances. It also includes practical, actionable steps that you can start implementing immediately. Each deliberate change will bring you closer to reclaiming control over your health and creating harmony between your mind, body, and environment.

At the end of the chapter, I introduce to two groundbreaking fields of research — psychoneuroimmunology and psychoneuroendocrinology — that shed light on the powerful, intricate connections between the mind, immune system, and hormones. Get ready to start making changes in your life in the most meaningful, lasting way possible.

Lifestyle Changes

REMEMBER

Modern *Homo sapiens* (that's us!) have thrived for thousands of years through movement, connection, and balancing short-term needs and long-term rewards. We hunted, gathered, and formed communities, and our bodies and brains evolved over time to function optimally when we have high levels of activity, close social bonds, and a natural rhythm between work and rest.

When you compare the way we live now to the lives of our ancient ancestors, it's clear these patterns have drastically shifted. We no longer need to chase or work hard for our meals or operate in tight-knit communities to make it through each day. Instead, we spend our time glued to screens, moving less, socializing virtually, and satisfying our every need with just a few taps of a device. While convenient, this way of life is making it harder for our ancient hormones to function at their best.

Exercise

We have long understood the connection between physical activity and overall health. Even Juvenal, the Roman poet and satirist of the second century, recognized that the "hard labors of Hercules" were far more effective than "banquets and downy cushions" in achieving his famous ideal of a "healthy mind in a healthy body." Due to the sedentary nature of modern life, most of us live far closer to leisurely style of living that Juvenal critiqued. In fact, the average adult in the U.S. now spends more than 10 hours a day sitting; only 23 percent of adults meet the recommended guidelines for both aerobic and muscle-strengthening activities.

Globally, the situation is similar, with the World Health Organization (WHO) reporting that one in four adults worldwide are not physically active enough. In countries like the U.K., approximately 75 percent of workers spend nearly six hours sitting each workday, the consequences of which go beyond just physical fitness or aesthetics. Regular inactivity disrupts essential biological functions that regulate your hormones, including the release of myokines — a fascinating class of signaling molecules released by the muscles during physical activity. These "messengers" play a vital role in regulating two crucial tier 1 hormones: insulin and cortisol, both of which are central to metabolic and stress-related processes in the body.

TECHNICAL STUFF

But how did this shift to moving less come about? Understanding the broader societal changes that have contributed to the decline in physical activity will help you start identifying practical strategies to overcome these barriers and reintegrate movement into your daily routine:

TIP

- **Sedentary work environments:** Sedentary jobs in the U.S. have increased by 83 percent since 1950. Most modern jobs now involve little to no physical exertion, but that doesn't have to be a barrier to incorporating movement into your day. Taking short, frequent breaks to stand up, stretch, or walk around can break up long periods of sitting and help combat the effects of a sedentary job. If walking or biking to work aren't options, consider setting up walking meetings or using a standing desk.
- **Technological distractions:** The average U.S. adult spends more than 7 hours a day consuming digital media, whether it's scrolling through social platforms, gaming, watching the news online, or binge-watching shows. However, instead of throwing your devices into a drawer and fighting against the use of technology, you can actually use them to your advantage. There are countless fitness apps, online exercise classes, and activity trackers designed to integrate movement in your life. Even setting a simple reminder to take breaks can help you shift you from a passive consumer to active engager.
- **Urbanization:** It's easy to see how urban sprawl, car dependency, and lack of green spaces can make incorporating physical activity a little trickier than it used to be, so you might have to get creative! Walking more during your commute (even parking further away or getting off public transport a stop earlier), exploring indoor fitness options, or seeking out local parks during weekends can make movement more accessible and enjoyable. Even short bursts of physical activity — 10 to 15 minutes at a time — can add up to big health benefits, so choose to climb stairs rather than getting the elevator, walk up escalators rather than riding them, walk in place or around the office while on calls, or stretch during TV breaks.

REMEMBER

» **Time constraints:** Effective time management starts with setting clear boundaries. If you constantly feel overwhelmed or stretched too thin, you need to reevaluate how you're protecting your time to make room for the things that truly matter. Prioritizing exercise not only boosts your energy and improves hormone balance but makes you more efficient and productive in the other areas of your life. Shifting your mindset to see exercise as investing in your future self rather than as time-consuming.

Loneliness

REMEMBER

Friendships activate the release of endorphins and other feel-good hormones, such as dopamine and oxytocin, which in turn stimulate your immune system's natural killer cells that target diseases and viruses. Studies also show that those with fewer or no close connections are more susceptible to psychological conditions like depression and are less equipped to fend off illness.

This concept of interconnectedness isn't new; it's a fundamental principle of nature. As the renowned astrophysicist Neil deGrasse Tyson put it while promoting his book *Astrophysics for People in a Hurry* (W. W. Norton & Company, 2017)"We are all connected; to each other, biologically. To the earth, chemically. To the rest of the universe, atomically." Interpersonal neurobiology, which I discuss toward the end of this chapter, shows how relationships and social interactions don't just affect your mental state but actively shape your brain and nervous system. Your hormones, environment, emotions, and social bonds are all intricately woven together to maintain balance and health.

The loneliness epidemic

Technology has made our world intensely hyperconnected. The paradox is that our constant connectivity has us feeling more isolated than ever and increasingly disconnected from meaningful human interactions. WHO now recognizes loneliness as a serious public health problem that's comparable in its health risks to smoking 15 cigarettes a day and obesity. In response, countries such as Japan and the U.K. have appointed "ministers of loneliness" who are tasked with developing strategies to combat the rising rates of loneliness and social isolation, particularly among younger citizens, older populations, and men.

Loneliness and pornography

REMEMBER

One underrecognized contributor to the growing loneliness crisis is pornography consumption. A study from the Institute for Family Studies revealed that daily pornography use among young adults is strongly linked to higher rates of depression and loneliness, underscoring the need for a broader conversation about how people interact with digital content, and more importantly, how people prioritize and cultivate meaningful human connections in an era where digital consumption often takes precedence over real-world intimacy.

Loneliness versus aloneness

Being alone doesn't always mean being lonely. In fact, solitude gives you wonderful opportunities for reflection, emotional processing, creativity, and mental restoration. Loneliness, in contrast, occurs when isolation is not a choice, or when there's a disconnect between how much social interaction you're craving or desiring and what is available for you.

REMEMBER

It's not just about physical isolation; you can feel lonely, disconnected, or unseen even when you're surrounded by other people. This happens when the social interactions you're having lack depth or meaning, when you don't feel emotionally connected to the people around you or you don't feel like you can be your true, authentic self. Loneliness then, is a deeply subjective experience. So for some, being physically alone doesn't result in loneliness at all, whereas others may feel profoundly lonely even though they have a huge family and social circle. The quality of your interactions matters far more than the quantity. People with closer friendships and higher quality relationships built on empathy and intimacy that allows them to feel seen and heard experience more life satisfaction and less loneliness and depression.

The hormonal impact of loneliness

On a physiological level, loneliness triggers elevated levels of stress hormones such as cortisol and norepinephrine, which can lead to a weakened immune system and a reduced sense of physical warmth. In 2023 the U.S. surgeon general highlighted that the absence of social connection can negatively affect cardiovascular health, neuroendocrine function, and the gut microbiome, all of which are linked to blood pressure, stress hormone circulation, and inflammation.

REMEMBER

In contrast to the quick dopamine hits we get from superficial interactions (for example, social media "likes"), meaningful in-person connections trigger the release of oxytocin, which fosters feelings of safety, connection, and stress relief. Without enough oxytocin-producing relationships, the body can remain in a prolonged state of stress.

Also, when people feel isolated or disconnected, they often turn to unhealthy coping behaviors to manage those feelings, such excessive alcohol consumption, binge eating, lack of exercise, social withdrawal, or even using social media as an emotional crutch. All these activities are linked to dysregulation in tier 1 hormones cortisol and insulin, compounding stress on the body and creating a vicious feedback loop that becomes tough to break.

Reclaim hormonal balance through connection

There is no need to feel ashamed about being lonely, and it's important to remember that each of us has the power to seek out and prioritize deeper, more meaningful relationships where we can express our authenticity. You can read in Chapter 9 about challenging negative thoughts or unkind beliefs about your worthiness, likeability, or lovability.

TIP

Taking steps to reconnect with your authentic self through creative outlets, nature, and mindfulness can have a profound impact on your hormone balance. Activities such as painting, drawing, journaling, or even walking in nature reduce cortisol levels and increase feel-good hormones like dopamine, endorphins, and oxytocin. They also enhance your resilience, giving you the emotional energy and capacity needed to put yourself out there and form genuine relationships.

TIP

Additionally, oxytocin — your bonding hormone — is released when you engage in real-world, meaningful interactions, even something small, like a friendly chat with your local barista. They don't need to be lengthy or profound conversations to positively impact your hormone levels. They just need to be genuine.

Disruption to traditional work models

REMEMBER

The workforce was once dominated by manufacturing, manual labor, and fixed office environments, but it's shifted toward knowledge-based, service-driven roles that are predominantly desk-bound, giving way to more flexible but less structured work environments that require people to have much greater self-awareness than was necessary for previous generations to manage our health effectively.

By being conscious of these modern challenges and making deliberate choices to prioritize your hormone health, you can transform your reality and thrive in this ever-evolving landscape. In the following sections, I outline the biggest hormone offenders so you can take steps to counteract them.

Exposure to artificial light

The invention of electric lighting has undoubtedly transformed our lives, enabling us to work, exercise, enjoy entertainment, and go about our daily routines well beyond daylight hours. However, widespread use of artificial light, particularly during winter months in the Northern hemisphere when the sun may set as early as 3:00 p.m., can disrupt natural circadian rhythms (refer to Chapter 2 for more information on your hormonal clocks). Among artificial light sources, blue light wavelengths are particularly problematic after sunset because they suppress the production of melatonin — your sleep hormone — delaying its release and making it harder to fall asleep and achieve restful sleep. Over time, poor sleep contributes to increased stress and worsens mood disorders, highlighting the need to minimize blue light exposure in the evening, such as from screens and LED lighting.

WARNING

The health risks of prolonged artificial light exposure are evident in research on night-shift workers, who face increased risks of metabolic disorders such as type 2 diabetes and obesity, menstrual irregularities, and a heightened risk of breast cancer. These effects are largely attributed to disrupted circadian rhythms and suppressed melatonin production.

Remote work and digitization

Research consistently shows that remote workers are generally more sedentary than their office-based counterparts which is a growing concern, as being sedentary impairs the body's ability to regulate key hormones such as insulin and cortisol and reduces the production of "happy hormones."

Chronic stress driven by poor work-life boundaries and increased feelings of loneliness are also issues. For instance, the American Psychological Association's 2024 *Work in America* survey highlighted significant concerns regarding workplace loneliness, particularly among younger employees. The survey found that 48 percent of workers aged 18 to 25 felt that colleagues not close to their age did not value their ideas, compared to 32 percent of workers overall and just 16 percent of those aged 65 and older.

TIP

If you find yourself feeling disconnected from colleagues, one option is to explore friendships in other environments. Engaging in communities outside of work can provide a sense of belonging and emotional fulfillment that may not always come from the workplace, especially if you're working remotely.

Embracing the evolution of work for better health

Remote work seems here to stay, which demands a new mindset about how you engage with your work environment and care for yourself in this evolving landscape. The following list looks at how you can approach this shift strategically, taking steps to ensure that while your work changes, your health remains a priority:

TIP

- **Incorporate movement into your day:** Physical activity doesn't need to happen all at once, so make time for short bursts that can have a cumulative effect o improving your energy levels, boosting productivity, and balancing hormones.

» **Prioritize work-life boundaries:** Set specific work hours, and when the workday is done, focus on activities that nourish your mind and body. This clear structure will not only improve your mental health and reduce stress but also allow your body to find its natural rhythm again.

TIP

» **Spend time in nature:** Spending at least 120 minutes per week in nature has been shown to significantly improve mental, emotional, and physical health, according to a study published in *Nature*. Those who spend time near blue spaces (bodies of water) report even greater benefits, including reduced stress, enhanced mental clarity.

» **Use technology to your advantage:** Just as technology has disrupted traditional work models, it can also be used to improve your health. If you're feeling stretched for time or struggle to remember to implement your healthy habits at first, technology is there to help you.

Social media and dopamine addiction

In a 2024 Senate judiciary hearing on "Big Tech and the Online Child Sexual Exploitation Crisis," Meta CEO Mark Zuckerberg addressed concerns about social media's impact on children's mental health. He stated that current scientific research had not definitively established a causal link between social media use and declining mental health among young people.

REMEMBER

Zuckerberg's statement was worded very carefully and a presented a view that has been widely contested by researchers. Studies continue to show a growing connection between social media use and declining mental health, particularly among teenagers. Currently, Facebook is the only platform available for long-term research given its early presence in the social media landscape, and one study by MIT economist Alexey Makarin revealed a clear correlation between increased usage on college campuses in the mid-2000s and a rise in mental health issues, including higher rates of depression and anxiety.

Researchers will continue explore the biological and psychological mechanisms driving trends such as the promotion of division, intolerance, and echo chambers through reinforcing algorithms. However, key questions still remain: why does social media appear to exacerbate mental health issues, and why do these effects disproportionately affect certain groups, such as teenage girls? What is increasingly clear is that the endless cycle of scrolling, liking, and refreshing is fueling a dopamine-driven feedback loop that can significantly impact your brain and hormones.

Defining dopamine addiction

Dopamine is a neurotransmitter that plays a key role in how people experience pleasure, motivation, and reward. Whenever you experience something pleasurable, dopamine is released in your brain. This reinforces the behavior, making you want to repeat it for another hit of satisfaction.

In Chapter 3, I classify dopamine as a tier 1 hormone. It motivates us to seek out experiences that trigger its release, driving many of our day-to-day actions that cultivate or disrupt hormone balance such as what we eat, how much we exercise and how much stress our body experiences.

WARNING

However, the idea of being "addicted to dopamine" is a bit of a myth. You can't be addicted to dopamine itself because it's just a chemical in your brain. However, you can become addicted to the activities or substances that cause the dopamine spikes, which then creates a cycle of craving that pleasure again and again. It's important to take back control of your dopamine feedback loop because over time, excessive stimulation can actually decrease the number of dopamine receptors in your brain. Consequently, things that used to bring you joy may start to feel less rewarding compared to the dopamine rush from your phone. Although you're not addicted to dopamine itself, you become addicted to the behaviors that give you that dopamine boost.

Breaking the cycle

TIP

- **Limit screen time:** Reducing your time on social platforms by small increments to work toward a goal of only 1 to 2 hours per day. Most smartphones offer screentime trackers to help with this.
- **Create a "dopamine menu":** In Part 4 of this book, you'll learn how to curate your daily activities to ensure you're getting dopamine from healthy and meaningful sources such as reading, exercising, self-care rituals, mindfulness, face-to-face interactions, art, and music.
- **Establish phone-free zones:** Create boundaries around your social media use by designating specific times or places where your phone is completely off-limits — in the bedroom, during meals, while exercising or working.
- **Take regular digital detoxes:** Consider going on short "digital detoxes" where you take a break from social media entirely for a few days or a weekend to help reset your brain's dopamine response.

Short versus long-term gratification

REMEMBER

The ability to deny yourself immediate pleasure for the sake of a greater long-term reward is strong predictor of your ability to achieve your goals. The reason so many of us struggle with this is not because we're "weak" or "undisciplined." Rather, it's due to the fact that we've been biologically hardwired to prioritize short-term gratification. For our ancient ancestors, rewards such as finding food or shelter were essential for survival, so our brains release dopamine when we experience these short-term rewards, reinforcing behaviors that lead to quick payoffs.

The modern challenge for us is that our prefrontal cortex — the part of the brain responsible for decision-making and long-term planning — has to work harder than ever to override our impulses for short-term rewards. In a world of convenience and instant gratification, everything is so easily accessible that it's become increasingly more challenging to prioritize long-term benefits over momentary satisfaction. This task becomes even more difficult when we're stressed, tired, or overwhelmed, which weakens the ability to delay gratification. This is why so many people struggle to make choices that support their long-term health.

Developing the ability to zoom out and make decisions that will benefit future you is the secret weapon to managing your hormone health. Opting for immediate pleasures — such as sugary foods — may feel rewarding in the moment, but over time, it can lead to weight gain, insulin resistance, and type 2 diabetes. Additionally, constantly chasing quick dopamine hits can raise cortisol levels, contributing to chronic stress and anxiety that can diminish your motivation and focus over time, making it harder to engage in activities that require sustained effort.

TIP

Delayed gratification requires patience and discipline. Think of it as "intelligent investing" — putting time in now for a reward later. Here are some steps you can take to intelligently invest in your future:

- **Set clear long-term goals:** Part 4 explains how to create a clear vision of what you're working towards.
- **Recognize the triggers:** Do you reach for your phone when you're bored or stressed? Do you grab a sugary snack when you're tired? Being aware of these moments and taking action to prevent them by putting your phone in the drawer or bringing healthy snacks will help you make more conscious decisions.
- **Reframe short-term gratification:** Instead of viewing long-term choices as a sacrifice, reframe them as investments in your future self. When you choose to exercise, go to bed early, or eat healthy, remind yourself that you're embodying your happiest, healthiest, highest self.

» **Create a supportive environment:** Surround yourself with people, resources, and tools that make it easier to focus on your long-term goals. Whether it's a workout buddy, a meal prep service, or a time management app, having supportive structures in place helps you stay on track even on the days when you're feeling a bit blah.

Lack of Purpose and Fulfilment

REMEMBER

At our core, we all deeply desire to contribute, to share our gifts, and to feel that our lives have meaning. We want to be needed, to be seen for who we are, feel that we belong, and know that we're making a difference. These are more than just lofty spiritual or philosophical ideas. When we have a clear sense of purpose, it signals to the brain that we are safe, secure, and moving in alignment with our values, which sending a positive ripple effect through your entire endocrine system.

But modern life, with its constant distractions, FOMO (fear of missing out), comparison culture and relentless pace, is pulling many people further away from a sense of purpose and fulfillment. Packed schedules and societal pressures to do it all and be it all for everyone, all the time can leave you overwhelmed. There's often little room for personal growth or connecting deeply with yourself and others, making it difficult to focus on what truly matters and will bring us long-term fulfillment.

The power of purpose

Purpose and fulfillment are essential for all people. Without a clear sense of purpose, you risk not only emotional dissatisfaction but also physical depletion. That said, purpose doesn't have to revolve around grand, life-altering missions (though if you have one, by all means, pursue it). More often than not, purpose is woven into the small, seemingly mundane decisions and moments of daily life.

While we all share a fundamental human need for meaning, belonging, and contribution, how each person finds and expresses purpose varies based on personal values, passions, life experiences, and strengths. Your purpose may also evolve and change throughout your life.

Purpose is powerful because it promotes the release of happy hormones. When dopamine is flowing, it's much easier to stay committed to goals, no matter how big or small. And serotonin helps us feel more positive, enabling us to handle challenges with greater ease. Purpose-driven living also fosters oxytocin production, the hormone responsible for social bonding and feelings of love and connection. When you're pursuing something meaningful, you tend to form deeper connections with those around you. Simply put, purpose builds a protective bubble around your emotional and physiological well-being, allowing your hormones to thrive.

REMEMBER

Think back to a time when you were truly passionate and lit up about something. You probably felt energized, optimistic, excited, and focused. Taking care of yourself likely felt very natural, you probably slept better and handled stress or challenges much more effectively. In Eastern medicine, this is known as "life force energy." When you feel fulfilled, your body moves toward balance, which translates into vitality and focus.

Importantly, purpose also acts as a powerful buffer against the body's stress response. When you live in alignment and pursue things you care about, your brain reduces the production of cortisol and adrenaline, which is why life feels so much smoother. You become more resilient in the face of stress, and you're better equipped to handle life's inevitable challenges.

Asserting your authenticity

REMEMBER

Authenticity is the foundation upon which purpose and fulfillment are built. To live in alignment with your purpose, you must first get clear on who you are and what matters most to you.

Living authentically isn't complicated, but in a world where you're constantly bombarded by external and cultural expectations, being true to yourself can sometimes feel like a radical act. Being authentic simply involves making choices that are aligned with your core values, passions, and strengths. You stop living for external validation from others or giving in to societal pressures and start consciously creating a life that reflects your true wants, needs, and desires. When you're no longer constantly battling internally between who you are and who you're expected to be, stress hormones naturally decrease, and feel-good hormones like serotonin, oxytocin, and dopamine rise, supporting hormone balance and your overall sense of fulfilment.

TIP

This way of life is about consistently choosing actions and environments that align with what's true or feels right for you, even in small ways. It's a process of learning and evolution — you certainly don't need to be perfectionistic about it or know your path right away. It can look like speaking up in a meeting, spending more time in places you love, carving out time for a passion project/side hustle that has nothing to do with your career, or setting boundaries with those around you concerning your diet or lifestyle choices.

When you become more authentic in your daily life, your energy will naturally increase. You'll find yourself more motivated, creative, and resilient. Sticking to your hormone-supportive habits will feel natural, and you'll find it easier to choose healthier coping mechanisms when challenges arise.

Speculating about the Increase in Hormone Imbalances

At the heart of the rise in hormone imbalances lies a fundamental issue: Our minds and bodies are under unprecedented levels of strain, and we have become disconnected from the signals our symptoms are trying to convey. Despite the substantial body of research, Western medicine has often fallen short in addressing hormone imbalances through a biopsychosocial lens — one that recognizes the intricate interplay between biological, psychological, and social factors. The approach to treating hormone-related conditions remains fragmented, treating isolated symptoms individually, often with medication. Healthcare professionals tend to overlook the broader, interconnected systems at work, missing opportunities to address the root causes of hormonal imbalances and to view the body as a holistic, integrated entity.

For instance, while stress is widely recognized as a key factor in hormone-related conditions like PCOS, missed periods, low testosterone, and insulin resistance, conventional treatments often focus on short-term solutions such as medication or supplements. These approaches typically target the symptoms but fail to address the deeper, underlying causes of the stress. This is where the biopsychosocial model offers a more comprehensive perspective, emphasizing the need to tackle not just the biological symptoms, but also the psychological and social drivers of hormonal imbalances for a truly holistic approach to healing.

REMEMBER

One of the key things I hope you take away from this book is that humans are deeply connected to our world. Your individual biology, psychological functioning, and interpersonal relationships all work together, each influencing the other. That means getting your body back to a true place of homeostasis requires addressing many different aspects of your life and coming back to a place of purpose and authenticity. No, this approach isn't as convenient as taking a pill. but a process that includes reflection, intention, and lifestyle shifts certainly leads to transformative, lasting change. The reward is a life that feels more vibrant, resilient, and authentic.

What's exciting is that emerging fields like psychoneuroimmunology and psychoneuroendocrinology are revealing just how deeply intertwined our mental, emotional, and hormonal health really are. The following sections dive deeper into these concepts, offering a pathway not just to symptom management but to truly reclaiming your hormonal health through a more integrative, holistic approach.

Other diseases and conditions linked to hormones

REMEMBER

Maintaining healthy hormone levels requires constant care and attention, just like a garden needs ongoing maintenance. There will always be weeds that threaten to disrupt your hormonal harmony. The key is learning how to tend to your hormones throughout all stages of life, ensuring they remain resilient and adaptable to whatever comes your way to reduce the risk of developing more severe diseases and conditions linked to hormonal dysfunction in the future. Here are just a few brief examples, though this list is by no means exhaustive and research continues to establish links between hormonal dysregulation and disease:

- **Autoimmune diseases:** Fluctuations in hormones such as estrogen and cortisol can trigger or worsen conditions like Hashimoto's, rheumatoid arthritis, and lupus.
- **Osteoporosis:** Declining estrogen levels weaken bones, especially after menopause, while cortisol imbalances exacerbate bone loss.
- **Breast cancer:** Elevated levels of estrogen, poor gut health, and exposure to xenoestrogens increase the risk of hormone-driven cancers.
- **Chronic fatigue:** Imbalances in cortisol, a key regulator of energy, often underlie persistent fatigue.
- **Cardiovascular disease:** Hormones such as estrogen, cortisol, and insulin affect heart health; imbalances increase the risk of high blood pressure and heart disease.
- **Digestive disorders:** Cortisol and insulin play a critical role in gut health, influencing conditions such IBS and leaky gut.

Psychoneuroimmunology

Psychoneuroimmunology (PNI) is an exciting and rapidly growing field co-founded psychologist Robert Ader and immunologist Nicholas Cohen in the 1970s. It explores the complex interplay between the nervous system, immune system, and psychological processes and offers a new lens through which we can understand the deep connections between our emotions, thoughts, mental health, and immune function. What makes PNI particularly promising for those seeking solutions for hormone balance — especially in conditions like endometriosis — is its recognition that stress, emotions, and behaviors directly influence immune responses. In turn, immune system activity can impact the brain and mental state.

REMEMBER

In the context of endometriosis, a condition marked by chronic inflammation covered more comprehensively in Chapter 6, PNI provides a framework to explore how unresolved emotional stress, low self-esteem, negative self-talk, or trauma may trigger or exacerbate the immune response, driving the condition forward. By understanding and addressing these psychosomatic pathways (physical symptoms caused or influenced by emotional or mental factors), PNI holds potential for helping explore integrative strategies that regulate both emotional and physical health to restore balance, ultimately offering new hope for better managing and even improving certain conditions.

TIP

For example, a study published in *Psychoneuroendocrinology* in 2019 demonstrated how mindfulness meditation could reduce inflammation and improve immune function by lowering cortisol levels. The research showed that regular mindfulness practice significantly decreased stress-related immune responses and regulated hormone levels in participants, illustrating the connection between mental states, immune health, and hormonal balance.

Psychoneuroimmunoendocrinology

Psychoneuroimmunoendocrinology (PNIE) is an extension of PNI that focuses on the crucial role hormones play in the complex interaction between the brain, immune system, and behavior. This emerging field delves deeper into how hormones act as key messengers, connecting the nervous, immune, and endocrine systems. By examining how these hormones modulate immune responses and how immune system activity can, in turn, affect hormonal balance, PNIE offers a more holistic perspective on hormone health.

For instance, sex hormones like estrogen and progesterone are known to regulate reproductive health, but they also influence immune responses. Hormonal fluctuations during the menstrual cycle, pregnancy, or menopause can alter immune function, leading to changes in inflammation and disease susceptibility. This means that immune system imbalances, such as chronic inflammation, can feedback into the endocrine system, further disrupting hormones like insulin, thyroid hormones, and sex hormones.

REMEMBER

Groundbreaking research, such as the 2021 *Nature Immunology* study on sex hormones and autoimmune diseases, highlights how estrogen can increase immune receptor expression, making women more prone to conditions like lupus, while testosterone offers a protective effect. These findings provide new insights into hormone-driven autoimmune diseases. As we better understand these interconnected systems, PNIE holds the potential to offer us solutions that address both the root causes and systemic impacts of hormonal imbalances.

3 Interpreting Your Symptoms

IN THIS PART . . .

Understand the unique rhythm of men and women's reproductive hormone cycles and align your lifestyle to unlock your body's full potential.

Uncover the often-overlooked signs of hormonal imbalances and learn how to be your own advocate by recognizing the signals your body sends to you.

Join the prevention revolution by empowering yourself with integrative and functional medicine approaches so you can avoid imbalances turning into something more serious.

Discover the pros and cons of different testing methods and learn to interpret your results with confidence so you can make informed, empowered choices — regardless of whether you have a diagnosis.

IN THIS CHAPTER

» Exploring how men can work with their 24-hour cycle

» Evaluating what's "typical" for a woman's monthly cycle

» Understanding how "cycle syncing" diet and lifestyle can optimize health

» Investigating the impact of birth control on women's health

» Clarifying perimenopause and menopause symptoms

Chapter 12
Understanding Your Reproductive Hormones

Hormones play a key role in the creation of new, human life. It's probably their single most important function. There would be no new life crested without hormones, and they have to work together meticulously in a complex network to make sure egg and sperm cells are created but also so to ensure the meeting between egg and sperm happen.

This chapter dives into the fascinating world of reproductive hormones — a specific subgroup of sex hormones — and the wider reproductive ecosystem in the body, with a focus on understanding reproductive hormone cycles, the impact of birth control, and midlife hormonal changes. You will discover practical strategies for men and women to optimize their reproductive hormone health by syncing their lifestyle with their hormonal cycles and learn to recognize signs of reproductive health imbalances so you can seek support.

TIP

If you'd like to know more about the various stages of sex hormone transformation that help men and women evolve from children to reproductive years and then midlife, read Chapter 4.

Examining the Male Hormone Cycle

Unlike women, whose hormone cycle typically lasts an average of 28 days during their reproductive years, men experience a 24-hour hormonal cycle. The star of the show is testosterone, supported by other key reproductive hormones such as follicle-stimulating hormone (FSH), luteinizing hormone (LH), and gonadotropin-releasing hormone (GnRH), which regulate sperm production, maintain overall reproductive health and play crucial roles in regulating processes such as muscle mass, mood, libido, and energy levels.

This 24-hour cycle can be broken down into several key phases:

- **Morning surge:** Testosterone levels are highest in the early morning, often peaking around 8:00 a.m. This surge, driven by the combined action of LH stimulating testosterone production and GnRH regulating its release, contributes to morning energy, alertness, and libido. FSH also plays a role during this time by working with testosterone to support the continuous production of sperm and cortisol is released to help you feel awake and alert.
- **Midday decline:** As the day progresses, testosterone levels begin to decrease, resulting in a natural dip in energy and focus in the afternoon. The body continues to produce sperm, with FSH and LH maintaining their roles in supporting spermatogenesis (the process by which sperm cells are produced).
- **Evening low:** Testosterone levels are at their lowest in the evening, which can result in reduced energy and increased relaxation, but the hormonal regulation of sperm production continues in the background.
- **Nighttime replenishment:** During sleep, the body works to replenish and balance hormone levels, preparing for the next day's cycle. This is a critical period where GnRH triggers the release of FSH and LH, which in turn stimulate testosterone production and support ongoing sperm production, ensuring that the cycle begins anew each morning.

TIP

Understanding these fluctuations can help you optimize your daily routine, aligning high-demand activities such as exercise or important meetings with peak testosterone levels and allowing for rest and recovery when levels are naturally lower.

Normal symptoms versus causes for concern

If the hormonal rhythm outlined in the preceding section reflects how you're feeling and how you experience each day, that's an encouraging sign that your hormones are behaving as they should. But how do you identify when your hormones need some love? The following symptoms are things to look out for:

TIP

- **Persistent fatigue:** Constant tiredness that doesn't improve with rest could signal low testosterone levels or another underlying condition.
- **Afternoon energy crashes:** While a slight dip in energy during the afternoon can be part of a normal circadian rhythm, significant or regular crashes — especially if they interfere with daily activities — could be a sign of hormonal dysregulation. This may include issues such as blood sugar imbalances, insulin resistance, or disruptions in cortisol and testosterone levels.
- **Mood changes:** Chronic irritability, depression, anxiety, or quickness to anger can be linked to hormonal imbalances, particularly low testosterone or elevated cortisol levels due to prolonged stress.
- **Decreased libido:** A significant and persistent drop in sexual desire could be a sign of low testosterone or elevated cortisol or estrogen levels.
- **Physical changes:** Unexplained weight gain, muscle loss, or changes in body hair may warrant a hormone check.
- **Cognitive issues:** Problems with concentration, memory, or mental clarity (often referred to as brain fog) could be related to hormonal imbalances, particularly in cortisol and testosterone levels.

REMEMBER

The tools and lifestyle shifts provided in this book will certainly help your body find its way back to balance, but if you're concerned or struggling with symptoms that are affecting the quality of your life, please consult a healthcare provider for an evaluation. Remember, you're the only expert in you and what "normal" feels like in your body, so follow your instincts.

Wired for childcare

While men's hormones also change as they hit mid-life, interesting shifts also occur in men's testosterone levels when they enter long-term partnerships, such as marriage, and when they become fathers. This doesn't mean you suddenly lose your "masculinity" but adapt biologically to be a caretaker.

REMEMBER

High testosterone levels make men more attuned to sexual cues from women and increases their libido, which can obviously be counterproductive when you're trying to build a healthy long-term relationship and care for young children who are dependent on you for safety, love and care. Fortunately, nature has a way of adjusting for this. When men enter long-term relationships, their testosterone levels decrease slightly, and this decrease becomes more pronounced if they have young children.

This post-birth reduction in testosterone is accompanied by changes in other reproductive hormones, such increases in oxytocin, the cuddle hormone, and prolactin (known for its role in stimulating milk production in women), which influences paternal behavior in men, promoting nurturing instincts and bonding with their children. Together, these hormonal adjustments lower men's interest in pursuing new sexual opportunities and helps them focus on caretaking responsibilities. Hormone balance returns to pre-birth levels long before your child takes their first steps, but this shift helps you transition from being just a partner to also becoming a parent, benefiting everyone involved.

Andropause, the "male menopause"

"Male menopause" is a common term for andropause or androgen deficiency in the aging male (ADAM), an age-related reduction of testosterone in cisgender males. The term *andropause* comes from the Greek words *andras* (male) and *pause* (cessation), literally meaning the decline of male hormones. While men's hormonal transition is not nearly as abrupt as women's experience, testosterone starts decreasing 1 percent each year from the age of 30. Signs include fatigue, insomnia, mood changes, loss of muscle mass and hair, decreased sexual function or fertility, and alterations in mental health and personality.

REMEMBER

Decreasing testosterone levels in middle-aged men is a natural part of the aging process — one that has been occurring for thousands of years. This gradual decline may actually serve important biological and sociological purposes. For instance, lower testosterone levels are associated with a reduction in reckless and impulsive behaviors, which can be beneficial as men take on more responsibilities within their families and communities. This hormonal shift also fosters more cooperative and socially attuned behaviors, allowing older men to take on roles as mentors and knowledge bearers within their communities.

WARNING

It's estimated that only 1 in every 50 men who report suffering from andropause actually has a significant shortage of male hormones, which is why testosterone replacement therapy (TRT) is often not the most appropriate solution. Although TRT continues to gain popularity, it comes with potential risks, including mood swings, irritability, increased aggression, and disruptions to the balance of other reproductive hormones, such as luteinizing hormone (LH) and follicle-stimulating hormone (FSH), which play essential roles in regulating natural testosterone production and overall reproductive health.

TRT has also been associated with complications such as cardiovascular issues and sleep apnea. While older theories suggested that high testosterone levels might also increase the risk of prostate cancer, more recent studies indicate that lower testosterone levels are often associated with more aggressive tumors. Therefore, given the nuanced risks and benefits of TRT, it's essential to carefully weigh your options under the guidance of a healthcare professional, particularly if you're older.

TIP

The healthiest conclusion in the research is that the best approach to managing andropause is following a healthy lifestyle and the guidance provided in this book about nutrition, stress, trauma, and emotional management. Mother nature is fair and gives men the skills and advantages they need to make the most of each phase of life.

Examining the Female Hormone Cycle

If you menstruate, you'll have about 400 menstrual cycles over roughly 35 to 40 years of your life. (I know, it's a lot!) Sadly, most menstruators know distressingly little about how this amazing process really works, why it's important to pay attention to it, and how to interpret the messages your body sends through symptoms. People in your life who don't menstruate should also educate themselves because understanding this powerful cycle fosters empathy, improves communication, and helps them support you better during different phases.

REMEMBER

Before we dive in, it's important to understand that the world is designed for men's 24-hour hormone cycle, following the circadian rhythm. If you think about the structure of the modern work day, you'll notice that meetings usually take place in the morning when testosterone and cortisol levels are high, making men energetic, communicative, and laser-focused. In the afternoons, declining testosterone puts them in the mood to socialize and connect; this is when they want to pitch to clients, network or go on dates.

As Figure 12-1 shows, those with menstrual cycles don't operate like that at all, and this way of life makes it harder for women to access the full strengths and superpowers of their unique biology. The infradian rhythm cycle (read more in Chapter 2) lasts 26 to 35 days on average, and it has four very distinct phases, mirroring mother nature's pattern of moving through spring, summer, autumn, and winter.

REMEMBER

If you menstruate, your hormones, particularly estrogen, progesterone, and testosterone, are meant to ebb and flow. As you cycle through the menstruation (bleeding), follicular, ovulatory, and luteal (premenstrual) phases, your body is changing nearly every week — and sometimes every day! Just as each season has distinct characteristics, the hormonal shifts occurring in each phase of your cycle create different physical responses and emotions.

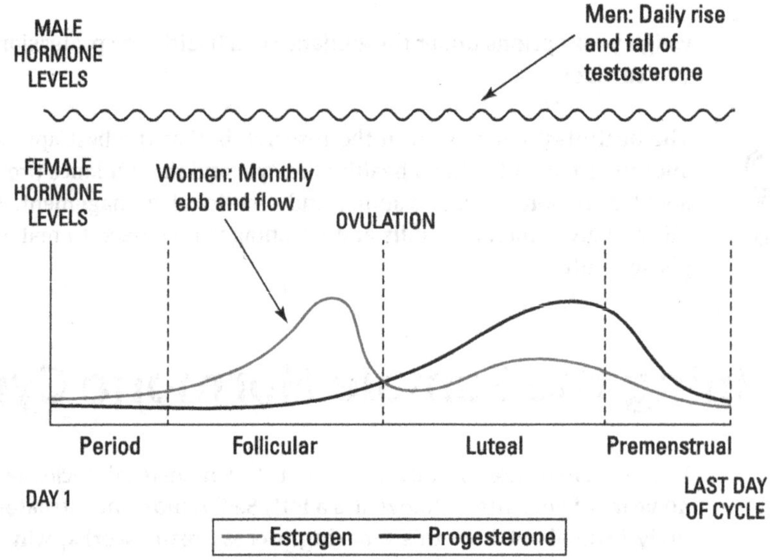

FIGURE 12-1: Male versus female hormone cycle.

TIP

So, if you don't feel like you're thriving the way you should be, or you're suffering from symptoms of hormone imbalances, then figuring out how to work with your cycle is going to be enormously supportive. But first, let's get to know the role of each of these phases:

- **Menstrual phase, inner winter** (3 to 7 days on average): This phase begins with the shedding of the uterine lining, known as the endometrium, which results in menstruation. During this time, estrogen and progesterone levels are at their lowest.
- **Follicular phase, inner spring** (7 to 10 days on average): During the follicular phase, the pituitary gland releases FSH, which signals the ovaries to begin producing multiple follicles. Each follicle contains an immature egg, but usually, only one becomes dominant and continues to mature. As this dominant follicle develops, it produces increasing levels of estrogen. The rising estrogen levels play a crucial role in thickening the endometrium, or the uterine lining, preparing it to potentially support a fertilized egg.
- **Ovulatory phase, inner summer** (days 14 to 16 on average): A surge in LH triggers ovulation, releasing the mature egg from the dominant follicle in the ovary. This egg then travels down the fallopian tube, where it may encounter sperm for fertilization. During this time, estrogen levels reach their peak, which has already helped the endometrium become thick and receptive. As ovulation occurs, progesterone levels start to rise, preparing the endometrium to further support a potential pregnancy by maintaining its thickness and ensuring a nutrient-rich environment.

- **Luteal phase, inner autumn** (days 17 to 28 on average): After ovulation, the empty follicle in the ovary transforms into the corpus luteum, which starts producing progesterone. This hormone plays a crucial role in preparing the endometrium, or uterine lining, to support a potential pregnancy by making it more stable and nutrient rich. If fertilization doesn't occur, the corpus luteum breaks down, leading to a sharp decline in both progesterone and estrogen levels. This drop in hormone levels signals the body that pregnancy hasn't occurred, resulting in the shedding of the endometrium, which leads to the start of menstruation. Then you move through the cycle again!

Normal symptoms versus causes for concern

Periods are such powerful indicators of your overall health that they're medically recognized as a sixth vital sign along with heart rate and blood pressure. Pretty cool, right? A recent study even linked irregular and long cycles with a shorter lifespan, showing how critical it is that you pay attention to your cycle and take care of your hormones. So, what does a healthy, normal menstrual cycle and period look like?

REMEMBER

Unfortunately it's not entirely straightforward because what's considered "normal" can vary due to various factors, but there are some basic guidelines for what's considered "typical" and what's cause for concern. Essentially, your cycle shouldn't disrupt the quality of your life. Any physical or emotional changes should all be very subtle.

A healthy cycle generally fits in these parameters:

- **Cycle length:** 26 to 35 days.
- **Period length:** Three to seven days.
- **Amount of bleeding:** No more than six pads or tampons per day.
- **Blood color:** It's normal for period blood color to vary, but if your period blood is very pale or light pink and watery, it could be a sign that you have low iron, which is worth having checked by a simple blood test.
- **Cervical mucus:** The week or so leading up to ovulation, cervical mucus or liquid becomes clear, watery, and stretchy and can look like egg whites.
- **Blood clots:** Occasional small clots, considered smaller than the size of a quarter in diameter, are normal. Larger clots or frequent or regular clotting with your periods can be a sign of hormone imbalance.

- **Pain:** Pain throughout your cycle shouldn't be more than occasional mild cramps. You shouldn't need pain medication, hot water bottles, or other comfort measures, but it's normal to sort of feel something going on in there.
- **Mood and PMS:** Any mild shifts in your mood or desire to socialize, your energy, sleep, and cravings are normal. However, they should not feel extreme, disruptive, or out of your control.

REMEMBER

Here are the symptoms that are cause for concern:

- **Long menstrual cycles:** Periods that occur 35 days or more apart.
- **Short menstrual cycles:** Periods that occur less than 25 days apart (meaning you have more frequent periods).
- **Skipped periods:** This is defined as missing more than three periods in a row. It's not uncommon to skip a period now and then due to stress, travel, or even a cold or nasty flu (and of course pregnancy), but skipping more than three periods in a row can signal that you're not ovulating; are experiencing PCOS, a thyroid problem, or hypothalamic amenorrhea, or be a sign of premature menopause.
- **Light periods:** Extremely scanty menstrual flow, or periods that last less than three days.
- **Bleeding between periods:** This can be due to uterine fibroids, cervical polyps, endometriosis, adenomyosis, or sexually transmitted infections (STIs) like chlamydia. If it persists throughout the month, it may also indicate a more serious issue, such as endometrial hyperplasia or even endometrial cancer. Postcoital bleeding (bleeding after sex) is a red flag and raises suspicion of cervical concerns, including cervical dysplasia or cervical cancer.
- **Period pain:** Your period should not make you spend days of the month on ibuprofen or other pain medication and should not make you cry because of the pain! If it does, there's likely more going on. While period pain is "normal" because it's so common, it's not "typical" or something you have to put up with.

The lesson here is that your menstrual symptoms, and bigger gynecologic concerns, are your body's way of sending direct messages. Communicating that something in your diet, environment, emotional world, mental well-being, or lifestyle is setting your ancient biological blueprint off track. If you don't listen to these messages, they just get louder and louder in the form of worsening symptoms or the onset of actual medical conditions that you're forced to pay attention to such as PCOS, infertility, thyroid issues, or endometriosis.

TIP

The mindset I invite you to adopt moving forward is that your menstrual cycles and ongoing gynecologic health gives you a monthly report card on how your diet, lifestyle, environment, happiness, level of stress, and emotions are affecting you. They are an opportunity every month to reflect and course correct with the tools provided in this book and if necessary, with the support of your healthcare team.

Pregnancy

During these fertile years, if her hormones are balanced, a woman ovulates approximately every 28 days, releasing an egg from the ovary. This egg, having developed within the protective confines of the ovary, makes its way to the fallopian tube, where it waits for sperm. Recent research from Stockholm University, Manchester University NHS Foundation Trust, and The University of Manchester reveals that as an egg slowly travels toward the uterus, it emits chemical signals to "choose" sperm. Sperm health and function are equally important in this process because they must respond effectively to these signals to ensure successful fertilization. (It takes two to create life!) If successful fertilization occurs, the egg and sperm merge, triggering the production of the pregnancy hormone human chorionic gonadotropin (hCG), which is essential for sustaining early pregnancy and signals the start of this transformative process.

REMEMBER

Progesterone has a very important role in this early stage. It needs to thicken the womb lining so that the fertilized egg can implant itself and grow there and also signal to the pituitary gland to decrease the production of LH and FSH to prevent multiple eggs from maturing. Low progesterone levels lead to reduced fertility in around one in seven women, including those who have PCOS and have a high number of follicles in the ovaries.

TIP

Women who deal with chronic stress, unresolved emotions, unresolved traumas (big *T* or little *t*; see Chapter 9), weight issues, or fears around pregnancy or motherhood or who don't feel safe or supported by their partner or support system may produce insufficient progesterone, increasing the risk of miscarriage. While progesterone supplements are an option, I've observed in my clients that naturally boosting progesterone levels by reducing cortisol (its precursor hormone) through emotional healing, cycle syncing, and dietary adjustments — as outlined in Part 4 of this book — can be highly effective. The first two months of pregnancy are the most critical; after that, the placenta takes over progesterone production.

Empowering Women to Cycle Sync

TIP

"Syncing" your life to your cycle and infradian rhythm is one of the most revolutionary and empowering biohacking tools available for women. *Biohacking* is the practice of making small, incremental changes to your lifestyle, diet, or environment to improve physical, mental, or emotional well-being. Sounds good, right? Living this way is the most effective way to nourish your two biological clocks and is the gateway to achieving peak feminine vitality. I've found with clients that it only takes two to three months of consistently and consciously considering what your brain and body are primed to do during each hormonal phase before syncing your life to your cycle becomes second nature.

TIP

Please note: If you're on synthetic contraceptives such as the pill, cycle syncing is a little different because you don't experience the ebb and flow of hormones I describe here, and the bleed you get isn't a real period. However, you still reap all the benefits of nutrition, engaging in different exercises, tuning into your body's signals, and bringing more intention to your life. It's a great idea to start cycle syncing before you transition off birth control, so the habits are second nature to you already.

Tracking your cycle

REMEMBER

Tracking your cycle is the essential first step. It helps you make informed decisions about your health, deepens your relationship with your body, and allows you to anticipate changes, manage symptoms, and optimize energy.

Tracking is also incredibly helpful when you're seeking support for hormone imbalances or planning for pregnancy. Tracking helps create a clear picture of your hormonal patterns, making it easier to identify any irregularities or trends that might indicate underlying issues. Whether you are dealing with PMS, irregular periods, or hormonal concerns or simply want to nurture your fertility, having this information at your fingertips allows a provider to pinpoint any potential root causes and recommend an effective treatment plan.

TIP

As you implement the cycle syncing tips I offer, you can use your tracking data to assess how these changes are impacting your cycle and overall well-being. Hormonal shifts don't happen overnight; they can take weeks or months to manifest noticeable changes. But by consistently recording your cycle details, you create a comprehensive log of your body's more subtle responses. This allows you to observe the shifts that might otherwise go unnoticed and keep you motivated to stay consistent with your new habits.

Follow these steps to track your cycle:

1. **Choose a tracking method.**

   Select an app (Clue, Flo, Moody, and Natural Cycles are highly recommended), a journal, or a calendar that you can keep easily accessible. You can also use a wearable device such as an Apple Watch or Oura Ring.

2. **Mark Day 1, which is** the first day of your period.

3. **Record daily (or as often as you can).**

   Keep track of the following things:

   - *Flow:* Track your menstrual flow when bleeding (light, medium, heavy) as well as the color of the blood (brown or bright red). If you have clots, note how frequent and big they were.
   - *Symptoms:* Note physical symptoms like cramps or bloating.
   - *Mood:* Log your emotional state (happy, irritable, and so on).
   - *Energy and sleep:* Track your energy levels and sleep quality.

4. **Monitor ovulation signs.**

   Track cervical mucus (clear, stretchy) and, optionally, basal body temperature (BBT) to confirm ovulation.

5. **Calculate cycle length.**

   Count the days from Day 1 of your period to the day before your next period starts. It's normal for your cycle length to vary by a day or two each month, but if you notice any significant changes or irregularities, it could be worth discussing with your healthcare provider.

6. **Use insights.**

   TIP

   Become your own cycle coach by tracking changes or improvements in your symptoms over time. For example, you might notice that you experienced more cramps during a month when your stress levels were high and you were sleeping less, perhaps due to a big work project. Use these insights to adjust your diet, exercise, lifestyle, schedule, self-care rituals, and emotional and nervous system work.

Syncing diet and lifestyle to maximize your cycle's superpowers

Whether you're looking to reduce hormone imbalance symptoms, boost your energy or productivity, enhance your workouts, or simply feel more in tune with

yourself, syncing with your cycle offers a holistic approach to living your best life, one phase at a time. See the cycle-specific shopping list I've provided on the *Hormone Balance For Dummies* cheat sheet at `www.dummies.com`.

WARNING

For women, the approach to intermittent fasting needs to be nuanced due to the cyclical nature of their hormones. Each phase of a woman's menstrual cycle requires different nutritional considerations, and strict intermittent fasting can disrupt hormone balance if not timed correctly. To find out more information on fasting for women, refer to Chapter 17.

Menstrual phase

While your energy levels may be lower, this phase offers an opportunity for introspection, self-care, and setting intentions for the month ahead. Here are some key ways to support yourself during this phase:

REMEMBER

- **Superpowers:** While you may feel withdrawn and less able to put up with other people's nonsense, this is a time for self-reflection to evaluate the last month of your life and check in on your thoughts, worries, and fears. What's going well, and where do things need to change? Solutions become clear in this phase, and your intuition and gut feelings are strong.
- **Food and nutrition support:** The process of shedding the endometrium (the lining of your uterus) is physically demanding on the body, so consuming nutrient-dense foods is crucial during this time. Foods that support the liver and kidneys are particularly beneficial, along with water-rich fruits, vegetables, and warming foods like bone broth and spices.
- **Body support:** You might experience fatigue, cramps, food cravings, no appetite, bloating, a lower back ache, headache, or migraine. Lean into your body's need for rest by hydrating properly, practicing yoga and stretching to promote circulation, walking rather than running, and doing gentle Pilates or foam rolling.

TIP

- **Lifestyle support:** Avoid big interviews or project launches if you can. This is the time to clear your calendar and prioritize rest, reflection, and rejuvenation. When your hormones kick back in, you can take action on all the solutions and clarity that came to you during this phase.

Follicular phase

With rising hormone levels, you'll feel your energy and motivation increase, making it the perfect phase for tackling challenges, connecting with others, and pursuing new opportunities. Here's how to make the most of this phase:

- **Superpowers:** As your hormones and energy ramp up, it's a great time to socialize, network, and try new or more challenging workouts. You'll have lots of motivation to get things done, and your creativity will be peaking, so try new things, brainstorm, and problem-solve. Tackle more mentally challenging tasks and initiate new projects at work or at home. This is an optimal time to put yourself out there in business and try new things in the bedroom.
- **Food and nutrition support:** You may be craving lighter foods, or you may want more robust meals. Honor what you're craving (using the blood sugar balancing tips in Part 3 of this book) and consume healthy carbohydrates such as legumes (it takes a lot of energy to ovulate), fatty fish, and protein.
- **Body support:** Enjoy your high energy levels and make the most of your workouts. This is the time when you can go for personal records or bests and life heavier weights!
- **Lifestyle support:** Connect with community (family, work, friends) and have important conversations to make the most of your heightened communication skills. This is a wonderful time to go on dates because those who naturally cycle usually feel naturally more attractive and confident during this phase!

TIP

Ovulatory phase

Your body is geared for connection and productivity during ovulation, making it a powerful phase for achieving goals, networking, going on dates and deepening relationships. Here's how to harness its strengths:

- **Superpowers:** This is your peak phase in terms of energy, confidence, and social interaction. Your communication skills are sharp, and you're likely to feel more outgoing, charismatic, and attractive (thanks, estrogen!). It's an ideal time for public speaking. Creativity is also heightened, so dive into projects that require innovative thinking.
- **Food and nutrition support:** This is a good time to focus on lighter, nutrient-dense foods. Consume plenty of vegetables and fruits, which are rich in fiber, to support your gut health and help your liver effectively metabolize and eliminate excess estrogen.
- **Body support:** Physically, you might feel your strongest and most resilient, making this a great time to push your limits in workouts or tackle high-intensity activities. However, be mindful of listening to your body's signals, especially if you experience any discomfort or pain during ovulation, when some women may feel slight twinges or cramps (known as mittelschmerz).

REMEMBER

TIP

» **Lifestyle support:** This is the optimal time to schedule important meetings, interviews, or social events. If you're in business, it's a great phase for launching projects or making key presentations or client pitches. Use this phase to make strides in both your personal and professional life.

Luteal phase

The luteal phase bridges the energy and productivity of ovulation with the restful introspection of menstruation, making it an ideal phase to focus on completing tasks and prioritizing self-care. Here's how to support yourself during this phase:

REMEMBER

» **Superpowers:** You may start with high energy levels, but as progesterone rises, you might feel the need for more rest and self-care. This is a great time for completing tasks, organizing, and preparing for the next cycle. Your attention to detail improves, making it an excellent phase for finishing projects and getting organized.

» **Food and nutrition support:** As your body prepares for the possibility of pregnancy, it's important to focus on nutrient-dense, grounding foods. Incorporate complex carbs like sweet potatoes, brown rice, and whole grains to sustain your energy levels. Magnesium-rich foods (like dark chocolate, leafy greens, and nuts) can help alleviate premenstrual syndrome (PMS) symptoms such as cramps, bloating, or mood swings. Continue to prioritize hydration and include foods that support digestion because bloating can be more common in this phase.

WARNING

» **Body support:** Begin with more intense workouts if you feel up to it; then when your energy dips as you move closer to your menstrual phase, you can transition to gentler exercises like yoga, Pilates, or walking. Pay attention to any signs of PMS and prioritize rest when your body calls for it. Pushing yourself in this phase is stressful on the body.

TIP

» **Lifestyle support:** This is a great time to focus on wrapping up projects, reflecting on what's been accomplished, and making plans for the next cycle. Consider clearing your schedule of high-stress or high-energy demands as you approach menstruation. Use this time for journaling and self-care rituals that help you transition smoothly into the next cycle.

Understanding the Impact of Birth Control on Your Hormones

The endocrine disruptor that may actually do the most harm is the one millions of women use to manipulate their hormones: synthetic (hormonal) birth control such as pills, patches, the vaginal ring, implants, intrauterine devices (IUDs), and injections. These are undoubtedly revolutionary developments that offer women unprecedented control over their reproductive health — protecting vulnerable populations, reducing the risk of unwanted pregnancies, and granting agency over their bodies in ways previous generations could only dream of. For many women, like me, hormonal contraception is not only a practical choice but a necessary one that provides life-changing relief for those with heavy or abnormal bleeding, endometriosis, or PCOS.

That said, while they can be supportive, they often serve as a quick fix for underlying root-cause issues that could be better addressed through diet and lifestyle changes. A more detailed and holistic investigation of these root causes should be undertaken by healthcare professionals before hormonal therapies are prescribed, ensuring that women receive the most appropriate and effective care for their individual needs.

WARNING

Informed consent means that your healthcare provider is supposed to give you information on the benefits and risks of options they recommend, as well as all the other existing options. Combined oral contraceptives, for example, are classified by the World Health Organization as Group 1 carcinogens for their possible relationship to liver cancer, in situ and invasive cervical cancer, and breast cancer. If you've been on synthetic hormone contraception before, did your doctor review these risks with you before handing you the prescription? And did you actually read that drug package insert? You can't achieve informed consent if you don't have the whole picture, and there is little doubt that, for many women (me included), the pill is the most pivotal prescription they'll ever fill.

REMEMBER

Although millions of women have been taking synthetic hormones daily for decades, we have embarrassingly little research on the range of effects that these hormonal contraceptives can have on women's bodies. The specific way that your body responds to hormonal contraception depends on a whole host of factors such as age, precontraception hormonal profile, general health, your brain's neurotransmitter profile, genetics, and probably lots of other things we don't know yet. Each of us is unique so what works for you might not work for your sister, coworker or best friend. That means if you're going to pursue hormonal contraceptive options, I encourage you to research, experiment and troubleshoot until you find the one that works the best for you. Ultimately, the only person who can decide whether the risks, side effects, or benefits of hormonal birth control are significant or meaningful to you is you. There are plenty of different hormonal or nonhormonal options available, and it's up to you to make choice that's best for you and your body.

Impact on the microbiome, immune system and metabolism

The side effects of synthetic birth control are wide-ranging, with research still in its early stages. These include potential changes such as shrinking of the clitoris (though evidence is limited), altering mate or partner selection on a genetic level (based on research into major histocompatibility complex (MHC) genes, which influence immune compatibility and mate preferences), and diminishing the benefits of the hormonal shifts associated with the menstrual cycle's different phases. In this section, I share what we know so far about the birth control and the brain, immune system, and metabolism.

Microbiome

REMEMBER

As explored in Chapter 10, your hormones are closely linked to the health and balance of your gut microbiome. The pill has been associated with various gut-related issues, including bloating, constipation, and IBS, all of which may indicate underlying gut dysfunction. However, research on the pill's direct impact on microbiome composition is still evolving; some studies show no change, whereas others suggest various effects on gut health.

TIP

Additionally, oral contraceptives have been linked to lower levels of essential nutrients such as vitamins B6, B12, and C, zinc, selenium, magnesium, and folate. These vitamins and minerals are crucial for many bodily functions, including energy metabolism, immune support, and mood regulation. It's imperative that you to monitor your nutritional intake and support gut health while using oral contraceptives to mitigate potential deficiencies and reduce the risk of more significant hormonal imbalances, if and when you decide to discontinue their use.

Immune system

Synthetic hormones have been shown in some research to affect your immune system and put you at risk of autoimmune diseases such as systemic lupus erythematosus (SLE), multiple sclerosis (MS), and rheumatoid arthritis (RA). Nearly 80 percent of people with autoimmune diseases are women, a disparity often attributed to the effects of estrogen on immune regulation. A 2019 study suggested that oral contraceptive use and hormone replacement therapies (HRT) used during menopause might increase the risk of autoimmune diseases, particularly SLE, in certain populations.

The exact mechanisms behind this relationship remain complex and are not yet fully understood. While the causative role of synthetic hormones in autoimmune disease development is still under investigation, their potential to influence immune function warrants careful consideration, especially in women with existing autoimmune conditions or those at higher risk.

Metabolism

While studies are mixed on whether synthetic birth control directly causes weight gain, according to Dr. Mary Pritchard, low-dose estrogen may increase ghrelin levels, potentially boosting appetite, and contribute to fluid retention. Evidence on changes to muscle mass is also conflicting, with some studies suggesting oral estrogen may reduce muscle gains in younger women and others showing neutral or positive effects. In aging women, HRT appears beneficial, helping preserve muscle mass and slow age-related loss. While these effects are complex and vary among individuals, it's clear that factors such as hormone levels, exercise, and nutrition all play vital roles in supporting a thriving metabolism and achieving fitness or weight goals.

Impact on brain, mental health, and the stress response

These hormones affect billions of cells in the body simultaneously, with their specific effects varying from person to person. This section is designed to help you better understand these impacts, explore your options, and navigate the often confusing process of trial and error to find what works best for you.

WARNING

It's important to note that while research on the effects of oral contraceptives on the brain is persuasive, the evidence remains modest, and many findings still require replication. Additionally, the mechanisms by which synthetic hormones influence brain function, mental health, and the stress response are not yet fully understood and need further investigation. As with much of women's health, there are significant gaps in research, but understanding the existing evidence can empower you to make informed decisions.

Brain

One review of scientific literature in 2014 showed that taking the pill is associated with changes in the brain's structure, neurochemistry, function, and mood modulation. The structural changes, which appear in brain's regions associated with emotion, get more pronounced the longer you take the pill and may not be reversable. Convincing findings from a large Danish study in 2016, which analyzed data from more than a million women, concluded the use of hormonal contraception, especially among adolescents, was associated with depression requiring antidepressant treatment. Since then, studies continue to associate the use of synthetic birth control, particularly the pill, with a poorer ability to regulate emotion and a higher risk of developing mental illness.

Mental health and stress response

One of the ways that scientists measure stress in the body is by registering the release of cortisol. In a nutshell, if cortisol was released, we know that person experienced stress or something meaningful happened. If cortisol wasn't released, we can assume they weren't stressed and nothing of consequence took place. Remember, stress isn't all bad: Stress responses are measured when we get exciting news like a job offer, have sex, or open presents on our birthday!

While too much stress is certainly bad, too little stress is also bad. Taking all those factors into consideration then, stress is never going to be something we want to completely eliminate, but it's certainly a response we want to experience when appropriate (such as real emergencies or when you're feeling sexually attracted to your partner) and in moderate doses.

So what does all of this have to do with birth control?

REMEMBER

Well, for nearly three decades, research has consistently shown that women on synthetic birth control, particularly the pill, exhibit altered cortisol responses to stress. Women taking the pill tend to have higher-than-average levels of total cortisol, elevated corticosteroid binding globulins (CBGs), and abnormal responses to externally administered cortisol. These findings are concerning because these types of patterns are usually observed when the body is overwhelmed by cortisol signalling, resulting in it shutting down the cortisol response entirely to protect the body from damage.

REMEMBER

Awareness of these effects at both a patient and provider level is vital. If dysregulated cortisol signalling can contribute to depression and anxiety, impaired learning, difficulty processing negative emotions, memory problems related to emotionally charged events, and metabolic disorders like obesity and insulin resistance, women and their healthcare teams need to know.

When you look at the impact these options can have on your endocrine system, it makes you wonder whether they're worth it. My point here is that although we don't yet fully understand the specific impact of the pill or other synthetic contraceptives (because dedicated research still in the early phases) it's important for you to become an expert on you and what works or feels good.

Natural birth control options

TIP

For those seeking contraception without hormonal disruption, nonhormonal options include barrier methods (condoms, diaphragms, cervical caps), fertility awareness methods (FAM), and copper IUDs. These options preserve the body's natural hormonal balance, maintain the microbiota, and avoid impacts on the HPA axis or cortisol levels.

WARNING

However, barrier methods require consistent use and have higher failure rates, particularly in vulnerable groups. FAM also depends heavily on being dedicated and consistent with monitoring, and it may not suit everyone. Copper IUDs, while effective and hormone-free, can increase blood loss and worsen period pain for some women, so weigh up your lifestyle, preferences, experiment and choose a method that best fits your needs.

Understanding Perimenopause and Menopause

REMEMBER

Modern life has significantly transformed women's experience of menopause. In the past, women often married and had children at a younger age and faced limited employment opportunities. By the time they approached perimenopause and menopause ("the change") their lives were generally less stressful, busy, and demanding than they are today. Now, many women are reaching the peak of their careers while also raising young children or caring for aging parents, all while navigating the physical and emotional challenges of this transition. (I know, exhausting!) A study published in October 2023 in the *Journal of Women's Health* reported that 37 percent of menopausal women said they felt shame related to their menopause symptoms, and 83 percent reported feeling stigma associated with symptoms. This combination of high responsibility, shame, low support, and hormonal shifts is making the menopause experience more complex than ever.

TIP

However, you also get to choose whether this transition becomes the ultimate portal for your personal growth and transformation. How? Well, one crucial aspect of managing this transition successfully is the importance of reducing — you guessed it — cortisol and insulin levels. Elevated cortisol and blood sugar roller coasters exacerbate menopause symptoms, making it essential to prioritize stress reduction, nervous system work, emotional release, and trauma healing during this time.

As I explain to my clients, the menopause transition is a powerful period for reclaiming personal power and setting boundaries. Learning to say *no*, doing more of what lights you up, and protecting your time, cortisol levels, and energy are vital steps I walk you through in Part 4. As you navigate this phase, it's important to recognize your worth and make choices that support a balanced, fulfilling life. There are also amazing advances in hormone replacement therapies that are revolutionizing care.

Demystifying the midlife changes

Perimenopause, the transitional phase leading up to menopause, is characterized by significant hormonal fluctuations and usually begins in a woman's 40s, although it can start earlier or later. During perimenopause, the levels of key sex and reproductive hormones — estrogen, progesterone, LH, and FSH — begin to change. The ovaries become less responsive to LH and FSH, leading to irregularities in the menstrual cycle and a gradual decline in the production of estrogen and progesterone.

REMEMBER

Menopause, which is defined as the point when a woman has gone 12 consecutive months without a menstrual period, marks the end of this transition. At this stage, the ovaries have significantly reduced their production of estrogen and progesterone, and LH and FSH levels remain elevated but ineffective in stimulating the ovaries. These hormonal shifts not only signify the end of a woman's reproductive years but also have broader implications for overall health, affecting bone density, cardiovascular health, and emotional well-being.

Normal symptoms versus cause for concern

REMEMBER

Menopause affects every woman differently, with symptoms varying not only from person to person but also across different ethnic groups. Recent studies highlight these differences, showing that Asian women, for example, are more likely to report body and joint aches as their most troublesome symptoms during menopause. In contrast, women of Afro-Caribbean origin tend to experience menopause earlier, with an average onset at 49.6 years compared to the overall average of 51 years. These women also undergo a longer menopausal transition and are more prone to severe and intense hot flashes and night sweats compared to women of other ethnicities.

These findings emphasize the importance of personalized approaches to managing menopause. Tailoring treatment and support to individual needs can significantly improve the quality of life during this transition and your experience of common symptoms such as the following:

- **Hot flashes/night sweats:** Common in up to 75 percent of women, triggered by fluctuating estrogen.
- **Irregular periods:** Signalling the ending of your reproductive cycle.
- **Sleep disturbances:** Often one of the earliest signs of entering perimenopause.
- **Mild mood changes:** Estrogen's decline affects serotonin levels.
- **Vaginal dryness:** Thinner, less lubricated vaginal tissues.

WARNING

Be aware of the following issues, which are causes for concern:

- **Excessive bleeding:** Very heavy, prolonged, or irregular bleeding may signal issues like fibroids or endometrial hyperplasia. Consult a doctor.
- **Post-menopausal bleeding:** Any vaginal bleeding occurring more than 12 months after your last menstrual period is always a red flag and should be evaluated promptly by a healthcare professional, as it may signal more serious concerns such as endometrial cancer.
- **Severe mood changes:** Persistent depression, anxiety, or irritability impacting daily life needs medical attention.
- **Bone loss:** Rapid bone density loss raises the risk of osteoporosis. Seek advice to manage and prevent fractures.
- **Heart health:** Declining estrogen increases cardiovascular risks. If you experience chest pain, shortness of breath, or unexplained fatigue, see a healthcare provider.

IN THIS CHAPTER

» Identifying if and when your hormones need some care

» Finding professional support for hormonal issues

Chapter 13

Preventing the Long-term Risks of Imbalance

In 1736, Benjamin Franklin famously emphasized the importance of prevention to fire-threatened Philadelphians, declaring that "an ounce of prevention is worth a pound of cure." Similarly, there's an ancient Chinese proverb that says ordinary doctors treat illness, whereas the best physicians focus on prevention.

While the concept of prevention is certainty not new, there's never been a more important time to prioritize it. Historically, Western healthcare has excelled in curative medicine, helping to treat and manage diseases. However, this focus has led to preventable or manageable conditions becoming more prevalent.

While existing preventive strategies — such as vaccination programs, routine screenings, and advances in sanitation — have significantly improved public health, modern life is presenting new challenges. The increasing complexity of hormonal imbalances, coupled with the strain on healthcare systems globally as populations live longer than ever before, makes it more important than ever to take personal responsibility for your health.

At its core, prevention is simply self-care on a deeper level. It's about giving yourself the attention and care you deserve before symptoms or issues arise. By taking proactive, preventative action, you're not just reacting to problems; you're nourishing and supporting your body every day to keep it in optimal condition. Think of it as investing in yourself, ensuring that your health is maintained in the same way you'd service a car before it breaks down. There's no need to wait for your body to signal that something is wrong before you start caring for it!

So, in this chapter, I familiarize you with signs and symptoms of hormone imbalance and disease, and then I take a deeper dive into the range of professional support available. Navigating healthcare systems and advocating for yourself isn't always easy, so I also provide strategies to effectively communicate your needs and ensure you receive the care you deserve.

Detecting Whether Your Hormones Need Attention

TIP

You are the only expert in you. Although medical tests and professional opinions are always valuable tools, please remember that no one knows your body better than you do. A key part of managing your hormone health is tracking your symptoms and regularly assessing how you feel each day, so please pay attention to patterns: energy fluctuations, mood swings, changes in sleep, digestion, or your menstrual cycle. These changes can often be early indicators that your hormones need care and attention.

As I discuss more in Chapter 14, blood tests are commonly used to assess hormone levels, but it's important to recognize that the reference ranges are typically based on population averages, which are not necessarily healthy. Just because your results fall within the "normal" range doesn't mean your body is functioning optimally for you. Additionally, hormones such as cortisol, estrogen, and testosterone pulse at different times throughout the day, meaning that a single blood test might not always give an accurate picture of what's really going on. Because of these natural pulses, relying solely on a one-time blood test could provide misleading or confusing results. So, if something feels off, honor that feeling and act (make the appropriate diet and lifestyle tweaks), even if your test results appear fine.

REMEMBER

Ultimately, true hormone balance is not based on numbers on a chart but in how you feel in your body. Balancing testing with self-awareness and symptom tracking is what enables you to take a more personalized, proactive approach to your health. And if you find yourself identifying with many of the symptoms discussed throughout this book, get excited! You now have the information and motivation you need to take action and begin implementing a root-cause prevention approach outlined in Chapters 16 and 17.

In the following sections, I outline key indicators of hormone disruption and imbalance, including chronic inflammation, common symptoms of imbalance, and the hallmark signs of hormone-related diseases. So, grab a notebook and jot down any symptoms that resonate with your experience to help you address them effectively in the coming chapters.

Chronic inflammation

WARNING

Chronic inflammation is both a symptom and a root-cause trigger for hormone imbalances and disease, which makes it crucial to recognize and address. Unlike *acute inflammation* — your body's natural and short-term protective response to injury or infection — *chronic inflammation* is a persistent, ongoing state that can last for months or even years. This prolonged inflammatory response not only signals an existing problem but also actively contributes to further hormone disruption and tissue damage, ultimately triggering or exacerbating conditions like heart disease; type 2 diabetes; autoimmune disorders such as Hashimoto's disease, rheumatoid arthritis, and lupus; and even cancer. It also worsens hormone-related conditions such as endometriosis and PCOS.

TIP

Recognizing chronic inflammation can be difficult because its symptoms are often subtle or can be mistaken for other issues. Common signs include persistent fatigue; frequent infections or slow recovery from illnesses; digestive problems such as bloating, gas, or constipation; joint pain or muscle aches; skin issues such as rashes, acne, or eczema; unexplained weight gain or difficulty losing weight; brain fog; and elevated blood sugar or insulin resistance. While it can sometimes be detected through blood markers, such as C-reactive protein (CRP), these markers may not always be elevated in people experiencing milder or nonspecific symptoms. Additionally, testing cytokines is not common in routine primary care; it's typically reserved for specific cases. Regardless of test results, adopting a low-inflammatory lifestyle is essential for supporting overall health and preventing long-term damage. This includes managing stress, consuming a nutrient-dense diet free from processed foods, and engaging in regular exercise. Everyone should be concerned about managing inflammation.

Signs and symptoms of imbalance

REMEMBER

This section covers the most common signs and symptoms of hormonal imbalance, focusing on key tier 1 players, the tier 3 thyroid hormones, and the reproductive hormones for both men and women (to learn how the hierarchy works, refer to Chapter 3). Remember, your endocrine system is highly interconnected, meaning you may experience symptoms across multiple hormones, which is why managing tier 1 of your hormonal hierarchy along with root-cause drivers such as inflammation and poor gut health is so effective.

REMEMBER

Hormonal imbalances can manifest in a variety of symptoms across different body systems. While the following lists aim to cover the most frequently encountered symptoms, they are not exhaustive. The purpose of these lists is to help you identify common patterns associated with specific hormones, as well as general symptoms of imbalance.

While some symptoms may indicate the need for medical testing, others serve as helpful markers for self-reflection. Not all symptoms require medical investigation, and routine hormone testing may not always detect imbalances, especially for hormones such as oxytocin or dopamine that influence your mood and behavior.

REMEMBER

It's important to note that symptoms linked to disease (covered later in this chapter in the "Signs and symptoms of disease" section) rather than general imbalances tend to be more serious and often signal underlying health conditions that may require prompt professional attention. In the following chapters, you'll find practical strategies to balance your endocrine system as a whole, rather than focusing on individual hormones. For more specific testing recommendations, refer to my detailed guidance in Chapter 14.

Tier 1 insulin: Mismanaged blood sugar and insulin levels

Many people may experience a combination of high and low blood sugar symptoms due to metabolic dysfunction, poor glycemic control, or prediabetes. Rapid fluctuations between high sugar spikes and low troughs can trigger a range of symptoms from both lists, reflecting the body's struggle to maintain stable blood sugar levels. To learn more about managing your blood sugar, refer to Chapters 16 and 17.

SIGNS OF HIGH BLOOD SUGAR (HYPERGLYCEMIA)

The following symptoms may indicated hyperglycemia:

- ☐ Trying to lose weight but finding that it just won't shift
- ☐ Having unexplained weight loss despite eating normally or more food than usual
- ☐ Feeling more fatigued than usual, even after a good night's sleep
- ☐ Feeling unusually thirsty throughout the day
- ☐ Needing to urinate more than usual, especially at night
- ☐ Experiencing blurry or cloudy vision

- ❑ Suffering from skin conditions like inflammation, acne, or slow-healing wounds
- ❑ Experiencing mood disorders, anxiety, or depression
- ❑ Frequently getting colds, flus, or yeast infections
- ❑ Feeling extreme hunger pangs
- ❑ Experiencing mid-morning and mid-afternoon energy slumps or feeling sleepy throughout the day
- ❑ Needing caffeine to boost your energy levels throughout the day
- ❑ Having insulin resistance, prediabetes, or type 2 diabetes
- ❑ Having heart disease or high blood pressure
- ❑ Having non-alcoholic fatty liver disease (NAFLD)
- ❑ Being told by a doctor that you need to lose some weight

SIGNS OF LOW BLOOD SUGAR (HYPOGLYCEMIA)

The symptoms of hypoglycemia include the following:

- ❑ Feeling shaky or jittery, especially if you haven't eaten for a while
- ❑ Experiencing sudden dizziness or lightheadedness, especially when meals are delayed
- ❑ Getting irritable or anxious more easily, particularly when you're hungry
- ❑ Needing to eat every few hours to maintain your energy
- ❑ Feeling confused or have difficulty focusing, especially when hungry
- ❑ Experiencing sudden cravings for sugary foods or drinks
- ❑ Having trouble sleeping or wake up with heart palpitations
- ❑ Experiencing energy crashes where you feel nauseous or sweaty
- ❑ Sweating excessively, even when you're neither exercising nor in a hot environment
- ❑ Noticing frequent headaches or difficulty concentrating
- ❑ Experiencing rapid mood swings or feelings of irritability

Tier 1 cortisol: Primary stress hormone

Chronic stress and irregular cortisol patterns often cause overlapping signs, reflecting the body's ongoing response to prolonged stress. These symptoms can manifest physically, mentally, and emotionally, and may feel confusing or contradictory. However, the key takeaway is the importance of addressing underlying stress, emotional resilience, and trauma healing (all outlined in this book) to restore balance and support overall health.

HIGH CORTISOL SYMPTOMS (CHRONIC STRESS OR OVERACTIVITY)

Do you struggle with any of the following issues?

- ❑ Having difficulty relaxing and finding it hard to unwind, even during downtime
- ❑ Having trouble falling or staying asleep, especially waking up between 2:00 and 4:00 a.m.
- ❑ Gaining weight, especially around the abdomen
- ❑ Experiencing digestive issues such as bloating, indigestion, or IBS-like symptoms
- ❑ Having high blood pressure
- ❑ Suffering from frequent colds or infections (due to weakened immune function)
- ❑ Feeling fatigued despite rest
- ❑ Being tired all day but wired at night
- ❑ Experiencing headaches or tension in the neck and shoulders
- ❑ Suffering from jaw, neck, or back pain
- ❑ Having tightness in the hips
- ❑ Feeling anxious or irritable
- ❑ Craving sugar and salt
- ❑ Being emotionally reactive
- ❑ Experiencing low libido
- ❑ Having brain fog or difficulty concentrating

Low cortisol symptoms (burnout or adrenal fatigue) can look like this:

- ❑ Feeling constant fatigue
- ❑ Having low motivation, drive, or energy to complete daily tasks
- ❑ Experiencing depression or flat mood or feeling disconnected
- ❑ Craving salt
- ❑ Having low blood pressure and feeling lightheaded or dizzy, especially when standing
- ❑ Experience frequent energy crashes
- ❑ Noticing unexplained weight loss
- ❑ Having a low tolerance for stress and being easily overwhelmed by situations that previously seemed manageable
- ❑ Experiencing muscle weakness or joint pain
- ❑ Having dark circles under the eyes

Behavioral coping patterns linked to cortisol dysregulation include

- ❑ Overworking or burnout
- ❑ Overexercising to manage stress
- ❑ Avoiding tasks or procrastinating
- ❑ Eating because of emotion, especially sugary or salty snacks
- ❑ Participating in numbing behaviors such as using alcohol or drug use, overworking, engaging in long social media scrolling, or TV binge-watching sessions
- ❑ Constantly feeling on edge or in a heightened state of alertness, which is known as hypervigilance
- ❑ Trying to be perfect and feeling like nothing is ever good enough
- ❑ Demonstrating people-pleasing behaviors, difficulty saying no, and putting others' needs ahead of your own, often to your detriment
- ❑ Being a "control freak" because of an overwhelming need to control situations or outcomes, leading to difficulty delegating tasks or accepting uncertainty

Tier 1 dopamine: The reward and pleasure hormone

REMEMBER

Balanced dopamine levels are crucial for overall well-being. High dopamine levels are often the result of activities or substances that overstimulate the brain's reward pathways — such as excessive social media use. Low dopamine levels are typically caused by a combination of lifestyle factors, mental health challenges, or neurochemical imbalances. Depression, anxiety, and ADHD are also commonly associated with low dopamine levels.

Signs of low dopamine include

- [ ] Feeling unmotivated or unenthusiastic
- [ ] Feeling fatigue or sluggish
- [ ] Difficulty focusing or concentrating (brain fog)
- [ ] Feeling apathetic or indifferent
- [ ] Experiencing low libido or sexual dysfunction
- [ ] Craving sugar or stimulants such as caffeine or nicotine
- [ ] Feeling emotionally flat or disconnected
- [ ] Procrastinating or avoiding tasks
- [ ] Increasingly using social media, mindless scrolling, or TV bingeing to fill a motivational void
- [ ] Experiencing an increased risk of addiction (for example, to food, social media, gambling)

Signs of high dopamine include

- [ ] Feeling excessively excited or impulsive
- [ ] Engaging in risk-taking behaviors
- [ ] Being anxious or restless
- [ ] Having difficulty sleeping (insomnia)
- [ ] Being overstimulated or easily overwhelmed
- [ ] Having heightened sensitivity to rewards, which leads to addictive behaviors like compulsive social media scrolling or binge-watching TV shows
- [ ] Feeling aggressive or having an irritable mood

Tier 1 oxytocin: The love and bonding hormone

REMEMBER

Oxytocin is considered a tier 1 hormone because it plays a critical role in regulating cortisol levels. While we often associate high oxytocin with positive feelings of love and connection, excessive levels can sometimes lead to emotional overdependence or challenges with setting healthy boundaries. Low oxytocin, on the other hand, can result from lifestyle factors such as poor diet, chronic stress, unresolved trauma, and existing hormone imbalances.

Signs of low oxytocin can include the following:

- ❑ Difficulty forming or maintaining close relationships
- ❑ Loneliness or social isolation
- ❑ Reduced empathy or emotional connection with others
- ❑ Difficulty trusting people
- ❑ Increased feelings of stress or anxiety in social situations
- ❑ Lack of emotional intimacy or difficulty connecting with a partner
- ❑ Postpartum depression (in new mothers)
- ❑ Reduced sexual satisfaction or interest

Signs of high oxytocin may look like this:

- ❑ Excessive attachment or dependence on others
- ❑ Overly trusting or failing to recognize unhealthy relationships
- ❑ Intense feelings of emotional closeness, even with strangers
- ❑ Heightened sensitivity to social rejection or conflict

Tier 3 thyroid hormones

Because these symptoms often overlap with other conditions, identifying a thyroid issue can be challenging. To understand if your thyroid might be contributing to your symptoms, refer to Chapter 14, where I outline helpful thyroid tests and how to interpret them.

Low levels of thyroid hormones (hypothyroidism) can show up with these symptoms:

- ❑ Fatigue or low energy

- ☐ Weight gain or difficulty losing weight
- ☐ Sensitivity to cold
- ☐ Dry skin, hair loss, or brittle nails
- ☐ Constipation
- ☐ Depression or low mood
- ☐ Brain fog or difficulty concentrating
- ☐ Slow heart rate
- ☐ Menstrual irregularities or heavy periods
- ☐ Muscle weakness or joint pain

Signs of high thyroid hormones (hyperthyroidism) can include the following:

- ☐ Unexplained weight loss despite increased appetite
- ☐ Nervousness, anxiety, or irritability
- ☐ Rapid heartbeat (tachycardia) or heart palpitations
- ☐ Heat intolerance or excessive sweating
- ☐ Tremors or shaking hands
- ☐ Difficulty sleeping (insomnia)
- ☐ Diarrhea or frequent bowel movements
- ☐ Thinning hair or hair loss
- ☐ Irregular or light menstrual periods
- ☐ Bulging eyes (in cases of Graves' disease)

Tier 3 reproductive hormones: Women

REMEMBER

The adolescent, reproductive, perimenopause, and menopause years often bring significant hormonal fluctuations as the body adapts to new physiological rhythms, and reproductive imbalances can present with a wide range of symptoms. For a more in-depth exploration of these transitional phases, refer to Chapters 4 and 12.

Common signs of reproductive hormone imbalance include

- ☐ Irregular or missed periods
- ☐ Painful or heavy periods

- ❑ PMS symptoms like mood swings, bloating, or cramps
- ❑ Premenstrual dysphoric disorder (PMDD), which is a severe form of PMS characterized by extreme mood changes, depression, and anxiety
- ❑ PCOS symptoms like facial hair growth, acne, or weight gain
- ❑ Endometriosis
- ❑ Fibroids
- ❑ Infertility or difficulty conceiving
- ❑ Low libido or sexual dysfunction
- ❑ Vaginal dryness or discomfort during sex
- ❑ Hot flashes and night sweats (primarily associated with perimenopause and menopause)
- ❑ Breast tenderness, the development of lumps or cysts, nipple sensitivity, breast swelling or heaviness
- ❑ Mood swings, irritability, or anxiety
- ❑ Fatigue or low energy
- ❑ Weight gain, particularly around the abdomen (primarily associated with perimenopause and menopause)
- ❑ Acne — often along the jawline or chin
- ❑ Hair thinning or hair loss, often associated with hormonal imbalances like elevated testosterone or thyroid dysfunction
- ❑ Sleep disturbances or insomnia, often linked to fluctuations in estrogen and progesterone
- ❑ Chronic bloating or digestive issues, sometimes linked to hormone-driven water retention
- ❑ Depression or persistent low mood, particularly around the menstrual cycle or during hormonal transitions
- ❑ Thinning of vaginal walls or loss of elasticity (typically associated with menopause and estrogen deficiency)

Tier 3 reproductive hormones: Men

TIP

For a more in-depth exploration of male hormonal transitional phases such as adolescence and andropause, refer to Chapters 4 and 12.

Common signs of reproductive hormone imbalance include

- ❑ Reduced sex drive or difficulties with erectile function
- ❑ Mood swings, irritability, or anxiety
- ❑ Depression or persistent low mood
- ❑ Loss of muscle mass or strength following a regular, multiple-day-a-week exercise regimen
- ❑ Increased body fat, particularly around the abdomen
- ❑ Hair thinning or hair loss
- ❑ Decreased bone density or increased risk of fractures
- ❑ Sleep disturbances or insomnia
- ❑ Sweating or hot flashes (as testosterone levels drop)
- ❑ Cognitive difficulties, such as difficulty concentrating or memory issues, often referred to as "brain fog"
- ❑ Infertility or reduced sperm count
- ❑ Gynecomastia (enlarged breast tissue)
- ❑ Frequent fatigue or energy crashes
- ❑ Reduced endurance or performance during exercise
- ❑ Sleep apnea, sometimes associated with hormonal changes
- ❑ Difficulty achieving or maintaining an erection
- ❑ Testicular atrophy (shrinking of the testicles)

Signs and symptoms of disease

REMEMBER

Recognizing the early signs and symptoms of hormone-related diseases is vital so that you can act before conditions worsen. Some symptoms may be mild or overlap with other imbalances, so it's best to seek professional help to prevent long-term health risks. Please also note that this section covers only the most common and prominent hormone-related diseases, not every possible condition.

Type 2 diabetes

Type 2 diabetes occurs when the body becomes resistant to insulin, or the pancreas doesn't produce enough insulin, leading to elevated blood sugar levels. Here are some symptoms:

» Frequent urination (polyuria)
- ❑ Excessive thirst (polydipsia)
- ❑ Increased hunger (polyphagia)
- ❑ Fatigue and low energy
- ❑ Blurred vision
- ❑ Slow wound healing
- ❑ Unexplained weight loss
- ❑ Numbness or tingling in hands or feet

Metabolic syndrome

Metabolic syndrome is a cluster of conditions that occur together, increasing the risk of heart disease, stroke, and type 2 diabetes. It's often linked to insulin resistance and high cortisol levels. The following symptoms may indicate the presence of metabolic syndrome:

- ❑ High blood pressure
- ❑ High blood sugar levels
- ❑ Excess abdominal fat (apple-shaped body)
- ❑ High triglyceride levels
- ❑ Low HDL cholesterol levels
- ❑ Fatigue, especially after eating high-carb meals
- ❑ Increased risk of heart disease and diabetes

Polycystic ovary syndrome

PCOS involves elevated levels of androgens (male hormones) and insulin resistance in women. There are four different types of PCOS, which you can find outlined in Chapter 6. Here are some symptoms:

- ❑ Irregular or absent menstrual periods
- ❑ Excessive facial or body hair (hirsutism)
- ❑ Acne or oily skin
- ❑ Weight gain or difficulty losing weight

- ❑ Thinning hair or male-pattern baldness
- ❑ Ovarian cysts
- ❑ Infertility or difficulty conceiving

Hypothyroidism

The thyroid gland is unable to produce sufficient levels of the hormones T3 and T4, leading to a slowdown in the body's metabolic processes. These symptoms can indicate hypothyroidism:

- ❑ Fatigue or constant tiredness
- ❑ Weight gain or difficulty losing weight
- ❑ Sensitivity to cold
- ❑ Dry skin, brittle nails, or hair loss
- ❑ Constipation
- ❑ Depression or low mood
- ❑ Slow heart rate
- ❑ Heavy or irregular periods

Hyperthyroidism

If the thyroid gland goes into overdrive, it produces too much T3 and T4. The leading cause of hyperthyroidism is Graves' disease, an autoimmune disorder that accounts for 70 to 80 percent of cases. Symptoms include these:

- ❑ Unexplained weight loss despite increased appetite
- ❑ Nervousness, anxiety, or irritability
- ❑ Rapid or irregular heartbeat (tachycardia)
- ❑ Heat intolerance or excessive sweating
- ❑ Tremors in the hands
- ❑ Difficulty sleeping
- ❑ Diarrhea or frequent bowel movements
- ❑ Thinning hair

Adrenal fatigue/insufficiency (Addison's disease)

Chronic stress can lead to reduced and insufficient cortisol production, commonly referred to as adrenal fatigue. Addison's disease, however, is a rare and more severe form of adrenal insufficiency that requires medical diagnosis and ongoing treatment. These symptoms may indicate adrenal fatigue:

- ☐ Chronic fatigue or low energy
- ☐ Muscle weakness
- ☐ Unexplained weight loss
- ☐ Low blood pressure or dizziness
- ☐ Salt cravings
- ☐ Darkening of the skin (in Addison's disease)
- ☐ Low blood sugar
- ☐ Mood swings, irritability, or depression

Cushing's syndrome

With Cushing's syndrome, the body is exposed to excessively high levels of cortisol for a prolonged period, either due to the use of corticosteroid medications or the presence of cortisol-producing tumors (often in the adrenal glands or the pituitary gland). People with Cushing's syndrome have the following symptoms:

- ☐ Weight gain, especially around the midsection, upper back, and face (moon face)
- ☐ Purple stretch marks on the abdomen
- ☐ Fatigue and muscle weakness
- ☐ High blood pressure
- ☐ Mood swings, anxiety, or depression
- ☐ Weak bones (osteoporosis) or fractures
- ☐ Thinning, fragile skin that bruises easily

Osteoporosis

Bones become weak and brittle due to a decrease in bone density that's often linked to hormonal imbalances, particularly low estrogen in women or low testosterone in men. Symptoms include

- ❑ Bone fractures from minor falls or injuries
- ❑ Loss of height over time
- ❑ Back pain from fractured or collapsed vertebrae
- ❑ A stooped posture (kyphosis)
- ❑ Weak or brittle bones

Infertility

Infertility is the inability to conceive after a year or more of regular unprotected intercourse, often due to hormonal imbalances affecting ovulation or sperm quality and production. In women, the symptoms can look like these:

- ❑ Difficulty conceiving after a year of trying
- ❑ Irregular or absent menstrual periods
- ❑ Painful periods or heavy bleeding
- ❑ PCOS symptoms such as excess body hair or acne

In men, symptoms include

- ❑ Low sperm count or motility
- ❑ Erectile dysfunction
- ❑ Low libido
- ❑ Testicular pain or swelling

Endometriosis

Tissue similar to the lining of the uterus grows I the uterus, often leading to pain and fertility issues. Symptoms associated with endometriosis include

- ❑ Severe menstrual cramps or pelvic pain
- ❑ Pain during or after sex
- ❑ Heavy menstrual periods or bleeding between periods
- ❑ Infertility or difficulty conceiving
- ❑ Painful bowel movements or urination, particularly during menstruation
- ❑ Fatigue, diarrhea, or constipation

Adenomyosis

Adenomyosis is often confused by with endometriosis, even by physicians, because both conditions share similar symptoms. However, adenomyosis occurs when tissue similar to the uterine lining grows into the muscular wall of the uterus. Distinguishing between the two typically requires medical imaging, such as an MRI or ultrasound, and sometimes additional tests or a biopsy to confirm the diagnosis. Here are the symptoms associated with adenomyosis:

- ☐ Severe menstrual cramps or chronic pelvic pain
- ☐ Heavy or prolonged menstrual periods
- ☐ Pain during intercourse
- ☐ Uterine enlargement or tenderness
- ☐ A feeling of pressure or bloating in the lower abdomen

Fibroids

Fibroids are noncancerous growths that develop in or around the uterus, often caused by imbalances in estrogen and progesterone. People with fibroids may experience the following symptoms:

- ☐ Heavy or prolonged menstrual bleeding
- ☐ Pelvic pain or pressure
- ☐ Frequent urination or difficulty emptying the bladder
- ☐ Constipation or bloating
- ☐ Pain during intercourse
- ☐ Lower back pain
- ☐ Infertility or recurrent miscarriages

Growth hormone deficiency

Growth hormone deficiency occurs when the pituitary gland doesn't produce enough growth hormone, impacting growth and metabolism. In adults, this condition is often due to pituitary damage from causes such as a pituitary tumour, surgery, or irradiation. It frequently appears alongside other symptoms of hypopituitarism, as multiple hormones may be affected by pituitary dysfunction.

Symptoms (in adults) include

- ❑ Decreased muscle mass and strength
- ❑ Increased body fat, particularly around the waist
- ❑ Fatigue or low energy
- ❑ Anxiety or depression
- ❑ Reduced bone density and increased risk of fractures
- ❑ Poor exercise tolerance

Symptoms (in children) include

- ❑ Slow growth rate (less than 2 inches per year after age 2)
- ❑ Short stature compared to peers
- ❑ Delayed puberty
- ❑ Increased body fat, especially around the abdomen
- ❑ Poor muscle development
- ❑ Immature facial appearance
- ❑ Low blood sugar (hypoglycemia)
- ❑ Delayed tooth development
- ❑ Fatigue or low stamina

Determining When to Seek Professional Help

TIP

Although most signs of imbalance can be managed or reversed completely through lifestyle and root-cause interventions, some situations exist where medical or functional expertise is necessary to prevent long-term complications. For example, if your symptoms are severe or persistent or suggest a more serious underlying condition is present, seeking help from a healthcare provider is critical for proper diagnosis and treatment. Even if professional support is needed, you should implement preventative and management diet and lifestyle strategies.

Joining the prevention revolution

REMEMBER

By joining the prevention revolution, you're making a choice to stop reacting to problems as they pop up and start preventing or proactively managing them instead. The reality is that hormonal imbalances and disease don't happen overnight. They're the result of years of decisions, environmental exposures and habits that either support or undermine your long-term health. By prioritizing prevention, you're not only working toward reducing your chance of disease but also the creation of a long, happy, and healthy life.

Epigenetics is an area of promise in the world of prevention, as advancements reveal how lifestyle factors — such as diet, toxins, trauma, and stress — can impact gene expression without altering DNA itself. This means our daily choices can influence which genes are turned "on" or "off," affecting long-term health. In the future, healthcare may use epigenetic data to personalize interventions based on individual risk factors. For example, changes in DNA methylation (a key epigenetic process) have been linked to chronic diseases such as type 2 diabetes, with potential applications in predicting and preventing this condition. While DNAm studies are beginning to identify subtypes of endometriosis, these insights may impact diagnosis and treatment options more than prevention.

Additionally, epigenetic testing has the potential to offer earlier detection and monitor risk factors over time. By integrating this with advanced hormone and toxin panels, healthcare professionals be able to create more effective, individualized health strategies that target prevention.

Advocating for yourself

TIP

Advocating for yourself means taking a proactive and informed approach to your healthcare. Prepare for your appointments by compiling a list of specific questions and concerns to address with your provider. You can use resources such as online forums or AI tools (for example, ChatGPT) to help you formulate questions and understand complex topics.

Also, make sure to track your symptoms consistently so you can paint a clear picture of your experience for your doctor. This helps your provider see patterns they may otherwise miss and gives you a solid foundation to discuss your concerns. Keeping a detailed record of things such as energy levels, mood changes, sleep quality, menstrual cycle fluctuations, and anything else that might be relevant to your specific experience will help you get the most out of your appointment.

REMEMBER

If a test result comes back "normal" but you still feel that something is wrong, don't hesitate to pursue further investigation. This could include asking for a more comprehensive test, discussing a referral to a specialist, or exploring options such as functional or integrative medicine. Healthcare providers are committed to supporting your well-being and want to hear your concerns. Your lived experience matters, and by collaborating with your provider, you can work toward the best possible outcome.

Evaluating benefits of integrative and functional medicine approaches

TIP

Integrative medicine combines conventional Western medicine with complementary therapies such as acupuncture, herbal medicine, and mindfulness practices. It treats the whole person — mind, body, and spirit — by blending evidence-based complementary treatments with standard medical care. This approach is particularly useful for supporting hormone health in a holistic way, without relying solely on medication. The following are some areas where integrative medicine treatments can be useful:

- **Stress-related hormone imbalances:** Techniques such as meditation, yoga, and acupuncture help support healthy cortisol levels and support adrenal health.
- **Reproductive health:** Herbal supplements and nutrition complement conventional treatments for conditions such as PCOS, infertility, and endometriosis to promote hormonal balance.
- **Menopause and perimenopause:** Natural remedies, such as mindfulness techniques, can help ease menopause and perimenopause symptoms, along with bioidentical HRT (hormone replacement therapy). Many first-line HRT prescriptions, such as transdermal estradiol (a type of estrogen) are also widely available through conventional medical practice and are no longer solely associated with integrative medicine.

In *functional medicine*, practitioners are primarily concerned with discovering and treating root causes. They view the body as an interconnected system, which means imbalances in one area can influence others. This approach is particularly helpful when dealing with hormone issues because it emphasizes understanding the entire hormonal network and the various factors that impact it. Functional medicine is helpful for the following issues:

- **Chronic or unexplained imbalances:** Conditions such as PCOS, thyroid disorders, or adrenal fatigue.

» **Hormonal transitions:** Dietary adjustments, supplements, and stress management support women experiencing PMS, PMDD, perimenopause, or menopause.

» **Thyroid health:** Functional medicine assesses gut health, nutrient deficiencies, and stress to better understand thyroid issues.

» **Blood sugar regulation:** Focuses on diet, exercise, and long-term strategies to manage insulin resistance and type 2 diabetes.

Deciding who to see for support

In this section, I describe the different situations when seeing a traditional general practitioner (GP) or endocrinologist (an expert in hormone-related diseases) is most appropriate as well as the circumstances when a functional or integrative medicine professional may be more appropriate.

TIP

See your GP or endocrinologist if your symptoms are acute (severe) or you suspect a significant hormonal disorder such as diabetes, infertility, PCOS, PMDD, endometriosis, adenomyosis, thyroid dysfunction, or adrenal insufficiency. They will likely recommend conventional diagnostic tests to identify or rule out medical conditions that need immediate attention.

If conventional tests don't provide answers or you prefer a more holistic approach, functional or integrative medicine can be helpful. These approaches often provide more illuminating insights because they aim to capture a more comprehensive picture of your health. For instance, functional medicine practitioners frequently use tests that go beyond standard blood panels, such as saliva or urine hormone testing, detailed gut health testing, hormone panels like the DUTCH (refer to Chapter 14 for more details), comprehensive thyroid panels (including T3, T4, and thyroid antibodies as well as thyroid-stimulating hormone), nutritional deficiency testing, and toxin screenings. These approaches can uncover imbalances or root-cause drivers and provide a customized, targeted plan.

TIP

Regardless of the type of medical professional you consult, make sure to check their qualifications and experience with hormone-related conditions. It's also important to choose someone who aligns with your approach and values when it comes to health. It's acceptable to shop around until you find someone who feels like the right fit for you. Remember, this is *your* journey, and working with a practitioner who understands your unique needs and respects your preferences is essential. Building trust and feeling supported are key factors in achieving the best results.

REMEMBER

You don't have to choose one approach or the other. In fact, a combination of conventional and holistic care often provides the best results and maximizes the strengths of both systems. Start with a GP for immediate concerns and then explore functional or integrative medicine to address lifestyle factors and long-term prevention.

IN THIS CHAPTER

» Making the most of available self-testing options

» Utilizing tests for comprehensive health insights

Chapter 14 Empowering Yourself with or without a Diagnosis

Hormone imbalance symptoms are surprisingly common in otherwise healthy individuals because they often serve as the body's early warning signals that something is off within its delicate internal systems. But what happens when you seek medical advice and your symptoms don't align with test results, or you don't receive a formal diagnosis? It's a frequent scenario that a person falls within the "normal range" on diagnostic tests or their symptoms aren't severe or consistent enough to meet traditional diagnostic criteria.

Even when you receive a diagnosis, tracking changes can be incredibly challenging. Measuring hormones and other biomarkers has historically been quite difficult. Relying on occasional doctor visits may not provide the continuous feedback needed to effectively manage your condition, and hormonal shifts often take time to manifest in noticeable physical or emotional changes, making it difficult to maintain motivation. This is where self-testing and monitoring your symptoms become powerful tools for real-time insights.

This chapter explains how to investigate your hormone health with or without a formal diagnosis, how to take charge of your well-being by using self-testing tools, and when to explore other diagnostic options that can ensure you get an accurate picture of your health and root-cause drivers.

Harnessing Self-Testing

In my experience with hormone imbalance, I went undiagnosed for over a decade despite experiencing debilitating mental, physical, and emotional symptoms. The symptoms I meticulously tracked and the medical test results I received never quite aligned, and doctors repeatedly assured me that I was "within the range of normal" or that my symptoms were "just part of being a woman." This approach left me feeling frustrated and dismissed because there was no viable treatment within conventional Western medicine apart from birth control, which only managed symptoms without offering a cure.

Though this explanation made sense in a medical context, it didn't ease my frustration or resolve my health issues. In my efforts to find solutions, I encountered an overwhelming number of products and books claiming to help, but I struggled to distinguish between effective advice and empty promises. Navigating this journey forced me to develop resourcefulness — an invaluable skill for all of us, especially as we stand on the cusp of a revolution in hormone testing and monitoring.

REMEMBER

What I learned is that achieving optimal hormone health and managing symptoms requires a multifaceted approach: a healthy lifestyle focused on prevention, tuning into your body's signals, addressing root causes of imbalance, and utilizing appropriate testing methods as needed. By educating yourself on innovative self-testing tools, you're positioning yourself to make the most of current and emerging opportunities.

Familiarizing yourself with different methods

Understanding how your body is performing or responding on a daily, weekly or monthly basis through self-testing is incredibly helpful. However, as with any tool, it's important to understand both the strengths and limitations to ensure you're getting the most accurate and meaningful information. First, I want to introduce some of the most common self-testing methods currently available.

REMEMBER

Whenever you're choosing a monitor or test in any of the following categories, ensure what you purchase is offered by a reputable company with good reviews and appropriate medical oversight.

Continuous glucose monitors

TIP

CGMs track glucose levels in real time, making them invaluable for those managing insulin resistance, prediabetes, diabetes, PCOS, or stubborn weight or anyone looking to understand how diet and lifestyle impact blood sugar regulation. While they can lead to tangible and sustainable changes and are enormously help with motivation, it's best to pair their use with professional help to interpret what you see, at least at first.

Look out for the following things:

- Ensure the CGM is FDA-approved in the U.S. or certified by relevant health authorities in your country, such as the CE in Europe.
- Make sure the device includes guidance on calibration and usage to avoid inaccurate readings.

Fertility- and ovulation-tracking tests

These tests help women understand their menstrual cycle, track ovulation, and optimize fertility. They measure hormone surges (such as in luteinizing hormone and follicle-stimulating hormone) through urine or saliva to predict ovulation windows.

Be mindful of the following things:

- Ensure the test is backed by clinical research and widely used by fertility specialists.
- Look for certifications or approvals from health authorities in your country.
- Consider tests with integrated app support for tracking and interpreting your results more effectively.

TIP

Saliva hormone testing

Saliva tests are commonly used to measure stress hormones such as cortisol throughout the day, as well as reproductive hormones during different phases of the menstrual cycle.

Look for the following things when choosing a test:

- Check for reviews or certifications that indicate the lab's accuracy.
- Make sure the test provides detailed instructions on sample collection. Poor collection technique can affect results.
- Consider tests that offer support for interpreting your results properly.

At-home blood spot tests

To measure key hormones such as thyroid (TSH, T3, T4), reproductive hormones (estrogen, progesterone, testosterone), and vitamin D levels, you send a blood sample from a small finger-prick to a lab for analysis.

Be on the lookout for these things:

- Ensure the company uses a certified lab (look for CLIA [Clinical Laboratory Improvement Amendments] certification in the U.S.).
- Review how the sample is handled and shipped. Prompt delivery and timeliness is crucial for accurate results.
- Choose tests that offer professional interpretation of the results rather than automated reports.

At-home thyroid testing kits

These tests help to detect hypothyroidism, hyperthyroidism, or autoimmune conditions such as Hashimoto's disease by measuring TSH, free T3, free T4, and sometimes thyroid antibodies in your blood.

Look for these things when you're buying a test:

- Look for tests that measure multiple thyroid markers (TSH, T3, T4) for a complete picture.
- Check that the company provides accurate and easy-to-understand instructions for sample collection.
- Choose tests that offer professional interpretation of the results rather than automated reports.

Comparing the pros and cons of self-testing

REMEMBER

Balancing the advantages of self-testing with its limitations is key to making it a valuable part of your overall health strategy. By choosing tests with a reputation of being reliable and interpreting your results with care — or having the help of a healthcare professional — you can harness the benefits while avoiding potential pitfalls.

Pros of self-testing include

- **Convenience:** Self-testing kits allow you to track your hormone health from the comfort of your home, avoiding the hassle of scheduling appointments, taking time off work, or waiting for lab results.
- **Affordability:** Many at-home tests offer comprehensive insights at a fraction of the cost of traditional diagnostic methods, making it a budget-friendly option.
- **Real-time monitoring:** Tools such as CGMs provide immediate feedback, helping you make lifestyle adjustments quickly and effectively and maintain motivation.
- **Empowerment:** Self-testing gives you greater control over your health, enabling you to take proactive measures based on your unique hormonal profile.
- **Prevention:** By detecting early signs of imbalance, you can intervene before symptoms worsen, potentially preventing more serious health conditions or hormonally driven diseases.
- **Preservation of privacy:** This option allows you to monitor your health discreetly, without the need to visit a doctor's office or share sensitive health concerns with others.
- **Personalization:** The data you gather allows you to tailor your health regimen specifically to your body's needs.

The cons of self-testing include

- **Risk of misinterpretation:** Interpreting test results can be challenging when you don't have professional guidance. Misreading data could lead to unnecessary worry or inappropriate actions. Plus, hormones fluctuate naturally throughout the day, and what may seem like an imbalance could be part of a normal cycle. This is why it's essential to understand the context behind the numbers and, ideally, consult with a healthcare provider to avoid overreacting to normal variations.

WARNING

- **Limited scope:** Some tests only measure specific hormones or may not provide a comprehensive view of your hormonal health, making it difficult to capture the full picture.
- **Obsession with tracking:** Self-testing can sometimes lead to an unhealthy obsession with monitoring every fluctuation. Constantly tracking hormone levels may cause stress, anxiety, or a desire for perfection, which can ironically disrupt hormone balance and is especially disruptive when you're trying to become pregnant. It's important to use these tools as part of a broader approach to wellness rather than becoming overly fixated on the data.
- **Accuracy issues:** Not all tests are equally reliable. Improper sample collection, timing errors, or unreliable labs can lead to inaccurate results. Additionally, conditions such as PCOS, which can cause chronically elevated LH levels, may lead to false positives when detecting an ovulatory phase LH surge.
- **No substitute for medical advice:** While self-testing provides valuable insights, it is not a replacement for professional medical evaluations. Hormonal imbalances are complex, and proper diagnosis and treatment often require expert interpretation of data.

Using CGMs

CGMs have become an invaluable and popular tool for people looking to manage blood sugar (and therefore insulin) levels more effectively. By providing real-time data on how blood glucose responds to your diet, lifestyle, and stress, CGMs cultivate a much deeper understanding of metabolic health and help you cultivate a hormone supportive lifestyle.

A CGM works by inserting a small sensor under the skin, which continuously measures glucose levels in the interstitial fluid. The device sends real-time data to your phone or another receiver, allowing you to track your glucose trends throughout the day and night. CGMs allow you to see the immediate impact of your meals, exercise, and even stress levels on your blood glucose. You can track which foods cause spikes and how long your blood sugar takes to return to normal and how your body responds to workouts. This real-time feedback is incredibly motivating, helping you understand how your daily habits are affecting your health and make adjustments accordingly.

While CGMs provide a wealth of data, interpreting the results can be tricky, especially when you're first starting out. It's helpful to work with a healthcare professional, such as a GP, dietitian, or endocrinologist, who can guide you through the initial stages, helping you understand what the numbers mean and how to adjust your lifestyle based on the trends you're seeing.

Make sure to set realistic goals when you use a CGM. Your blood sugar will fluctuate naturally throughout the day, and your aim should be to maintain healthy ranges rather than focusing on individual spikes or drops. A healthcare professional can help you identify your target range based on your health goals and existing conditions.

Anyone can benefit from understanding their blood sugar trends. The following sections take a closer look at how CGMs can benefit different individuals.

Type 1 diabetes

If you have type 1 diabetes, your body struggles to produce insulin because the immune system mistakenly attacks and destroys the insulin-producing beta cells in the pancreas. For them, monitoring blood glucose levels is a daily necessity because insulin is required to replace and mimic the body's natural response to fluctuating blood sugar levels. Too little insulin leads to high blood sugar (hyperglycemia), which can cause long-term damage to organs and tissues. On the other hand, too much insulin can cause dangerous drops in blood sugar (hypoglycemia), which may lead to severe health risks like seizures or unconsciousness. CGMs help to reduce the risk of extreme highs and lows by offering real-time feedback, allowing for better insulin management.

Type 2 diabetes/insulin resistance

In individuals with type 2 diabetes or insulin resistance, the body doesn't use insulin efficiently, leading to elevated blood sugar levels. CGMs allow these individuals to track how different foods, exercise, and stress impact their blood glucose in real time so they can create personalized dietary and lifestyle changes to keep blood glucose levels stable.

Polycystic ovary syndrome

Polycystic ovary syndrome (PCOS) often involves insulin resistance, making blood sugar regulation more challenging. Using a CGM can help women with PCOS see how their blood glucose is responding to their lifestyle so they can make informed decisions regarding meal timing, carbohydrate intake, and exercise, helping to improve metabolic function and reduce PCOS symptoms.

Anyone looking to optimize metabolic health

Even if you don't have a formal diagnosis, a CGM can offer valuable insights into how your lifestyle is impacting your blood sugar. For example, if you're experimenting with a new diet or trying to shift stubborn weight, a CGM gives you real-time feedback on how well your body is managing blood sugar, which can help with making more sustainable changes and identifying areas where your metabolism might need support.

Decoding what your symptoms are telling you

Your body is constantly sending you signals, often long before a formal diagnosis can be made through testing methods. Whether they manifest as fatigue, mood swings, low libido, afternoon energy crashes, irregular periods, or changes in weight, these signals are your body's way of communicating that something may be off with your delicate endocrine system. Tracking your symptoms regularly (using the guidelines provided in Chapter 15) and familiarizing yourself with what they may mean is the most crucial tool in understanding and managing your hormone health.

REMEMBER

Body awareness and symptom tracking is the missing link that connects the data from tests with how your body actually feels, helping you fine-tune your treatment, management, or prevention plans. No test will ever be able to offer the full picture without the context of how you feel on a daily basis. So, by keeping a log of your symptoms (you can refer to the guide in Chapter 15), you begin to build a map of your body's natural rhythms and responses to your diet, lifestyle, time of the month (for women) or stress. It also helps you identify patterns that might be missed in a one-off doctor's visit or a single lab test, giving you a much clearer understanding of what might be driving your symptoms and how best to address them.

Using Other Key Tests

REMEMBER

Despite significant advances in laboratory methods over the past 50 years, conventional hormone tests remain susceptible to interference or inaccuracies that may produce incomplete or misleading results. Many tests fail to account for the dynamic nature of hormone fluctuations, or they focus on single hormone levels without considering the broader context, such as the balance between key hormones. This can leave individuals without a clear diagnosis or with symptoms that persist despite "normal" test results.

Preventative screenings

Preventative hormone screenings are not just for people experiencing symptoms. They can also be an essential part of staying proactive about your long-term health. Hormones fluctuate naturally with age, stress, or lifestyle changes, and identifying imbalances early can help you take steps to restore balance before more significant health issues arise.

TIP

Incorporating hormone screening through at-home testing kits or regular check-ups with your healthcare provider into your routine allows you to maintain optimal health and proactively navigate shifts such as perimenopause, menopause, and andropause. I recommend the key preventative screenings in this section to help monitor and assess hormone imbalances.

Please note: The recommendations provided are based on guidance from specialists, such as endocrinologists, and standard practices in some healthcare systems. However, access to regular testing may vary depending on your location and healthcare provider. For example, in systems such as the NHS in the U.K., repeated thyroid function testing may only be offered if you have a diagnosed thyroid disorder, borderline results, or a relevant family history. Likewise, repeated hormone blood tests are not generally part of HRT management, unless you're taking testosterone. Standard practice may vary, so always consult with your healthcare provider. These guidelines are intended to offer proactive advice but may align more with private healthcare access or self-testing in some regions.

Thyroid function tests

I recommend these tests every one or two years, or more frequently if you have symptoms such as fatigue, weight changes, or mood swings or if you're at high risk for thyroid issues:

- **TSH (thyroid stimulating hormone):** This is often the first test ordered to assess thyroid function. Elevated TSH levels can indicate an underactive thyroid (hypothyroidism), whereas low levels may indicate an overactive thyroid (hyperthyroidism).
- **Free T3 and Free T4:** These hormones provide more insight into how the thyroid is functioning. T4 is converted to T3, the active hormone that the body uses for metabolism and energy. Testing can help identify conversion issues or pinpoint the stage of thyroid imbalance.
- **Thyroid antibodies:** For autoimmune thyroid conditions such as Hashimoto's disease or Graves' disease, testing for antibodies (TPO and TgAb) is crucial for early detection and intervention.

Sex hormone panel

Have a sex hormone panel annually or every 6 months if you're experiencing symptoms such as irregular periods, low libido, or mood changes, or are undergoing hormone replacement therapy (HRT).

- **Estrogen and progesterone:** Tracking the estrogen-to-progesterone ratio is particularly important for assessing overall reproductive health.
- **Testosterone (free and total):** Testosterone is not just important for men but also plays a role in women's health. Low levels in men can lead to low energy, reduced muscle mass, and decreased libido, whereas high levels in women may contribute to PCOS and other hormonal issues.

Cortisol levels

I suggest testing cortisol levels annually, or more frequently if you experience high levels of stress or symptoms such as chronic tiredness, anxiety, and difficulty waking.

Please note that while cortisol testing can provide insights into stress levels, it's important to distinguish between recognized medical conditions such as Cushing's syndrome (high cortisol) or Addison's disease (low cortisol) and less defined concepts like "adrenal fatigue," which is not widely accepted as a medical diagnosis. You may gather some helpful information from testing but, instead of focusing solely on cortisol results, it's more effective to prioritize general stress-balancing measures, as discussed in Part 4.

Saliva or blood cortisol tests measure cortisol levels at different times throughout the day, offering insight into how your body handles stress. Abnormal fluctuations may indicate heightened stress responses or medical conditions such as Addison's disease.

Insulin and blood glucose tests

If you're at risk of diabetes or have conditions such as PCOS, you should be tested annually. If you're prediabetic or diabetic, you should test more frequently, every three to six months, or, as directed by your healthcare provider.

- **Fasting insulin and glucose:** These tests can help identify insulin resistance, a precursor to type 2 diabetes or PCOS. However, fasting insulin tests may not be used in standard practice in some regions, even in diabetes clinics, but fasting glucose and Hemoglobin A1c (detailed below) are both widely utilized.

» **Hemoglobin A1c:** This test measures your average blood sugar levels over the past two to three months and is commonly used to screen for prediabetes and diabetes.

Vitamin D levels

Vitamin D plays a significant role in hormone production, especially for the thyroid and reproductive hormones. Low levels of vitamin D have been associated with hormone imbalances, hypothyroidism, fertility issues, bone loss, mood disorders, and immune system dysfunctions.

Testing annually with a 25-hydroxy vitamin D test may be considered, especially in winter months or for individuals who have limited sun exposure. However, where testing is not routinely available, it is a good idea to take vitamin D supplements during the winter months and potentially year-round for individuals with darker skin tones or low light exposure (for example, Hijab wearers).

Lipid panel

While a lipid panel is traditionally used to assess cardiovascular health and menopause, it's also relevant for hormone balance. High levels of LDL cholesterol and triglycerides can indicate issues with thyroid hormones or insulin regulation, for example.

Testing frequency depends on your individual risk factors, age, and healthcare system guidelines. Annually may be appropriate for those who have a higher risk of cardiovascular issues; for those at low risk, testing every five years is typically sufficient.

Bone density screening

Osteoporosis is often linked to hormone imbalances, particularly in postmenopausal women due to declining estrogen levels. Bone density screenings, such as DEXA scans, can help detect early signs of bone loss and take preventive steps to maintain bone health. Women older than 50 or who are postmenopausal should check every two years. Men over 60 should also be on this schedule. If you have risk factors for osteoporosis, you should begin checking before you reach these ages.

Prolactin levels

Prolactin is a hormone primarily involved in lactation, but high levels in nonpregnant women or men can indicate hormonal imbalances. Elevated prolactin can lead to irregular periods, infertility, or prolactinoma (a benign pituitary tumor).

A simple blood test can screen for abnormal prolactin levels, but you need to do it only if symptoms occur (for example, irregular periods, infertility, or unusual milk production outside of pregnancy).

Saliva hormone testing

Unlike blood tests, which measure hormone levels in the bloodstream, saliva tests assess the levels of free, bioavailable hormones, meaning the hormones that are not bound to proteins and are actively available for use by the body's tissues. This makes saliva testing particularly valuable for monitoring cortisol, progesterone, estrogen, and testosterone levels over a 24-hour period, offering a more dynamic picture of your hormonal profile. Testing may be considered annually, or every six months if you're addressing specific hormone imbalances (menopause, PCOS) and are interested in tracking your individual patterns. However, this is typically a personal choice for those seeking deeper insights rather than a routine medical recommendation.

One of the key benefits of saliva testing is its convenience. Samples can be easily collected at home, making it less invasive and less stressful compared to blood draws, which is important when measuring hormones such as cortisol that are sensitive to stress.

REMEMBER

However, interpreting dynamic cortisol levels from saliva tests outside the context of overt adrenal dysfunctions, such as Cushing's or Addison's disease, lacks clear consensus in the medical community. While saliva cortisol patterns can provide useful insights for understanding stress-related health trends, they should be evaluated alongside clinical symptoms and lifestyle factors, rather than as standalone diagnostic markers.

For the most reliable interpretation and guidance, saliva testing should be integrated with other assessments and discussed with a healthcare provider who is experienced in hormone health.

Blood tests

REMEMBER

Blood tests are a widely used method for assessing hormone levels and are commonly used to diagnose conditions such as hypothyroidism, diabetes, and reproductive disorders. However, they have their limitations. Because hormones fluctuate naturally throughout the day, a single test provides only a snapshot of hormone levels at the time of collection, which may not reflect daily or cyclical variations. Timing is critical, especially for hormones such as progesterone, estrogen, and cortisol, where results can be misleading if not tested at the right time. They also typically measure active hormone levels without evaluating how hormones are being metabolized in the body, limiting the full picture of your hormone health.

Common hormone-related blood tests include thyroid panels (TSH, Free T3, Free T4) to assess thyroid function, sex hormone panels (estrogen, progesterone, testosterone) to monitor reproductive health, and cortisol tests for adrenal function. Other valuable tests include FSH and LH for fertility issues, and insulin and glucose for metabolic health (though insulin testing is not routinely performed in many systems). Prolactin may be tested for suspected pituitary disorders, and SHBG helps understand sex hormone binding. Vitamin D testing is also useful in certain contexts, particularly in individuals with limited sun exposure or symptoms of deficiency.

While blood tests provide essential information, combining them with other testing methods such as saliva, urine (for example, the DUTCH), or continuous monitoring (for glucose) give you a more complete picture of your hormone health. Always consult with a healthcare provider to ensure tests are timed correctly and interpreted in the context of your overall health.

The DUTCH

The DUTCH (dried urine test for comprehensive hormones) test is a well-known tool for assessing hormone levels, offering a detailed and comprehensive view of your hormonal health. However, while it is widely used by some practitioners, including many doctors, it has not yet achieved universal clinical acceptance. Many practitioners find its potential intriguing but agree that more research and evaluation are needed to clarify its uses and the interpretation of results.

The DUTCH helpfully measures sex hormones such as estrogen, progesterone, and testosterone, along with adrenal hormones like cortisol and DHEA and their metabolites (the byproducts of hormone processing in the body). By evaluating both hormone levels and how they are metabolized, the DUTCH might provide a more in-depth understanding of imbalances and metabolic issues and help identify root causes of certain symptoms.

WARNING

This test does require you to pay very careful attention to the collection process because it involves urine samples taken at multiple points throughout the day. Following the instructions precisely is crucial to ensure accuracy. Additionally, the accuracy of the results depends on using an accredited laboratory. Due to the complexity of the data, it's also important to have the results interpreted by a healthcare professional experienced in hormone diagnostics.

Overall, the DUTCH can be valuable for those seeking a comprehensive view of their hormone health, offering actionable insights to guide tailored treatment plans. However, its current use in clinical settings often relies on practitioner expertise and patient interest rather than widespread clinical consensus, and further evaluation of its applications and limitations is needed.

Gut health testing

TIP

Optimizing your gut health can improve hormonal regulation (such as estrogen, blood sugar control, and stress hormones), reduce inflammation, and support nutrient absorption. Please be aware that the current crop of available gut health tests vary in their level of evidence, ranging from well-established diagnostic tools to tests with more limited research support. Available gut health tests include

- **Comprehensive stool analysis:** Assesses gut bacteria, yeast, parasites, and inflammation markers. Useful for detecting imbalances that might increase estrogen or disrupt gut health, providing insights that can be particularly valuable when evaluated in conjunction with your hormone test results.
- **SIBO breath test:** This test is widely used by gastroenterologists to diagnose bacterial overgrowth in the small intestine that causes bloating and nutrient malabsorption, which can impact hormone production and regulation.
- **Organic acids test (OAT):** Measures byproducts of gut bacteria and yeast, revealing possible fungal or bacterial imbalances linked to inflammation and oxidative stress.
- **Zonulin test (leaky gut):** Checks for intestinal permeability. High levels can allow toxins into the bloodstream, raising inflammation and disrupting cortisol. However, there is limited confidence in Zonulin tests within the research literature, and their clinical application remains debated.
- **IgG food sensitivity test:** Identifies food triggers that cause low-grade inflammation, which strains the adrenal glands and interferes with hormone regulation.

TIP

You can obtain gut health tests through functional medicine practitioners, naturopaths, or specialized labs such as Genova Diagnostics and Doctor's Data. Many of these tests are also available through direct-to-consumer health platforms, making them super convenient if you prefer at-home testing and simple reporting.

However, it's important to integrate gut health test results with medical advice because some of these tests are primarily recommended by functional medicine doctors and naturopaths rather than being widely endorsed by conventional medical specialists such as gastroenterologists. At the moment, microbiome testing is not part of routine health screening due to the significant variability in individual microbiomes and the lack of consensus on what actually constitutes a healthy microbiome.

Nutrient and mineral testing

TIP

While often overlooked in standard check-ups, deficiencies in essential nutrients and minerals can drive hormone imbalances, affecting metabolism, reproductive health, and energy levels.

For example, magnesium supports blood sugar regulation and stress resilience, which are crucial for managing insulin resistance and reducing symptoms of PCOS. Vitamin D, essential for immune health and thyroid function, also influences fertility, with low levels often linked to menstrual irregularities and metabolic disorders. Vitamin B12 helps lower homocysteine levels, which is beneficial for adrenal health and insulin sensitivity. Iron, vital for oxygen transport and energy production, is particularly important for women because low iron can lead to fatigue and hormonal disruptions impacting fertility. Zinc, essential for immune function and hormone production, influences testosterone and estrogen balance.

TIP

Current healthcare practices in many Western systems prioritize evidence-based testing for specific medical conditions rather than broad nutritional screening, due to resource constraints and a lack of consensus on the clinical utility of routine nutrient testing in asymptomatic individuals. A full nutritional assessment may not be offered in the absence of symptoms or a clear clinical need. So, if you're interested in a deeper look at your nutrient status, consider asking your healthcare provider about testing, but know you may need to look elsewhere.

Specialized labs, such as Genova Diagnostics or SpectraCell, offer more detailed intracellular tests, assessing not only circulating nutrient levels in your blood but also how effectively your body is utilizing them. These options may be useful if you want to explore more comprehensive insights into your nutrient and mineral status, but their availability and cost should be considered.

Inflammatory markers

TIP

Chronic inflammation is a widespread issue, with studies estimating that up to 60 percent of adults worldwide have some degree of chronic inflammation linked to lifestyle factors such as poor diet, stress, lack of exercise, and environmental exposures. While tests like CRP and ESR can help detect systemic inflammation, they may not be significantly elevated in this context and are more typically used by doctors to diagnose specific conditions — for example, inflammatory arthritis or inflammatory bowel disease.

If you suspect chronic inflammation, you should consult a doctor who can assess your symptoms and recommend appropriate tests if necessary. However, regardless of test results, addressing your diet and lifestyle will be crucial. Focus on anti-inflammatory foods (such as fruits, vegetables, omega-3-rich fish, and whole grains), exercise, stress management, and adequate sleep. Taking proactive steps to support your overall health is often the most effective way to manage inflammation.

Toxin screening

Toxin exposure, particularly from mold mycotoxins and endocrine-disrupting chemicals (EDCs), are sneaky hormone saboteurs. Mycotoxins, the toxic byproducts of mold found in damp environments, can elevate cortisol levels, strain the adrenal glands, and contribute to symptoms like chronic fatigue, immune suppression, and hormonal imbalances. Urine tests from specialized labs can measure mycotoxin levels. Testing for exposure to EDCs through urine or blood also helps identify specific toxins, allowing for targeted reduction strategies like choosing organic oats and grains to reduce exposure to glyphosate, a commonly used herbicide with hormone-disrupting effects.

Thyroid testing

WARNING

Thyroid function testing remains one of the most common laboratory assessments for hormone imbalances. However, despite the widespread use of thyroid tests — particularly thyroid stimulating hormone (TSH), T4, and T3 — there are still significant limitations in how they are used and interpreted. The American Thyroid Association (ATA) and international organizations like the U.S. Centers for Disease Control (CDC) and the International Federation of Clinical Chemistry and Laboratory Medicine (IFCC) have made ongoing efforts to standardize and improve thyroid testing, but even with advancements, the interpretation of thyroid test results can still be ambiguous, and routine tests remain prone to analytical interference.

REMEMBER

Standard testing for thyroid function typically focuses on TSH as a primary marker, but TSH alone may not provide a comprehensive view of thyroid health. TSH is a signal from the pituitary gland to the thyroid, and while it indicates how hard the thyroid is working, it does not reveal how well the thyroid is converting and utilizing its hormones. T4 and T3 levels are often measured as secondary markers, but even these tests have limitations, particularly in how they account for daily hormonal fluctuations and the influence of external factors like medications, stress, or underlying health conditions.

TIP

Holistic and integrative approaches try to address these limitations by recommending a full thyroid panel, which includes not only TSH, T3, and T4 but also Reverse T3 and thyroid antibodies like TPO (thyroid peroxidase) and TgAb (thyroglobulin antibodies). However, the inclusion of Reverse T3 remains controversial due to a lack of clear evidence or consensus on its clinical interpretation. Thyroid antibodies are essential for diagnosing autoimmune thyroid conditions such as Hashimoto's or Graves' disease, but they may not need to be part of routine thyroid screening and are typically ordered when thyroid function abnormalities are identified or if there is a family history of autoimmune thyroid disease.

One of the key issues with current testing methods is the variation in results due to geographical, physiological, and pathophysiological factors. This means that while a person may have "normal" thyroid hormone levels in one location or under certain conditions, these same levels may indicate an issue elsewhere or in a different context. For example, people living at high altitudes often have slightly higher TSH levels due to the body's response to lower oxygen levels. In this case, what might be considered a normal TSH range at sea level could indicate suboptimal thyroid function for someone living at a higher altitude. Similarly, women in different stages of their menstrual cycle may have fluctuating thyroid hormone levels, meaning that a blood test performed at one point in the cycle could show "normal" levels, even though they may experience symptoms of thyroid dysfunction at other times. These geographical and physiological factors must be considered for accurate diagnosis and interpretation of thyroid function.

Moreover, despite advancements in laboratory assessments, many tests are still prone to analytical interference, which can lead to inaccurate or misleading results. Technologies such as mass spectrometry, while promising, are not yet widely available for routine thyroid testing.

TIP

It's also important to note that in conventional practice, treatment decisions, such as prescribing thyroxine therapy, are typically based on abnormal test results rather than symptoms alone. Collaborating with a healthcare provider to order and interpret the right tests within the context of your overall health will be helpful, especially if your test results do not align with how you're feeling. Continue to advocate for yourself!

Interpreting your results

TIP

When navigating the different hormone testing methods, it might be helpful to have tools that help you understand your results with clarity and accuracy. The Omni Calculator (`www.omnicalculator.com/`) is a highly valuable resource widely used by health professionals and educators that relies on established medical guidelines, studies, and standards. While it's always a good idea to consult a healthcare professional, Omni's following calculators can be a reliable starting point for understanding basic health metrics:

TIP

- **Estrogen and Progesterone Ratio Calculator:** The Omni pg-e2-ratio calculator looks at the ratio between your estrogen and progesterone levels, which many healthcare practitioners overlook. Instead of focusing solely on whether individual levels fall within the "normal" range, this calculator emphasizes the importance of a healthy ratio, which can provide some additional information on hormone balance.

REMEMBER

For example, during reproductive years, an optimal estrogen-to-progesterone ratio for women is typically between 100:1 to 200:1 (measured in pg/mL). As menopause approaches, this ratio naturally decreases due to hormone fluctuations. Tracking this ratio gives a more precise picture of your hormone health, enabling you to make personalized adjustments.

- **Blood Sugar Converter:** Ideal for anyone using CGMs or managing blood sugar levels. It allows you to convert readings between mg/dL (used in the U.S.) and mmol/L (used in other countries) which makes it easy to compare and understand glucose data across different devices and ensures you're interpreting glucose levels correctly.
- **Pregnancy Weight Gain Calculator:** For pregnant women, this calculator estimates healthy weight gain based on prepregnancy weight, BMI, and pregnancy stage. Maintaining appropriate weight gain during pregnancy is key for balancing hormones, minimizing the risk of gestational diabetes, and promoting overall health for both mother and baby.

TIP

The Macronutrient Calculator helps determine the ideal balance of proteins, fats, and carbohydrates based on your body composition and goals, and the Body Fat Calculator estimates body fat percentage using measurements like waist circumference and height. Both provide a wealth of insights that can empower you fine-tune your lifestyle.

4

Create Your Hormone Balancing Action Plan

IN THIS PART . . .

Turn your intentions into action by creating your personalized plan, setting goals, building lasting habits, and designing a lifestyle that works for you.

Address the root causes of your imbalance so you can build a resilient hormonal foundation and unlock the power of your tier 1 hormones.

Master the art of hacking your hormone hierarchy with simple yet powerful tools to stabilize blood sugar, reduce stress, and elevate your "happy" hormones, all while supporting your body's natural detox systems.

Inspire and equip teenagers to embrace their hormone health with confidence, fostering open communication and stress resilience.

Maintain your vibrancy in later life by exploring solutions such as hormone replacement therapy and nurturing your emotional health.

IN THIS CHAPTER

» Embracing your body's amazing ability to self-repair

» Setting up your personalized, actionable plan for success

» Tailoring your strategy to fit your unique needs and goals

Chapter 15
Turning Intention into Action

Congratulations! You're ready to turn your knowledge and insights into meaningful action. In this chapter, I explain how to set up the solid, unshakable foundation you need to create (and most importantly, execute!) your personalized hormone health plan. This chapter is all about designing a new lifestyle and mindset that genuinely works for you and supports your unique health journey. So whether you need to develop awareness about your current routines, set achievable goals, figure out how to create new habits that stick, or find a supportive accountability buddy, this chapter lays the groundwork for real, tangible results.

REMEMBER

Health is deeply personal, and although everyone (regardless of gender or age) can follow the root-cause approach, there's no one-size-fits-all way of applying it. For instance, each person likes to take care of their mental health in different ways, has a unique work schedule, and prefers different types of exercise. The key is to focus on creating a plan that feels accessible while inspiring you to reach for more. You should create something that energizes you and helps you step into the best version of yourself rather than taking on something you dread and eventually avoid. So, grab your journal or notepad, and let's dive in!

Knowing You're Not Broken

REMEMBER

The first mindset shift that needs to happen when you're working on your hormone health is recognizing that Western medicine has largely been designed to treat disease and manage symptoms rather than prevent them from occurring in the first place. This means that when it comes to hormone imbalances or their related conditions, conventional approaches often focus on addressing the immediate symptoms.

These treatments are undeniably valuable in managing and alleviating symptoms, particularly in acute or severe cases. However, over recent decades, we, the general public, along with medical professionals, have increasingly lost sight of the personal power we hold to prevent hormonal imbalances and address root causes when diagnosed. Our fast-paced, convenience-driven lifestyles have led to a reliance on quick fixes — something that offers immediate relief — but the inescapable truth is that the pressures of modern life place significant strain on our bodies. People can no longer afford to be thoughtless about their health, expecting Western medicine to simply patch things up. Although medications can play a critical role in a treatment plan, they often serve as temporary solutions because they mask deeper imbalances caused by stress, poor lifestyle choices, and exposure to environmental toxins.

REMEMBER

Tangible transformation occurs only when you prioritize prevention and address the root causes of your health issues. By leveraging the strengths and superpowers of Western medicine and focusing on the basic fundamentals of hormone imbalances and environmental factors, you can reclaim control and steer yourself away from the brink of hormonal chaos.

REMEMBER

As healthcare systems around the world become increasingly strained, the urgency for a shift toward personal responsibility has never been greater. While it remains critical to hold corporations and industries accountable for their contributions to the decline of public health, the power to initiate meaningful transformation ultimately rests in your hands.

REMEMBER

The truth is that your body is not betraying you; it's merely responding to the environment and circumstances in which it has been placed. Yes, modern life has put incredible strain on your hormones. Yes, the information out there is often very confusing. And yes, it's easy to feel lost in a medical system that often treats your body as a series of isolated parts rather than an interconnected system. However, you have endless opportunities in front of you to use what you've discovered and listen to your body, identify root causes, and begin making necessary changes.

Taking advantage of your self-repairing body

REMEMBER

What many of my clients find reassuring is that the human body possesses a remarkable ability to regenerate itself, which is a powerful asset when it comes to supporting the endocrine system. Although not all diseases or more serious conditions can be entirely reversed, some can, and these interventions will certainly help alleviate symptoms and optimize your health. This means that hormonal imbalances are not necessarily permanent conditions — only signals that your body is striving for equilibrium.

For example, skin cells renew every 27 days, and the lining of your gut renews in just 2 to 5 days. More complex tissues, like liver cells, take a bit longer, regenerating in 300 to 500 days, and red blood cells are fully replaced within 120 days. Even your reproductive organs undergo constant renewal: Women regenerate their uterine lining monthly, and men produce new sperm every 72 to 90 days.

TECHNICAL STUFF

This regenerative capacity is the foundation of an emerging field called *regenerative medicine* in which researchers are exploring how the body's ability to regenerate cells and tissues can be harnessed for therapeutic purposes. Although still in its early stages, scientists are experimenting with stem cells, tissue engineering, and even gene editing to encourage the body to repair damaged tissues and organs more effectively, offering potential new treatments for conditions such as diabetes and endometriosis.

Sleeping: Your secret weapon

TIP

Research continues to reinforce that deep, restful sleep allows your body to perform essential repair and regeneration work. Without enough of it, not only will your body be deprived of the time it needs for these healing processes to complete, but your immune system becomes compromised, leaving you more susceptible to illness and injury. Consequently, your body has to divert its healing energy to fight off illnesses instead of maintaining and repairing the damage that comes from modern life.

REMEMBER

The key takeaway is that you're not stuck in the state you're in now. Healing, improving, and optimizing your hormone health and the functioning of your endocrine system is possible, and it begins by working with your body's natural regenerative capacity, returning to the basics, and implementing the root-cause interventions covered in the rest of Part 4.

Riding the healing roller coaster

REMEMBER

The sooner you accept that the healing process is far from linear, the sooner you'll be on the path to success. Growth, like life, often feels like being strapped into a roller coaster: exhilarating highs where you can see your progress and feel amazing and frustrating lows of setbacks or no evidence of any tangible changes despite your hard and consistent effort.

Humans are wired to seek stability and familiarity over discomfort. However, healing requires a lot of temporary discomfort for future gains. An essential part of this journey is creating new habits that stop you from seeking safety in habits you're familiar with, especially if those patterns contributed to your imbalance in the first place.

TIP

Keep reminding yourself of the truth that sustainable progress is never about perfection but about resilience and adaptability in the face of challenges. Perhaps even draw a roller coaster on a sticky note and leave it somewhere you can see it each day!

Harnessing the power of self-compassion

If something doesn't challenge you, it doesn't change you, and remember that you certainly aren't going to get it "right" every day. You'll make mistakes and revert to old habits as you proceed on your path to improvement. Practice self-compassion rather than beating yourself up for every perceived failure or slip-up. (Spoiler, there are none if you just keep going!) Treat yourself with the same kindness and patience you'd offer a friend, and remind yourself that healing is an act of courage. Your willingness to show up for yourself, even when things get tough, is the most important thing. Your progress might look squiggly, like the line in Figure 15-1, or it might even feel like you're going backward, but over time, you will trend upward.

Taking radical responsibility

You're the author of your own life story. You have the power to alchemize your past and present into a powerful, healthy, and vibrant future. You get to decide what actions to take, what decisions to make, and what habits you form. When you start focusing on your ability to shape your life, you place yourself in the driver's seat, and you're capable of steering your life in the direction you desire. External circumstances will undoubtedly challenge you on this journey (I can guarantee it!), and whether you get to where you want to go is entirely determined by how you respond to those circumstances.

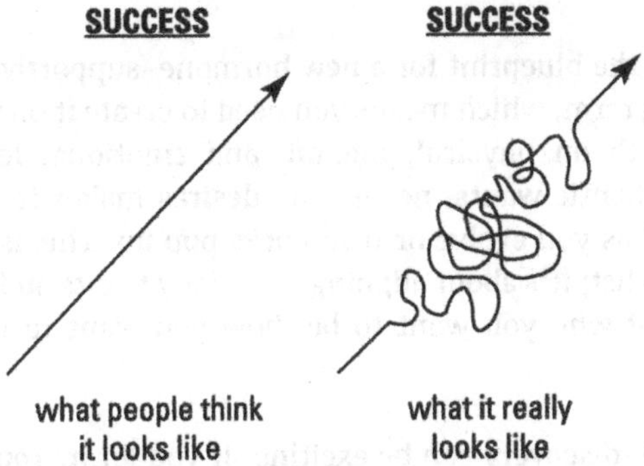

FIGURE 15-1: The journey to success isn't a straight line.

REMEMBER

Taking radical responsibility isn't about blaming yourself. (You're trying to reduce stress, and blaming yourself won't do that!) It's about owning your power in every situation and seeing obstacles not as reasons to give up or as evidence that it won't work out for you, but as opportunities to rise. Every time you choose to act instead of react, to persist instead of quit, you are taking control of your narrative and raising your self-esteem.

When you approach your life from this perspective, challenges become stepping stones instead of roadblocks. You begin to see setbacks as feedback and opportunities to adjust and grow. When you hit a plateau or regression, ask yourself these questions:

- What's the lesson here?
- What adjustments can I make?
- How can I be kind to myself while I course-correct?

In taking radical responsibility, you free yourself from waiting for circumstances to change and realize that you have the power to create your own hormonal breakthroughs. You are no longer at the mercy of life's ups and downs; you are actively creating the health, vitality, and balance you desire.

Creating Your Action Plan

This approach is not another cookie-cutter, copy-and-paste "plan" for you to follow. It's an invitation to craft an action plan that becomes an extension and expression of who you are at your core. It's an opportunity to set goals and routines that truly excite and inspire you. As covered in Chapter 11, purpose and fulfilment are two of the ultimate nervous system (and therefore, hormone) regulators. When you intentionally put supportive structures in place, you're setting yourself up for long-term success.

REMEMBER

Your action plan is the blueprint for a new hormone-supportive lifestyle you can stick to for the long term, which means you need to create it on your own terms to nurture your growth on physical, mental, and emotional levels. A plan that expresses your authentic wants, needs, and desires makes it much easier to be adaptable and fluid as you evolve or roadblocks pop up. This is not about ticking off tasks on a to-do list; it's about aligning your daily habits and choices with your long-term vision of who you want to be, how you want to live, and how you want to feel.

REMEMBER

This journey of self-discovery can be exciting, if you let it. You can use trial and error to find out what resonates with and works for you. You are wonderfully unique and shaped by a complex interplay of factors — your genetic blueprint, life experiences, diet, environment, and lifestyle preferences. This individuality extends to your hormonal profile, which is as distinct as the patterns of a snowflake (no two are ever the same!). So even though the principles of root-cause healing apply universally, how you respond to or choose to implement these principles may be different than what other people do, and that's completely OK!

Developing an action plan involves four steps, which I outline in the following sections:

1. **Develop awareness.**
2. **Setting long- and short-term goals.**
3. **Create effective habits.**
4. **Find an accountability buddy.**

Developing awareness

Awareness is the foundation for any meaningful change. To get to where you want to go, you need to understand where you're starting, what got you there, and what roadblocks you need to overcome to move forward.

TIP

The first three parts of this book are about cultivating a deeper awareness about your endocrine system and hormones — how they work and communicate with you. In Part 4, you get to be the observer of your own life and reflect on whether your behaviors, habits, and thoughts are setting you up for optimal hormone health. Are there patterns that show up repeatedly and sabotage your progress? Are there triggers that consistently derail you? Be curious, not judgmental, about your experiences.

Awareness also means paying closer attention to your physical, mental, and emotional symptoms and identifying the messages your body is sending you through issues such as painful periods, digestive discomfort, low moods, hormonal acne, or fatigue. Every symptom is feedback.

Set some time aside to grab a journal or notepad, put on some music, make a nice warm drink, and work your way through the following 10 journal prompts:

- What physical symptoms have you been experiencing regularly? For example, do you experience fatigue, painful periods, difficulty sleeping, digestive issues, muscle aches, low libido, or sleep disturbances? Refer to Chapter 13 for more signs and symptoms.
- When do these symptoms tend to flare up? Are there specific triggers, such as when you're stressed or eat particular things? For women, are these related to a specific time of the month?
- What emotional symptoms do you notice throughout the week? Examples include irritability, mood swings, anxiety, or a sense of overwhelm.
- What are the patterns in your energy levels throughout the day? Do you notice a slump in energy at certain times in the morning or afternoon? Does your energy fluctuate based on what you eat or your daily routines?
- What are your typical responses when you feel stressed or overwhelmed? Do you turn to food (over- or underconsumption), withdraw from exercise, avoid by overworking, or experience changes in sleep habits?
- Do you need to follow up on your symptoms and get any testing done?
- What behaviors do you engage in that may be hindering your progress? Are there certain people, environments, or situations that lead you to make unhealthy choices?
- What habits do you want to change but find difficult to let go of? For example, do you procrastinate or engage in late-night scrolling, snacking, or negative self-talk? Do you overwork, stay busy, and avoid emotions?
- What thoughts or beliefs tend to arise when you feel stuck in a rut or overwhelmed by your health challenges? Are these thoughts supportive or limiting? How might they be affecting your actions and decisions?
- What are signs that indicate you're making progress, even if they feel small?

Setting short- and long-term goals

The second step is to shift your focus toward the future by envisioning your healthiest, happiest self. You need to set intentional, clear goals that will serve as your "North Stars" to guide you over the bridge between where you are now and where you want to be.

Refer to your answers from the journal questions in the preceding section and use them to set both short- and long-term goals. Focus on one goal at a time, and apply the SMART (specific, measurable, attainable, relevant, and time-bound) method. (Read more about SMART goals in the next section.) This will help you create goals that challenge you while still being realistic and manageable. Start with your big vision for the long-term and break it down into actionable, short-term steps that will set you on the path to success.

REMEMBER

I want to share an important point: Many people make the mistake of setting goals that are either too vague or too grandiose, so they set themselves up for failure. For instance, a goal such as "I want to feel better" lacks specificity and direction, whereas a goal along the lines of "I want to lose 50 pounds in a month" is unrealistic and unsustainable. What's much more effective is setting SMART goals, which challenge you but are achievable enough to foster momentum and keep you motivated.

Setting SMART Goals

The SMART method is a well-established framework for effective goal setting. It originally developed in the business world to enhance productivity and focus. Over time, it has proven highly valuable for personal development, helping people to create clear, achievable, and motivating goals. Each aspect of SMART — specific, measurable, attainable, relevant, and time-bound — ensures that goals are both actionable and realistic, paving the way for consistent, meaningful progress.

TIP

- **Specific:** Make sure your goals are clear and well-defined. Rather than saying, "I want to be less stressed," be specific: "I want to lower my stress levels at work by practicing mindfulness meditation for 10 minutes every morning and going for a lunchtime walk."
- **Measurable:** Make sure you have a way to track your progress. Instead of setting a vague goal such as "I want to have more energy and sleep better," you might say, "I want to increase my daily energy levels by wearing my blue light-blocking glasses in the evening 3 hours before bed."
- **Attainable:** Your goals should be realistic and manageable. They should stretch you but not so far that they feel impossible. For instance, setting a goal to reduce sugar intake by 50 percent within the next month is more attainable than trying to cut out all sugar overnight.

TIP

Drastic changes, especially with things you crave, can backfire. Your brain often responds to restriction with an even stronger desire for the thing you're trying to avoid, which leads to more intense cravings.

» **Relevant:** Make sure your goals align with your long-term objectives and values. Ask yourself, "Is this goal going to get me closer to the person I want to become?"

» **Time-bound:** Give yourself a deadline to work toward. A time frame gives your goal structure and prevents you from procrastinating. One example is "I will practice breathwork before bed for the next 30 days."

Long-term goals paint a picture of where you want to be in the months and years ahead and require sustained effort and commitment over the long term, so you first decide what your ultimate goal is. Once you have it established, you can then break it down into smaller, actionable, achievable steps so you don't get overwhelmed.

Setting long-term goals

To set your long-term goals, consider what the happiest and healthiest version of you looks and feels like. What would your daily routine be? What environments would you spend time in? What people do you surround yourself with?

Your goals will be specific to you, but here are some examples:

» Wake up feeling energized, excited, and optimistic

» Get a regular period with no severe PMS

» Exercise every day within a supportive gym community and look forward to it

» Find new friendships or a community I can plug into who motivate me and who want to go on hiking trips

» Feel confident in my body and clothes

» Have more purpose and fulfillment in my life

» Boost my metabolism, heal my insulin resistance, and lose weight

Setting short-term goals

Once you have your big vision down, you can create stepping stones to help you get there. They can be actions or changes that you're able to realistically achieve within a few days or weeks. They're meant to give you quick wins. Some examples include joining a gym and committing to classes by adding them to your diary. If necessary, you may also want to set the goal of getting testing done to assess your hormone levels, gut health, or nutrient deficiencies. If you're seeking comprehensive tests that aren't specified under health service guidelines or available for ordering in standard labs, you can always consider reputable private services that offer relevant tests and provide reliable results. Refer to Chapter 14 for testing advice.

Creating effective habits

REMEMBER

This step is where real transformation begins. In his bestselling book, *Atomic Habits* (Avery, 2018), James Clear explains that small, consistent behaviors, when repeated regularly, compound to create significant, lasting change. The key, Clear emphasizes, is not solely to fixate on the goals you want to achieve, but rather to focus on building the systems and structures that support those goals. While goals define the desired outcome, it's the habits — the daily processes and actions — that drive you toward those outcomes.

Read through the rest of this section to familiarize yourself with the frameworks for successfully building and breaking habits. Then, as you continue through the upcoming chapters — particularly Chapters 16, 17, 20, and 21 — consider which hormone-supportive habits you need to implement and use the habit loop framework to help you craft your new habit and adding it to the habit tracking log provided later in this chapter. You can also apply this framework to breaking your current habits that are misaligned with your goals.

TIP

You don't have to overhaul your entire lifestyle at once; instead, start small and focus on incremental changes. Choose one or two habits that feel most accessible for you and begin with them. Once you've established consistency with those, you can gradually layer in more habits so they build over time. This way, you create sustainable change that supports your goals without feeling overwhelmed. Remember, the goal is progress and consistency, not perfection.

Creating new habits

Forming lasting habits requires more than just willpower; it involves understanding the cues, cravings, and rewards that drive your behavior. By designing habits that align with your lifestyle and making them enjoyable and easy to integrate, you're more likely to stick with them in the long term. In this section, I walk you through the steps of making habits stick.

TIP

1. **Make it obvious (cue).**

   Identify the cue or trigger that initiates the habit loop. A time of day, a location, or even an emotional state could all be cues. For example, if your goal is to engage in regular physical activity, you could set a cue by placing your workout clothes in a visible spot the night before. The idea is to remove barriers between you and the habit, making the desired action as seamless as possible.

TIP

One technique to use is habit stacking, which means you attach your new habit to an existing one that's already firmly established. For example, you could pair your morning dog walk with a mindfulness practice you find on YouTube. This way, you're pairing a new behavior with something you already do automatically, creating a natural flow.

2. **Make it attractive (craving).**

   If a habit feels like a chore then it's unlikely to last without a motivator. It's helpful to find ways to make your new habit something you look forward to. James Clear suggests using "temptation bundling" — linking something you want to do with something you need to do. For example, if you enjoy listening to podcasts but struggle to make time for daily walks, you can bundle them together. This pairs an attractive reward with the behavior you want to reinforce.

3. **Make it easy (response).**

   The easier a habit is, the more likely you are to stick with it. This means scaling down behaviors to something manageable, such as doing one push-up or meditating for one minute. By removing the friction, you create momentum. Once you get started, it becomes easier to do more.

4. **Make it satisfying (reward).**

   To effectively reinforce habits, your brain requires a sense of immediate gratification, which enables you to tap into the dopamine-reward loop. One way to do this is by tracking your habits. Create a visual cue, such as marking an X on a calendar each time you complete your habit. Doing this creates a sense of accomplishment and taps into the very human desire not to break the streak.

Breaking old habits

REMEMBER

Certain habits, such as skipping exercise to sleep in or picking up a ready-made meal on the way home rather than using the healthy food you have in the fridge to whip up a healthy dinner, undermine your progress. You can take the following steps to combat that tendency.

1. **Make it invisible (remove the cue).**

   Remove the triggers that initiate the behavior. (The journaling in the "Developing awareness" section earlier in this chapter helps with this, so go back to that section if you haven't already done that activity.) Bad habits thrive on cues, just as good habits do. To eliminate bad habits, make sure to distance yourself from the cues that spark them.

TIP

For example, if you tend to overindulge on sugary, carbohydrate-heavy, or processed snacks while watching football with your family on Sundays, start by removing them from your home and replacing them with healthier (yet still delicious) alternatives. Or try substituting a different activity during commercial breaks, such as taking a brief walk or stretching. You could even shift the focus to sharing a healthy meal or snack together before the game starts. The goal here is to make it more difficult to indulge in the behavior by removing its triggers from your environment and replacing them with more supportive cues for healthier choices.

2. **Make it unattractive (reframe the craving).**

   Habits usually persist because you associate them with some level of reward, even if the reward is fleeting or damaging in the long run. To break a habit, reframe the behavior and make it unattractive. One great way to do this is by focusing on the negative long-term consequences of the habit.

   TIP

   For instance, if you find yourself reaching for soft drinks or sodas for energy, reframe that craving by visualizing how it could be affecting your health and hormone balance. Imagine the long-term effects, such as increased inflammation, energy crashes, or disrupting your sleep cycles. Associating the habit with these undesirable outcomes can make the habit feel less rewarding and help you resist it more easily.

3. **Make it difficult (increase friction).**

   The more difficult you make a habit, the less likely you are to follow through with it. For example, if you check your phone the moment you wake up each day, make it harder to do that by leaving your phone in another room or in the hallway overnight. The extra effort of having to get up to retrieve your phone increases friction and makes the habit less tempting.

4. **Make it unsatisfying (create accountability).**

   TIP

   One of the most powerful tools for breaking a habit is accountability. When your actions have consequences beyond yourself, it becomes much harder to justify continuing the behavior. One way to harness this is by setting up a system where there's a real consequence for your actions. For example, if you're trying to cut down on smoking, you could commit to donating a significant amount of money to a cause you *don't* support every time you smoke a cigarette.

The power of identity in breaking habits

REMEMBER

Breaking habits is about so much more than willpower or discipline. Every time you resist the urge to engage in a bad habit, you're casting a vote for the person you want to become. You're not simply trying to stop a behavior; you're focusing on aligning with your new identity, which it much more powerful.

For instance, instead of saying, "I'm trying to stop overeating," shift your mindset to, "I'm someone who respects their body's fullness cues and nourishes themselves with healthy, balanced meals." This mental shift toward seeing yourself as someone who naturally makes decisions that aligns with their goals and values is transformative.

Finding an accountability buddy

Humans are inherently social creatures, and the ability to create meaningful, lasting change is magnified when we're supported and surrounded by others. As the famous African proverb says, "If you want to go fast, go alone; if you want to go far, go together." Therefore, the last step of your action plan is to find an accountability buddy.

Taking advantage of social contagion

One of the most significant ways the people around us influence our health is through social contagion — the idea that behaviors, emotions, and habits can spread through social networks. For example, if your close friends, family, or coworkers prioritize healthy habits such as regular exercise, a balanced diet, or mindfulness practices, you're far more likely to do the same. Studies have demonstrated that eating habits, smoking, drinking, and even sleep patterns are often mirrored within social circles. This extends to emotional health as well. Positive and negative moods can be "contagious," and your emotional environment can greatly affect your mental health. You become who you surround yourself with!

Understanding the importance of norms and expectations

REMEMBER

Another reason why the company we keep matters for our hormone health is that we are deeply influenced by social norms. What's considered "normal" behavior within a particular social circle or community tends to set a baseline for how the people in those groups behave as individuals. So if you're surrounded by a group that drinks, smokes, or eats processed foods, it can become more difficult to resist those behaviors yourself because the behaviors have become normalized within that social context. Conversely, in a group that prioritizes fitness, sobriety, healthy diets, trauma recovery, or mindfulness, those behaviors become part of the expected routine, which subtly encourages everyone to align with the group's norms.

Powering up with accountability

One of the key psychological theories behind accountability is the concept of "commitment devices." These are external motivators or agreements that encourage you to stick to your goals because you feel a greater sense of responsibility. For example, signing up for a charity run to motivate yourself to exercise works because you've made an external commitment to a cause. When you share your intentions and progress with someone else, you're far less likely to let things slip through the cracks. In fact, you get to harness the positive energy and momentum that comes from knowing someone else is invested in your growth and cheering you on.

REMEMBER

Having someone who understands your journey and regularly checks in on your progress can help alleviate the loneliness that often accompanies personal transformation. Change isn't easy — especially when it requires sacrificing short-term comforts, summoning grit, and drawing on determination. An accountability buddy can provide the extra push you need when your motivation slips (or your old patterns and behaviors creep back in). This person can also offer fresh perspectives when inevitable challenges arise and celebrate your wins with you. They may help you see progress you might otherwise overlook. Plus, by supporting each other, you create a positive feedback loop of encouragement, pushing each other to new heights.

Building your support network

REMEMBER

It's important to acknowledge that not everyone around you may fully understand the hormonal and health challenges you're navigating. The reality is that much of the way modern people are living their lives is the reason so many are suffering from hormonal imbalances. People who aren't as educated about these issues may not make the connection between lifestyle and hormone health, and that's okay.

If you find yourself without someone in your immediate circle or community who "gets it," don't hesitate to find your people in online communities. Social media groups and wellness forums are great places to find an accountability buddy and connect with like-minded individuals.

TIP

Put yourself in new environments where you'll be surrounded by people who share similar goals or lifestyles. Most people genuinely want to help and uplift others, especially when they see someone working hard toward their goals. Try joining a local group to help build your network of people you can rely on for motivation and accountability.

The following journal prompts can help you reflect on what you need in an accountability buddy:

- What kind of support do I want to receive from an accountability buddy? What kind of support can I offer in return?

» Who in my life could be a great accountability partner for my health and hormone goals?

» How will I maintain a positive and encouraging relationship with my accountability buddy?

» How can I put myself in environments where I'm surrounded by like-minded people who help me normalize this new way of living?

Identify at least one person in your life who could be your accountability buddy. If no one immediately comes to mind, explore options in online communities or consider enlisting a professional, such as a personal trainer, nutritionist, or therapist. When you've found your person (or people), initiate a conversation with them about your mutual goals and how you can keep each other on track. Then, plan your first check-in within the next week to set your accountability system in motion!

Customizing Your Action Plan

After you've done the deep work of reflecting on your symptoms, habits, and behaviors and set meaningful long- and short-term goals, built a strong support system, and know how to create hormone-supportive habits and break the less desirable ones, it's time to put all of your knowledge and preparation into action by weaving together the threads of your hormone health journey. In this section, I tell you how to customize your action plan.

Becoming an expert in you

No one knows your body better than you. You are the expert in your own lived experience, and even though doctors, specialists, and health practitioners have invaluable knowledge to share, they can only work with the information you provide them. Taking an active role in your health, regardless of whether you have a formal diagnosis, ensures you're equipped with the insights and understanding needed to monitor your progress and adapt as you go.

REMEMBER

Tracking your symptoms, noting changes in your body, and documenting how you feel over time is incredibly valuable, not only to guide your own decisions but also to share with a doctor or specialist should you need to seek professional guidance down the line. By keeping an account of your experiences, you're building a comprehensive picture of your health that helps any practitioner better understand your unique situation and tailor their advice accordingly.

TIP

It's also incredibly helpful to be able to look back in times of doubt or low motivation. A tracking document serves as a reminder of how far you've come and the progress you've already made. On challenging days, your record can provide clarity, reaffirming that even small, gradual improvements add up over time. It's also a powerful tool for celebrating your wins — big or small — which keeps you motivated and connected to your goals.

REMEMBER

Hormone imbalances are notoriously tricky to diagnose because the symptoms can be subtle and complex; they can also vary greatly from person to person. As covered in Chapter 14, even if your hormone levels fall within the "normal" range on a test, you may experience symptoms of imbalance such as fatigue, mood swings, weight fluctuations, or irregular periods. The standard ranges are based on averages, which don't always reflect what's optimal for your body and life circumstances. In fact, you might feel far from "normal" while still being told that nothing is wrong on paper. Plus, just because there may not be anything officially "wrong," doesn't mean there isn't room for improvement!

Continue to trust your intuition and tune in to the signals your body is sending you. If something feels off, it probably is. Your body has an incredible capacity to communicate its needs. Often, subtle symptoms or gut feelings are its way of letting you know that adjustments are needed. Going on a hormone-balancing journey means being proactive, taking the time to educate yourself, listening to your body, taking action, and staying consistent with an approach that works for you.

Table 14-1 shows an example of a symptom tracking log that you can customize to suit your unique needs. Take some time to create a template on your computer or in your journal that you can easily fill in. You don't need to obsess over tracking every single day (it's not about micromanaging your life). However, make it a habit to jot down notes on the days when you experience symptoms worth mentioning or when you feel really good! Over time, you'll begin to identify patterns that help you make adjustments that align with your goals.

Creating a habit tracking log and action plan

TIP

Table 14-2 shows an example habit tracker that serves as the foundation for your action plan. You can begin using it now and refine it as you read through the final chapters of this book. By tracking your daily habits along with how you're feeling, you'll start to identify patterns in which behaviors are helpful and which may be holding you back. This insight will empower you to assess and adjust using the habit-building framework described in the "Creating Your Action Plan" section earlier in this chapter. For instance, you might discover that getting consistent sleep significantly boosts your energy the next day or that eating a protein-rich breakfast stabilizes your mood and keeps you feeling full throughout the day, preventing overeating. Once you gain clarity on what works for you, sticking to your chosen habits becomes far more intuitive and rewarding.

TABLE 14-1 **Example Symptom Tracking Log**

Date	Symptoms Noticed	Suspected Triggers	Time of Day/Phase of Cycle (for women)	Notes about Energy, Mood, and So On
October 1	Bloating, fatigue, irritability	Not sure. I've been stressed at work and my period is due soon.	Day 28 of cycle	Energy dip mid-afternoon
October 7	Felt amazing today!	Went to bed early, wore my blue light blocking glasses before bed, ate a protein-heavy breakfast and did a 5 minute meditation.		Mindfulness in the morning really helps
October 14	Difficulty sleeping	Stayed up late watching Netflix/gaming and didn't wear my blue light blocking glasses.	Evening	Woke up feeling sluggish, skipped workout due to fatigue and grabbed an energy drink on the way to work
October 28	Afternoon energy crash, irritability	Poor sleep the night before, skipped breakfast.	3:00 p.m.	Snacked on sugary foods to boost energy, felt worse later

The log in Table 14-2 is structured around the root-cause approach to hormone balance, with a focus on habits that support cortisol regulation, blood sugar balance, happy hormones, hormone detoxification, and overall health. However, there's no rigid formula; it's a flexible guide. If you're not sure where a particular habit should fit, that's perfectly fine. You can customize the tracker to suit your unique needs and goals, so please feel free to adapt it by adding categories that are specific to you or tracking different habits that resonate with your personal journey.

TABLE 14-2 Example Habit Tracker

Habit	MON	TUE	WED	THU	FRI	SAT	SUN
Tier 1 Insulin: Blood Sugar Balancing							
Strength training to build muscle	X		X		X		
Protein-rich breakfast	X		X	X	X	X	X
Walked after dinner	X		X	X	X		X
Hit my daily protein goal (e.g. 30g with each meal)	X		X	X	X	X	X
Tier 1 Cortisol and Nervous System Support							
Listened to a mindfulness audio on my commute	X			X			X
Healthy coping mechanisms at work — for example, walk around the block or deep breathing	X	X	X		X		X
Yoga class 3 times per week		X		X			X
Tier 1 Dopamine and Other Happy Hormones (e.g., Oxytocin)							
Didn't check my phone first thing in the morning. Put music on instead!		X		X	X		
Purpose and fulfillment hobbies — for example, volunteering, mountain biking						X	X
Supporting Hormone Detoxification and Elimination							
Adequate water intake	X	X	X		X		X
Lymphatic support — for example, rebounding or dry brushing			X		X		
General Health and Well-being							
Wore my blue light blocking glasses a few hours before bed	X	X		X	X	X	X
Gut health: adding herbs, nuts and seeds to my meals to hit 30 different plant-based foods a week	X		X		X		
Sleep (7–8 hours)	X	X	X		X		
Took my probiotics, supplements, and medication	X	X	X	X	X	X	X

Individual approaches to diet and exercise

It seems like there's a new diet or exercise trend emerging every month with each promising rapid results and revolutionary benefits. All have their merits, but the relentless cycle of trends and comparisons can leave many people feeling compelled to jump on the latest bandwagon (or stressed if they can't), often without regard to whether it aligns with their personal needs, preferences, or long-term sustainability.

REMEMBER

Ultimately, the most effective approach to diet is one rooted in simplicity and consistency. The focus should always be on quality, whole, nutrient-dense foods. Think colorful vegetables, healthy fats, lean proteins, complex carbohydrates, herbs, spices, and whole grains. The closer these foods are to their natural state, the better to help minimize the intake of unnecessary additives and preservatives and the more supportive they are for your gut health. (Refer to Chapter 10 for more gut health–specific tips.)

When it comes to nutrition, there is no "one-size-fits-all" approach. If certain foods don't agree with you or you're seeking more personalized guidance, consulting with a dietician or nutritionist can provide valuable insights into what works best for your body.

As for exercise, the key is to find activities that not only benefit your body but also bring you genuine enjoyment. If you don't find joy in your workouts, it's unlikely you'll stick with them long term. Movement should be something you look forward to, and it can be yoga, running, swimming, weight lifting, Pilates, or simply a walk in nature or from the office to your home.

REMEMBER

That said, building muscle should be nonnegotiable for everyone as muscle is a vital endocrine organ. As covered throughout the chapters of this book, muscle tissue plays an essential role in hormone regulation, including insulin sensitivity, cortisol balance, and overall metabolic and reproductive health. So, whether you build muscle through strength training, bodyweight exercises, or other forms of resistance work such as Pilates, the important thing is to integrate muscle-building exercises into your routine at all life stages in a way that feels aligned with your goals and preferences.

IN THIS CHAPTER

» Creating a positive "domino effect" within your hormone hierarchy

» Appreciating what supplements can and can't do

Chapter 16
Taking a Root-Cause Approach

We are all life artists. Consciously or unconsciously, we take the raw material of our lives — our diet, lifestyle, environment, challenges, relationships, jobs, genetics, wins, and opportunities — and create with them. Each day, we pick up a paintbrush and get to continue creating the masterpiece that is our lives. But what happens when the colors on our canvas don't reflect the life or health we truly want? Often, it's because we've only been working on the surface to address symptoms when they pop up rather than proactively tackling the underlying causes.

In this chapter, I share how to take a root-cause approach, getting to the heart of what's really going on so you can fully harness the raw material of your life. The key to success is realizing that it's not about the resources you have but about your resourcefulness in shaping the outcome in your favor.

Hormone imbalances are not isolated occurrences; they are powerful signals from the body that alert you that something deeper is out of alignment. Whether it's chronic stress, unresolved trauma, environmental toxins, poor nutrition, or a disruption in your natural rhythms, your hormonal health is intricately tied to every aspect of your mind, body, and environment. Addressing these imbalances requires that you look at the body holistically, understanding that when one system is out of balance, it affects every other system.

Setting the "Domino Effect" in Motion

In Chapter 3, I explain that hormones work in hierarchical structure, and I suggest you imagine setting up a line of dominoes: Each piece is standing upright, aligned perfectly, ready to cascade at the touch of a finger. The moment one domino falls, it knocks into the next, setting off a chain reaction.

REMEMBER

In the world of hormones, a very similar scenario unfolds when an imbalance occurs because hormones operate within a finely tuned structure in which each one influences and is influenced by others. This interdependence means that a disturbance in one hormone can cause imbalances in others, much like a toppling line of dominoes. Because your tier 1 hormones are the primary regulators of many physiological processes, imbalances in tier 1 can create a domino effect, disrupting the entire hormonal system.

REMEMBER

The opposite is also true, when your tier 1 hormones are healthy and functioning optimally, they create a stabilizing effect that reverberates throughout the entire hormonal hierarchy. By addressing the root cause of imbalances in these influential hormones, you can prevent a cascade of negative effects before they can reach deeper into your system, potentially contributing to the development of chronic conditions and diseases rooted in hormonal disruption. The result is a healthier, more resilient body and mind — one capable of handling life's challenges without spiraling into the cycle of hormonal imbalance that can underlie many common health issues.

Remember, your endocrine system is a nearly perfect machine that works hard to keep you alive and thriving, but it needs your support – it has more than 50 hormones to manage! So, by focusing on the most influential ones, as I describe in this chapter, you craft a stable foundation that supports the entire hormonal hierarchy, making sure that you produce the right number of hormones at the right time and create a positive domino effect.

Prioritizing insulin

REMEMBER

Insulin is the main hormone that regulates your blood sugar levels throughout the day by acting as a key that unlocks cells, allowing glucose to enter. Here's the process in a nutshell: After you eat and your blood sugar rises, the pancreas releases insulin into the bloodstream. Insulin binds to receptors on cells, opening glucose channels so that cells can absorb glucose for energy or store it for later use. This process (shown in Figure 16-1) ensures that blood sugar levels stay balanced while providing fuel for the body's cells.

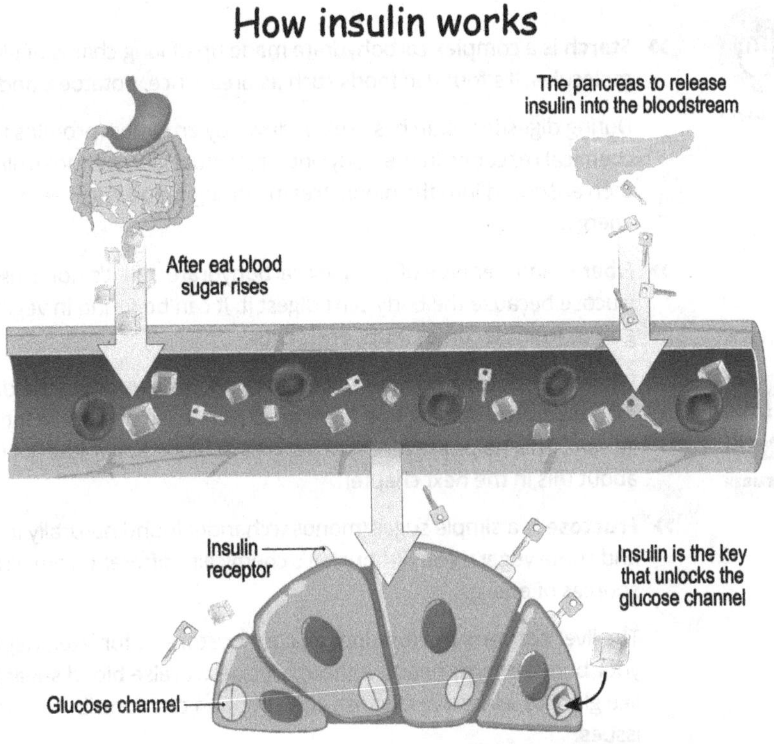

FIGURE 16-1: How insulin works.

designua/Adobe Stock Photos

Your body burns an astonishing eight billion molecules of glucose every second. For perspective, imagine every glucose molecule as a drop of water. In just 10 minutes, your body would use up enough glucose to fill an entire Olympic-sized swimming pool. Basically, humans need a lot of fuel to function properly.

REMEMBER

Glucose is a type of simple sugar (or monosaccharide) that serves as the primary source of energy for your body. Different types of carbohydrates, such as starch, fiber, fructose, and sucrose, are broken down in various ways to release glucose into the bloodstream. (The online appendix at `www.dummies.com/go/hormonebalancefd` includes a list of healthy sources for each type of carbohydrate.) It helps to imagine them as four siblings on a family tree (see Figure 16-2) with different personalities who share the same parent.

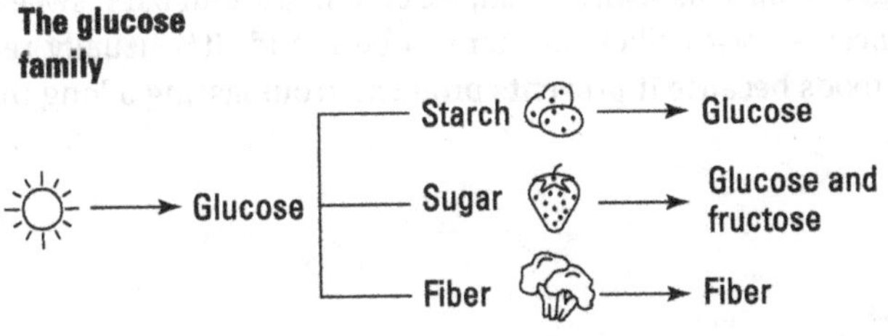

FIGURE 16-2: The glucose family tree

REMEMBER

- **Starch** is a complex carbohydrate made up of long chains of glucose molecules. It's found in foods such as bread, rice, potatoes, and pasta.

  During digestion, starch is broken down by enzymes (proteins that speed up chemical reactions in the body) into individual glucose molecules, which are then absorbed into the bloodstream, raising blood sugar levels and providing energy.

- **Fiber** is another type of complex carbohydrate, but it's not broken down into glucose because the body can't digest it. It can be found in vegetables, whole grains, fruits, legumes, nuts, and seeds.

  REMEMBER

  While fiber doesn't provide glucose directly, it slows down the digestion of carbohydrates, leading to a more gradual release of glucose into the bloodstream. This helps prevent sharp spikes in blood sugar levels. I talk more about this in the next chapter.

- **Fructose** is a simple sugar (monosaccharide) found naturally in fruits, honey, and some vegetables. Although it's chemically different from glucose, both are sources of energy.

  The liver converts fructose into glucose or stores it for later, depending on your body's energy needs. Although it doesn't raise blood sugar levels directly like glucose, excessive fructose consumption can contribute to metabolic issues.

- **Sucrose** is a disaccharide, meaning it is made up of two simple sugars: one molecule of glucose and one molecule of fructose. It's commonly found in table sugar, as well as in many processed foods.

  During digestion, sucrose is broken down by enzymes into its two components: glucose and fructose. The glucose is absorbed into the bloodstream, and the fructose is processed by the liver, as explained earlier.

REMEMBER

Nature is clever and designed glucose to be consumed in a very specific way — in plants, where it's paired with fiber. This is key, because as noted earlier, fiber helps slow down your body's absorption of glucose into the bloodstream, preventing a rapid spike.

One of the big reasons we're experiencing a global metabolic health crisis is the fact that our supermarket shelves are now lined with products filled with starch and sugar — such as white bread, ice cream, protein bars, sweetened yogurts, and fruit juices — with fiber nowhere to be found. It's usually removed from processed foods because it prevents products from lasting a long time on the shelves.

REMEMBER

Here's an example: If you take a fresh, firm banana and pop it in the freezer overnight, will it still have the same texture when it thaws the next morning? Nope! If you try to eat the banana after it's defrosted, you'll find both the banana and its skin are mushy because the fiber has been broken down by the freezing and thawing process. The fiber and its health benefits are still there, but the texture won't be the same, which is a problem for processed foods that need to be frozen, shipped around the country/world, thawed, and stored on shelves without losing their texture.

We've also turned up the dial on the sweetness of foods. A chocolate bar from the 1970s was certainly not like what we get today. The basis of modern food processing is to first strip away the fiber, and then ramp up the starch and sugars so that foods become hyperpalatable, triggering a stronger dopamine response in the brain so we keep consuming more.

REMEMBER

Why do we love sweetness so much? Well, there are no natural foods that are both sweet and poisonous, so sweet foods (which were rare finds for our ancestors) were a safe option. In periods where food wasn't readily available, eating all the fruit before anyone else could get to it was a massive advantage, so we evolved to feel pleasure (hey there, dopamine!) whenever we eat something sweet. We eat more and more because it's really difficult for our brains to curb cravings for things that taste like fruit. Sweetness and dopamine feel incredibly rewarding. This is reason number one why willpower isn't the issue with overeating or indulging in sweet foods. We have ancient evolutionary programming telling us that chocolate at 3:00 p.m. is a brilliant survival strategy!

Dealing with excess glucose

REMEMBER

When there's more glucose in your bloodstream than your body needs for immediate energy, you store it for later use in two main forms:

- **Glycogen:** Some of the extra glucose is converted into glycogen and stored in the liver and muscles. Glycogen acts as a quick-access energy reserve that can be broken down and used when your body needs fuel between meals or during exercise.
- **Fat:** Once glycogen stores are full, any remaining excess glucose is converted into fat and stored in adipose tissue for long-term energy. Building muscle is especially important because muscles have a greater capacity to store glycogen, which can help prevent excess glucose from being converted to fat. This process explains why consuming more sugar and carbohydrates than your body can use for energy often leads to weight gain.

When glucose levels in the bloodstream exceed what the body can effectively use or store, this condition is known as hyperglycemia. If hyperglycemia becomes chronic, it can contribute to serious health issues such as insulin resistance, type 2 diabetes, and systemic inflammation.

TIP

As I mention earlier, fructose is metabolized differently and can't be stored as glycogen. Instead, it's processed in the liver, but if you consume too much, it's directly converted into fat. This is why high levels of fructose, often from added sugars in processed foods like high-fructose corn syrup, are linked to increased fat storage and metabolic issues. Avoiding sources of added fructose, especially in sugary drinks and processed foods, can help reduce the risk of fat accumulation and support healthier metabolic function.

What's very important to understand here is that glucose isn't the problem, and you don't need to eliminate carbohydrates completely. There is an amount of glucose that is just right for you and your hormones. There is space on your plate for a little bit of everything, including sugar/glucose.

Understanding healthy blood sugar levels

When blood sugar and insulin levels are stable, the body is much better able to burn fat. A 2021 study of 5,600 people by Canadian scientists found that weight loss is always accompanied by a decrease in insulin levels, while another review found that insulin levels rise before obesity is developed. The key takeaway here is this: When insulin levels are high, fat storage is promoted, making weight gain more likely. Conversely, lower insulin levels signal the body to burn stored fat for energy, leading to more effective and sustained weight loss, which helps maintain broader hormonal balance and positively impacts estrogen levels.

The flat horizonal line in Figure 16-3 is your ideal blood sugar status line. With mismanaged blood sugar, your glucose levels soar high above that line and then drop down way below it over and over again throughout the day (which is why it's often referred to as riding a "blood sugar roller coaster"). While it's pretty much impossible to ride that flat line at all times, when you learn how to manage your blood sugar, your levels will gently rise and fall above and below the line while remaining in the healthy range. The benefit of flattening the glucose curves is that you also flatten your insulin and fructose curves.

REMEMBER

I cover the step-by-step process for managing glucose in the Chapter 17. For now, I want to make it clear that managing your glucose (and therefore insulin levels) doesn't require sophisticated testing, a glucose monitor, or calculations (unless you're diabetic, of course). But, if you haven't been paying attention to your blood sugar, then your levels probably need some love and a glucose monitor might be helpful for you to learn more about how different foods impact your body. (Read Chapter 14 for more information.) Even people with the best intentions and who are health conscious can throw things out of whack with juice cleanses and avoiding food groups. In a world flooded with processed foods and misleading diet advice, maintaining healthy, stable blood sugar levels is nearly impossible without proactively educating yourself and making intentional efforts.

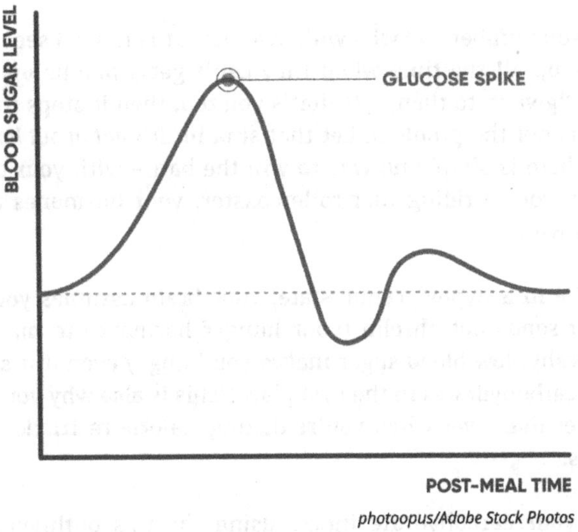

FIGURE 16-3: The blood sugar roller coaster.

Hypoglycemia (low blood sugar)

REMEMBER

So far in this chapter, I've primarily talked about elevated blood sugar levels that can lead to insulin resistance and hyperinsulinemia (excess insulin in the bloodstream). These, in turn, can contribute to conditions such as PCOS, reproductive hormone imbalances, and, if left untreated, type 2 diabetes. But we haven't addressed low blood sugar levels, known as hypoglycemia, which is just as detrimental to your health and hormones and usually occurs through two different pathways:

- You're constantly dieting, skipping meals, or consider coffee and a muesli bar to be enough for you. If your body lacks adequate food and carbohydrate intake, your blood sugar levels can become chronically low. Glucose is your brain's primary source of fuel, so without it, you'll feel moody, tired. and lethargic and even struggle to concentrate and take on new information.
- The second, more complex route begins in overindulging in carbohydrates. Anything more than half a cup of mashed potatoes or rice is enough to skyrocket your blood sugar and get your pancreas pumping out insulin to bring your blood sugar levels back down by taking the sugar (in the form of

glucose) to the cells where it can be stored for future use. What happens here is that your pancreas miscalculates the amount of insulin it needs and produces too much, so instead of bringing your blood sugar back to its baseline, it takes too much glucose, reducing your blood sugar levels too low. This is why you might feel the urge to snack on something sweet even though you had lunch an hour ago. Your body is trying to get your blood sugar levels up to where they should be.

REMEMBER

This is reason number two why willpower isn't the issue. I see my clients beating themselves up all the time when they can't get a handle on their cravings or when they "give in to them." If that's you too, then it stops today because your willpower is not the problem. Let that sink in: *It's not about how much willpower you have.* There is simply no way to win the battle with your biology and blood sugar when you're riding that rollercoaster; your hormones are powerful and will always win.

When you're in a hypoglycemic state, your brain assumes you're in starvation mode, so it sends out ghrelin (your hunger hormone) to make you want food again. Basically, low blood sugar makes you hungry even if it's the result of you overeating carbohydrates in the first place! This is also why you might find yourself hungrier than ever when you're dieting, calorie restriction, and cutting out food groups.

TIP

Managing your carbohydrate intake using the tips outlined in Chapter 17 is crucial. Keeping it stable at every meal, every day will make sure your pancreas produces the amount of insulin you need to escort the glucose you've consumed to where it needs to go, preventing excessive blood sugar spikes or dips and keeping your mood, emotions, cravings, and hormone hierarchy on a nice even level. For more on how continuous glucose monitoring (CGM) devices can provide insights into your blood sugar trends and help fine-tune your diet and lifestyle, refer to Chapter 14.

Insulin and reproductive health

REMEMBER

For both men and women, insulin levels are an important piece of information used by your brain and gonads (sex organs) to decide whether your body is a safe environment for reproduction. When insulin is out of whack or you're riding blood sugar rollercoasters, it causes a domino effect and negatively affects the rest of your hormonal hierarchy. Essentially, it suggests to the body that you're not healthy, which is why men and women with high insulin levels are more likely to be infertile.

For men, elevated glucose levels are associated with reduced semen quality (fewer viable candidates) as well as erectile dysfunction. For women, polycystic ovary syndrome (PCOS; read more in Chapter 6) is often driven by too much insulin, and they have a difficult time losing weight as high insulin levels make it hard to burn fat effectively. Insulin tells the ovaries to produce more testosterone and interrupts the natural conversion of male to female hormones, which leads to even higher testosterone levels.

Insulin and estrogen have a closely connected relationship; when insulin levels are consistently high, estrogen can become unbalanced, potentially leading to symptoms such as irregular cycles, painful or heavy periods, weight gain, and mood swings.

Prioritizing cortisol

If you haven't read earlier chapters that cover the role and effects of cortisol extensively, you may want to visit them to better understand this hormone. Here, I want to focus on cortisol's relationship with its fellow tier 1 hormone insulin. You can think of these hormones as two sides of a seesaw, working together around the clock to keep your body's energy in balance.

REMEMBER

For example, when cortisol levels rise in response to stress, one of its primary functions is to raise blood sugar levels to ensure your body has enough energy to respond to the stressor by fighting or fleeing. That's really smart! Cortisol signals your liver to release stored glucose (glycogen) into the bloodstream, giving your body a quick energy boost. However, the increase in blood sugar also triggers a rise in insulin to help move the extra glucose into cells, bringing your blood sugar back down.

If you're dealing with chronic stress, this constant fluctuation in blood sugar can lead to insulin spikes and drops, which leaves you craving quick energy in the form of sugary or fatty foods like chocolate or cookies because when your blood sugar drops after the initial insulin response, your body craves fast-digesting carbohydrates and fat to replenish those energy levels quickly.

The cortisol-insulin cycle and weight gain

REMEMBER

Elevated cortisol not only increases blood sugar and insulin but also signals the body to store fat, particularly around the abdomen, so you have energy for future stressors. This system made sense in the context of our ancestors who needed to store fat during periods of famine or danger, but it's less helpful for us now. With food readily available, chronic stress often leads to overeating, meal skipping, weight gain, and fat storage.

Cortisol, insulin, and estrogen excess

Fat cells, particularly those in the abdominal area, secrete estrogen, which means weight gain due to elevated cortisol and insulin levels can lead to an excess of estrogen in the body. For women, excess estrogen may result in worsening PMS symptoms and increased risk of reproductive health issues such as fibroids and endometriosis.

In men, it can lead to reduced libido, erectile dysfunction, fatigue, weight gain, and an increased risk of conditions like gynecomastia (enlarged breast tissue), infertility, and prostate issues. Crucially, it can also disrupt the balance of testosterone, which can further exacerbate these symptoms.

REMEMBER

The key takeaway is that managing stress is a vital part of metabolic health by preventing insulin spikes, cravings, or meal skipping.

Managing dopamine and oxytocin

REMEMBER

Dopamine and oxytocin are often overlooked yet essential tier 1 hormones. Dopamine governs motivation and reward, driving behaviors that shape overall hormonal health, whereas oxytocin regulates social bonding and trust, deeply influencing emotional resilience and connection (refer to Chapter 2 for more details). These two hormones may not be as associated with stress-response or metabolic pathways as insulin and cortisol, but their profound ability to shape how we think, feel, and act underscores their foundational importance in overall health and makes them deserving of their tier 1 status. Without taking steps to nurture and regulate these hormones, achieving true hormonal resilience is impossible.

TIP

When your dopamine system is functioning well, engaging in behaviors and habits that support hormone health — such as exercising, eating nutrient-dense, protein-rich meals, or completing tasks like identifying and replacing household products that contain endocrine disruptors — feels much more manageable and rewarding. If it's dysregulated, you're more likely to struggle with procrastination and give in to instant gratification, emotional eating, reduced motivation, addictive behaviors, social withdrawal, excessive social media use, or difficulty sticking to healthy routines.

The dopamine-insulin relationship

Dopamine has an indirect but important role in regulating insulin sensitivity and glucose metabolism. You can think of dopamine as the strategist of your metabolic team: It helps the brain send signals to the pancreas to release insulin at the right times, which ensures that glucose is properly absorbed into cells.

REMEMBER

But here's where it gets tricky. Indulging in sweet treats and processed foods cause a surge in dopamine, lighting up your brain's reward center like it's the Fourth of July. It feels great in the moment, but over time, your brain starts craving those quick hits of pleasure more often, and suddenly you're reaching for that bag of cookies much more often than you'd like. This creates a feedback loop, where sugar cravings drive insulin spikes and insulin works overtime to clean up the aftermath.

When dopamine pathways are overstimulated due chronic stress, excessive use of social media, or diets high in processed foods, it contributes to metabolic dysregulation. Eventually, the cells become tired of all the insulin knocking at their doors and stop responding. This is where insulin resistance comes into play, which can eventually lead to a cascade of metabolic issues such as PCOS, obesity, and type 2 diabetes.

REMEMBER

This relationship is a two-way street. Dopamine influences how your body processes insulin, and insulin also modulates dopamine. Research shows that insulin can lower dopamine levels in specific regions of the brain. By reducing dopamine in these areas, insulin helps temper cravings and eating behaviors. However, when insulin signaling is impaired — whether through stress, poor diet, or insulin resistance — dopamine can go unchecked, leading to increased cravings for high-sugar, high-fat foods and contributing to a feedback loop of overindulging or persistent cravings.

The dopamine-cortisol-insulin loop

The brain's dopamine system interacts with cortisol to help regulate how you respond to stress. In normal conditions, dopamine helps buffer the negative effects of stress, maintaining a sense of motivation and reward when you face challenges.

REMEMBER

However, when cortisol levels remain elevated due to prolonged stress, it depletes dopamine levels, contributing to feelings of low motivation, fatigue, and even depression. Lower dopamine levels can drive cravings for quick dopamine hits — often in the form of sugary or fatty foods — and that leads to insulin spikes and further blood sugar imbalances. The result is a vicious cycle where stress, dopamine, and insulin become interlinked, disrupting metabolic health and hormonal balance.

REMEMBER

Here's an important point: Dopamine isn't just about feeling good. It's about learning to stick with healthy habits and prioritizing long-term gratification over short-term pleasure. Sure, skipping your workout to watch the latest episode of your favorite show might give you a brief dopamine rush, but long-term, it can wreak havoc on your hormone hierarchy and metabolism. The trick is balancing those dopamine-driven impulses and choosing behaviors that promote lasting well-being.

Oxytocin

The unsung hero in the tier 1 group is oxytocin. While often dubbed the love or bonding hormone and most famous for its role in facilitating childbirth, oxytocin has some serious tier 1 status that affects everything from relationships to eating habits and cortisol levels. Nourishing connections and feelings of love and belonging are not just "nice to haves," they're essential components of our hormonal health.

The following are ways oxytocin plays an important role in your overall health and well-being:

REMEMBER

- **Regulation of eating behavior and metabolism:** Recent studies have illuminated oxytocin's capacity to enhance insulin sensitivity (improving the body's response to insulin), which significantly impacts how your body processes glucose. Oxytocin plays a crucial role in regulating eating behaviors and maintaining energy balance. Research has demonstrated that it can suppress food intake, particularly reward-driven eating (the consumption of food based on its pleasurable or rewarding qualities rather than hunger or nutritional needs), which is easily triggered by the abundance of hyperpalatable, highly processed foods in our environment. By moderating the desire for these foods, oxytocin helps maintain healthier eating habits and supports long-term metabolic health.
- **Influence on body composition:** Oxytocin plays a multifaceted role in regulating body composition by supporting muscle maintenance and regeneration, preserving lean body mass, promoting bone mineralization, and minimizing the accumulation of adipose (fat) tissue. All these contributions are critical for enhancing metabolic health. By fostering muscle growth and repair, oxytocin helps preserve lean body mass, which is essential for maintaining a higher metabolic rate.

REMEMBER

- **Enhancement of cognitive control:** Research suggests that oxytocin administration can enhance brain activity in areas associated with cognitive control and decision-making in relation to food. For example, oxytocin has been shown to suppress neural responses to palatable food stimuli, which may help individuals exert better control over their eating behaviors. This enhancement of cognitive control can be instrumental in managing overeating and promoting healthier dietary choices.

TIP

- **Mitigation for the effects of cortisol:** Most importantly, oxytocin plays a crucial role in mitigating the effects of cortisol. In moments of social bonding, oxytocin curbs the hypothalamic-pituitary-adrenal (HPA) axis (responsible for the release of cortisol), leading to a calmer physiological state and promoting feelings of safety and trust.

The relationship between your hormones and detox organs

Once hormones have served their purpose, they need to be efficiently broken down and removed from the body to avoid buildup, which can lead to imbalances. For example, if cortisol isn't efficiently cleared, it can make it difficult to regulate other hormones (such as insulin and estrogen).

This is where your body's detox team — your liver, kidneys, lungs, skin, and lymphatic system — comes in. They work hard to filter out toxins, endocrine-disrupting chemicals, excess hormones, and other waste products. Taking care of these organs (as I outline in Chapter 17) is a key part of the root-cause approach.

IN THIS CHAPTER

» Figuring out how to manage your blood sugar levels and metabolism

» Learning how to finally get your stress hormones under control

» Giving your happy hormones a boost

» Taking care of your body's natural detox system

Chapter 17 Hacking Your Hormone Hierarchy

Congratulations, you made it! You're about to dive into page after page of actionable advice that you can use to begin filling in the custom hormone balance action plan you started putting together in Chapter 15. If you haven't already read that chapter, you should read it and then return here.

In this chapter, I guide you through the root-cause approach to hormone balance, equipping you with the diet and lifestyle fundamentals you need to get your blood sugar and metabolic health under control, bring your stress hormones back to a healthy and resilient place, boost your happy hormones, and take care of your body's natural detoxification to avoid the buildup of excess hormones and pesky hormone-mimicking toxins. In a nutshell, you build the foundation for optimizing the entire hormonal hierarchy, including reproductive health and beyond.

REMEMBER

Everyone's hormonal profile and ecosystem is completely unique, so please don't feel like you need to implement absolutely everything outlined in the following pages. Instead, focus on what resonates most with you and what seems applicable to your individual health needs.

Getting Your Blood Sugar under Control

You can achieve wonderfully stable blood sugar or glucose levels when you consciously and consistently implement the tips and tools in this section with every meal, every day. This isn't a diet. It's a way of eating that needs to become entrenched as part of your lifestyle over time because your entire endocrine system relies on your glucose levels staying well-regulated. Once you start eating in a way that supports your hormones, you'll free up so much energy and mental bandwidth you can channel into living your life and having more fun.

TIP

You don't have to use the following tips all at once or all the time. Think of this list as a toolkit you can draw from: Pick the strategies that fit best into your lifestyle or meal situation and start building them into your routine gradually. For more resources on this topic, I suggest checking out *Diabetes For Dummies*, 6th Edition by Dr. Simon Poole and Amy Riolo (Wiley, 2023) the work of Jessie Inchauspé (The Glucose Goddess), Dr. Mark Hyman, and Dr. Casey Means.

Getting off the blood sugar roller coaster

If you're striving for weight loss, it's time to shift your mindset from obsessing over calories to focusing on the quality of the food you consume. Focusing on reducing calories alone is an outdated, oversimplified approach because we now know that not all calories are created equal. Although 100 calories of sugar, protein, or fat may provide the same amount of energy, they each impact your body in very different ways. Research increasingly proves that managing glucose levels by minimizing spikes and dips is far more effective in promoting sustainable weight loss while positively benefiting your overall health. A win-win!

TIP

Even though stabilizing your glucose levels is crucial, consuming excessive calories, even if they come from low-glucose-impact foods, still leads to weight gain. The takeaway Is that you need to prioritize balanced eating with whole foods in a nutrient-dense diet that flattens your glucose spikes, using the guidelines I recommend in the following sections.

Consuming foods in the optimal order

TIP

The order in which you eat your food significantly impacts blood glucose levels. By consuming fiber first and then protein and fat, leaving starches and sugars for last, you can reduce your overall glucose spike by up to 73 percent and insulin spike by 48 percent. When you eat starches or sugars first, they are quickly broken down into glucose, which floods the bloodstream and causes a rapid glucose spike. The faster and more concentrated the load of glucose, the larger the spike. However, when you eat fiber first, it forms a mesh in the intestine that slows down the digestion and absorption of sugars and starches that follow, leading to a much steadier glucose release.

Think of it like playing Tetris: when the blocks (glucose) come down slowly, they're easier to manage. Eating in the right order effectively slows down the speed at which glucose enters the bloodstream, making the process more manageable for your body. This reduces the demand for insulin, allowing the body to switch back to fat-burning mode faster.

TIP

When eating dishes such as a curry or casserole where proteins, fats, vegetables, and carbs are all mixed together, separating everything can feel tricky, but don't worry. I suggest you have a few bites of nonstarchy vegetables first and then enjoy the rest of the meal as it is.

Going green first

A longstanding tradition across many cultures is to begin meals with vegetables — an intuitive practice that aligns with how different foods affect the body. In regions like the Mediterranean, meals often start with marinated vegetable dishes. Similarly, in parts of the Middle East, fresh herbs and salads like tabbouleh are common openers. These fiber-rich starters help keep you fuller for longer and prevent the glucose spikes and dips that can lead to cravings later on.

REMEMBER

The key is to embrace a variety of vegetables — whether it's grilled zucchini, roasted broccoli, or a simple green salad — but be mindful of the form. Whole or lightly cooked vegetables retain their fiber, which plays an essential role in slowing the release of glucose. Soups can offer a healthy option packed with nutrients, but they often lack the fiber that curbs blood sugar spikes — especially if they're processed or made primarily from starchy vegetables like potatoes. Similarly, avoid juicing or mashing vegetables because this process can break down or remove much of the helpful fiber.

TIP

When dining out, I often start with a salad or order a vegetable-based side to enjoy before my main course. If I'm unsure of the options, I'll eat a handful of nuts before I head into the restaurant. Even these small adjustments can significantly impact your glucose levels!

Prioritizing high-quality protein every meal

Protein is your blood sugar's best friend. It stabilizes insulin, reduces cravings, and keeps you full longer. As the building blocks of hormones, proteins are essential for balanced hormone function. While protein needs vary by a person's size, age, activity level, and lifestyle, a general recommendation is 20 to 30 grams per meal for women (60 to 100 grams daily) and 30 grams per meal for men. For a list of high-quality protein sources, refer to the online appendix at www.dummies.com/go/hormonebalancefd.

Starting the day savory

WARNING

Many people assume that starting the day with something sweet gives them the energy boost they need. However, 2018 research from Stanford shows that eating a sugary breakfast can send glucose levels soaring to levels as high as those with diabetes, even if a person doesn't have the condition.

When you eat sugar-and starch-heavy foods on an empty stomach, they're quickly broken down into glucose, and your body is especially sensitive to glucose in the morning. Your breakfast can result in the highest glucose surge of the day, setting the stage for a roller coaster of sugar highs and crashes.

Starting the day with a savory, balanced meal that includes protein, healthy fats, and fiber helps flatten the glucose curve, providing more stable energy levels. Popular savory breakfasts around the world — eggs with vegetables in Turkey, the classic English breakfast with protein and fats, or omelets in the U.S. — provide you with a much better foundation for keeping blood sugar steady.

TIP

For the best results, aim for a breakfast that combines protein (such as eggs, Greek yogurt, or tofu), healthy fats (like avocado or nuts), and fiber (from vegetables or whole grains). For example, an avocado and eggs on whole-grain toast or a veggie-packed omelet. However, if you prefer something sweet in the morning, you don't have to give it up entirely to begin with. The trick is to eat it after your savory items. So have some eggs or Greek yogurt first, then enjoy a small portion of fruit, granola, or your favorite pastry afterward. This way, you get to enjoy your sweet treat without the extreme blood sugar spike.

Even smoothies can work for breakfast, but it's important to include the right ingredients. Add protein (a high-quality protein powder without hidden sugars or artificial additives), healthy fats (seeds or coconut oil), and fiber (from vegetables like spinach or avocado). Berries are always a great fruit choice because they're lower in sugar and higher in fiber compared to other fruits.

Partnering your carbs with protein, fat, or fiber

TIP

When you're out and about or in a situation where carbs and sugars are unavoidable, you can still make smart choices by pairing carbs with protein, fat, or fiber to slow down the glucose absorption into your bloodstream. For example, if you're reaching for a croissant in a meeting, go for the ham and cheese variety. If you're celebrating a colleague's birthday with chocolate cake in the office, add some Greek yogurt or nuts. You can do the same at home: Add avocado or cheese to your toast or crackers. If you're serving something sweet for dessert, top it with cream or yogurt.

REMEMBER

When it comes to whole grains such as brown rice or whole wheat pasta, they offer only a slight improvement in glucose response compared to refined grains, mainly due to their slightly higher fiber content. So, you also need to pair them with protein, fiber, or fat.

When selecting fats, prioritize healthy options such as olive oil, butter, ghee, coconut oil, or those from nuts, seeds, and avocados. If you're concerned about seed oils, recent evidence suggests that the worry around them may be overstated, but it's still best to avoid highly processed options such as soybean, corn, or rapeseed oils. For fiber, focus on vegetables, nuts, and seeds, or consider supplements like psyllium husk when on the go. For protein, aim for sources such as eggs, meat, dairy, nuts, seeds, or protein powders (without artificial sweeteners; check the online appendix for a helpful guide on how to choose your protein powder).

Sipping and stabilizing with vinegar

TIP

One of the simplest ways to reduce glucose spikes is by drinking a glass of water with one tablespoon of vinegar diluted in it before a meal, especially if you'll be eating something sweet or high in carbs. Research shows that vinegar can significantly flatten glucose and insulin spikes because its acetic acid slows down the rate at which food enters your small intestine, giving your body more time to digest and absorb glucose at a steadier pace. It also reduces the amount of insulin needed after eating.

TIP

Common vinegars such as apple cider, balsamic, red wine, and white wine vinegar are all effective, though apple cider vinegar is the most popular choice because of its milder taste when diluted in water. You can drink the mix up to 20 minutes before your meal, which is helpful when you're going out. I also like to carry a small bottle of apple cider vinegar with me in my bag to make sure I'm prepared.

If drinking vinegar doesn't sound appealing, you can start by using smaller amounts and gradually increase it. Alternatively, eating fermented vegetables soaked in vinegar as a starter will offer similar benefits. Cultures in the Mediterranean have long used vinegar in their cuisine for both flavor and its health benefits, often adding it to salad dressing or marinades (which you're welcome to do, too).

REMEMBER

Although vinegar is an easy and affordable tool for curbing glucose spikes, it's not a magic solution for an unhealthy diet. Additionally, although diluted vinegar isn't usually strong enough to harm your teeth, using a straw to drink the mix can help minimize any risk to your enamel.

Walking it off

Whenever your muscles contract during physical activity, they help burn glucose, making exercise a powerful tool for managing glucose levels. By simply walking for 10 minutes after a meal, you can lower your glucose spike by 3 to 27 percent. If you prefer more intense exercise, like resistance training or hitting the gym, that's even more effective, though some people find strenuous exercise right after eating uncomfortable.

The key is timing. Glucose spikes typically peak around 70 minutes after a meal, so moving your muscles before this peak is ideal. Resistance exercises in particular have been shown to reduce glucose spikes by as much as 30 percent immediately after a meal and can further reduce spikes over the next 24 hours by 35 percent.

Even small efforts make a difference. Walking after a meal, performing squats during a TV break, or doing calf raises at your desk can all help flatten your glucose curve. Research shows that short, frequent bursts of exercise seem to be more effective than longer isolated chunks of exercise when it comes to glucose regulation, so try to be active as possible throughout the day.

Building strong muscles and stablizing sugars

TIP

Building muscle is one of the most effective ways to support glucose regulation because muscles act as glucose storage tanks, soaking excess glucose from your bloodstream when needed. The more muscle mass you have, the more efficiently your body can clear glucose, reducing blood sugar spikes and improving insulin sensitivity.

Snoozing to lose the spikes

No matter how balanced your diet is, good sleep (seven to nine hours per night for most adults) is essential for managing glucose levels. One study found that just a few days of inadequate sleep led to glucose spikes up to 40 percent larger after meals. The good news is that just two nights of sufficient sleep can help restore you to normal glucose regulation.

Giving up the snacking

When you finish a meal, your body immediately enters what's called the postprandial state, which can last up to four hours as your organs work to process the nutrients from your food. During this time, blood rushes to your digestive organs, hormones are released, and your body prioritizes systems such as fat storage, while others, such as your immune system, take a back seat. This post-meal state can be demanding on the body, especially when your meal causes a significant glucose spike.

TIP

Historically, people often didn't snack between meals, meaning their bodies spent far less time in this postprandial state. Today, thanks to frequent snacking, most people spend up to 20 hours in this state, which increases stress on the body. When you give your body a break between meals, insulin levels drop, and your organs can shift into "clean-up" mode, removing damaged cells and repairing tissue. This also allows your body to start burning fat instead of storing it.

REMEMBER

This ability to easily switch between burning the glucose from your last meal and burning stored fat is called metabolic flexibility. You can boost it by eating larger, more balanced meals so you don't feel the need to snack constantly, or you can try intermittent fasting, which helps extend the periods when your body is out of the postprandial state and can support fat-burning and cellular repair. Keep in mind that fasting is based on gender and age, as explained later in this chapter in the "Considering gender differences for intermittent fasting" section.

Savory snacking

It's easy to reach for something sweet when you're feeling stressed, tired, or sluggish. But when you must have a snack, savory choices are much smarter for maintaining stable energy levels throughout the day, especially if you experience an afternoon slump.

Go for choices that provide the necessary fats, proteins, and fiber to keep your glucose levels stable. Examples are a spoonful of nut butter, Greek yogurt with nuts or seeds, carrots with hummus, almonds paired with a square of 90 percent dark chocolate, or veggie slices dipped in guacamole. You can also opt for a boiled egg to help curb your hunger while avoiding the energy dips that come with sugary snacks.

Saving your sweet treat for dessert

TIP

Instead of snacking on sweet treats throughout the day, try enjoying them as part of your dessert at the end of a meal. This approach helps keep your body out of the postprandial state for longer and reduces the glucose spike that sugary snacks can cause when eaten on their own. Also, adding cinnamon to your meals has been shown to help reduce glucose spikes, making it a simple and natural tool for improving metabolic health. So, try using Ceylon cinnamon, often called "true cinnamon," in your sweet treats!

SETTLING THE SWEET DEBATE

Many people believe that honey is a healthier alternative to sugar, but on a molecular level, there's essentially no difference between the two. Both honey and table sugar are made up of glucose and fructose molecules but are packaged differently. So, whether you're using honey, agave syrup, brown sugar, maple syrup, or even coconut sugar, the basic composition remains the same, and each causes the same blood sugar spikes regardless of whether they offer trace minerals or antioxidants (like those found in raw honey or maple syrup). Even so-called "natural" sweeteners such as molasses or evaporated cane juice are still forms of sugar and have similar effects on your glucose levels as table sugar. Interestingly, some artificial sweeteners can spike insulin levels, which may prime the body for fat storage and encourage weight gain. Therefore, the best sweeteners are natural alternatives such as monk fruit, pure stevia extract, and allulose.

Considering gender differences for intermittent fasting

Humans have historically thrived in a fasted state, with examples such as Ramadan demonstrating how the body can adapt to extended periods without food. Fasting is a useful tool because it taps into two primary energy systems: the sugar-burning system, which is activated after eating, and the fat-burning system, which kicks in about eight hours after your last meal. When fasting, the body depletes glycogen stores in the liver and begins to metabolize stored fat, making it a powerful tool for weight loss and metabolic health.

REMEMBER

Fasting triggers a host of beneficial processes, including insulin regulation, increased ketone production (which enhances fat-burning), improved gut health, and cellular repair. Studies even suggest that fasting can reset dopamine pathways and enhance immune function. However, it's important to acknowledge that intermittent fasting (IF) affects men and women differently due to hormonal differences, as described here:

- **Men:** Men tend to respond well to IF because their hormones are relatively stable throughout the month. A common approach is the 16:8 method (16 hours fasting, 8 hours eating), which has been shown to improve both metabolic health and fat loss.

REMEMBER

- **Women:** For women, the approach needs to be more nuanced due to the cyclical nature of their hormones. Each phase of a woman's menstrual cycle requires different nutritional considerations, and strict intermittent fasting can disrupt hormone balance if not timed correctly. To find out more information on fasting for women, I highly recommend the free YouTube content by Dr. Mindy Pelz.

Here are some general guidelines for naturally cycling premenopausal women. Refer to Chapter 12 for more information about the various phases of the menstrual cycle:

- **Menstrual phase:** All forms of fasting are suitable. Your longest fasts should take place during this phase because estrogen and progesterone are at their lowest levels.
- **Follicular phase:** This is a good time for intermittent fasting, but it's advised you keep fasts shorter than 15 hours and eat dinner earlier rather than skipping breakfast.
- **Ovulation phase:** You can do some fasting, but if you have lower progesterone levels, it's better to focus on eating hormone-supportive foods (such as carbohydrates, healthy fats, and proteins). Long fasts are generally not recommended during this phase.
- **Luteal phase:** Minimize or avoid fasting as the body prepares for menstruation. Focus on nutrient-dense foods to support hormone production and energy.

There's less variation in the fasting recommendations for menopausal and postmenopausal women:

- **Menopausal women:** During this transition, women should avoid extreme fasting windows and start with shorter fasting windows, such as 13 to 15 hours, which helps support blood sugar stability and promotes metabolic health without overly stressing the body.
- **Postmenopausal women:** Once women enter menopause, their hormonal fluctuations level out (making their response to fasting more similar to men's) so they can engage in longer fasts more regularly. Fasting windows of 15 to 24 hours (or Dr. Pelz suggests even 36 to 48 hours) can be incorporated.

FASTED WORKOUTS

While they can promote fat burning and metabolic flexibility, their suitability varies by gender and age. Experts such as Dr. Stacy Sims caution that, for women, fasts may increase cortisol levels and disrupt hormone balance, particularly if poorly timed. Alternating fasted and nonfasted workouts or avoiding them during certain menstrual phases can help support overall health and fitness.

Improving your gut health

TIP

Nurturing a healthy, varied gut microbiome helps you maintain better blood sugar stability. For example, when you're fasting, these beneficial microbes send signals that encourage the liver to switch over to burning fat for energy. However, if your gut lacks diversity — often due to factors such as multiple rounds of antibiotics — it can interfere with this signalling, making it harder to stay in a fasted state or regulate blood sugar effectively.

TIP

Luckily, it's possible to restore and diversify your gut microbiome relatively quickly. By incorporating gut-friendly foods, eating a whole food nutrient-dense diet free processed foods, and following the strategies outlined in Chapter 10 promotes better gut health and, in turn, improves your body's ability to manage glucose, estrogen, cortisol, and serotonin production, supporting overall hormone balance.

Regulating Your Stress Hormones

REMEMBER

Stress is often thought of as something that happens to you, triggered by external events, people or circumstances. However, the truth is that stress is largely an inside-out job, shaped by how you interpret and respond to the world around you. Your internal dialogue, thoughts, beliefs, and perceptions all have a profound influence on how stress manifests in your body. Remember, you can't control what happens to you, but you can control how you respond. Simple strategies, like wearing blue light-blocking glasses before bed, can help lower cortisol levels and promote a sense of calm, supporting the deeper work suggested in the following section (refer to Chapter 20 for a deeper explanation).

Meeting your inner voice

Your inner voice — the constant mental dialogue everyone has — is one of the most powerful forces in shaping your experience of life. It's primarily based on a combination of your past experiences, beliefs, subconscious patterns, and the meanings you have attached to various events throughout your life. You can reshape how your inner voice speaks to you as part of your stress-management response.

Adjusting your focus

TIP

The first step to meeting and mastering your inner voice is becoming aware of where your focus lies. Are you constantly fixated on potential problems, shortcomings, or failures? Or do you make room for positive outcomes and possibilities? For example, focusing on worst-case scenarios amplifies your body's stress response, triggering higher cortisol levels. Focusing on the most likely or best-case scenarios, solutions, or gratitude can promote relaxation and, therefore, better hormone balance. Journaling and meditation are great practices to connect you with your inner voice.

Interpreting the meaning

Once you've identified what you're focused on, determine what do you decide it means. A missed opportunity might mean failure to one person, but it could also mean a chance for growth or learning to another who views failure as a stop along the journey to inevitable success. When your inner dialogue frames situations as threats or failures, it activates your body's stress responses. However, when you reframe these moments as growth opportunities, you can dampen the intensity of the stress reaction or avoid it all together.

Taking action

REMEMBER

Finally, consider how your inner voice shapes your actions. When you're stressed, you might fall into patterns of avoidance or overreaction. These behaviors, in turn, reinforce the stress response, creating a vicious cycle. By consciously shifting your inner narrative — changing how you talk to yourself — you can take more empowered, grounded actions. This might mean practicing mindfulness, choosing healthier coping mechanisms, or simply pausing before reacting. Therapeutic solutions outlined in Chapter 9 can also be enormously helpful in shifting your inner dialogue on a subconscious level.

Understanding your body's signals

Understanding your personal stress signals — both in your body and behavior as outlined in Chapter 9 — can help you manage it more effectively. This means tuning in to how your body responds under different states of your nervous system. For example, when you're in a sympathetic (fight-or-flight) state, you might feel your heart racing, notice shallow breathing, experience muscle tension, start scrolling on social media, or feel agitated. Conversely, when you're in a parasympathetic (rest-and-digest) state, your body feels relaxed, breathing becomes deeper, your heart rate slows, and you may experience a sense of calm and desire to connect deeply with others.

TIP

As you become aware of your patterns and triggers, you can start using stress management techniques such as deep breathing to shift yourself back into a more relaxed, parasympathetic state. Additionally, understanding your patterns gives you the option to explore therapeutic treatments outlined in Chapter 9 that can help rewire how your brain and body respond to different situations, reducing the intensity of your reactions as your brain creates new pathways.

Removing conscious stress

Conscious stress refers to the stressors you're fully aware of, such as looming work deadlines, family conflicts, financial worries, or juggling multiple responsibilities. They can easily overload your nervous system, but you have the power to address them and create more nervous system capacity by delegating tasks, detoxing unnecessary obligations, and letting go of what's not serving you:

» **Delegate:** Not everything on your to-do list has to be done by you (seriously, it doesn't) so start identifying tasks or responsibilities that can be passed on to others. Delegating not only reduces your mental, emotional, and physical stress load but also allows you to focus on what truly matters and where your expertise is most needed, which boosts your sense of fulfilment and purpose.

REMEMBER

» **Detox:** Some stressors come from internal expectations or patterns of behavior that can be adjusted. Detoxing from perfectionism, people-pleasing, or overcommitment will help clear mental and emotional space. For example, reframe negative thoughts or let go of the need for everything to be perfect. Simplifying your schedule by cutting out unnecessary commitments creates more time for rest and recovery and restores the capacity of your nervous system so you can pour into the people you love from a place of overflowing energy and presence.

REMEMBER

» **Ditch:** Evaluate your responsibilities and stressors and identify which can be eliminated entirely. Look for tasks that don't serve your personal or professional growth or well-being. Ditch the things that create stress but don't contribute to your goals or happiness.

Releasing unprocessed emotions and historical stress

TIP

Exercise is one of the most potent avenues for processing unprocessed emotions and releasing historical stress, which is why you may find yourself getting emotional during or after a workout. Fascinatingly, both strength training and dance have been shown to rival the effects of antidepressants, such as selective serotonin reuptake inhibitors (SSRIs), by significantly improving mood and alleviating depression. Starting your day with exercise, music, or dance will have a profound impact on your emotional health by releasing endorphins and fostering joy.

If you're seeking more targeted practices, here are four somatic emotional release techniques you can easily do at home or in any space where you feel safe and comfortable:

TIP

- **Rocking:** In a seated or lying position, gently rock your body back and forth for two to five minutes. This rhythmic, repetitive motion soothes the nervous system, releasing stored emotional tension. Allow the movement to be slow and calming. This is a great one to do in bed as you prepare for sleep.
- **Shake and twist:** Stand tall and tune into your body. Begin shaking your hands, legs, arms, and feet for two to three minutes, as if you're shaking off water. Then plant your feet wider than your shoulders and twist your torso from side to side, letting your arms swing freely for three to five minutes.
- **Breathwork:** Inhale slowly and fully through your nose, expanding your abdomen, and exhale fully through your mouth until you empty your lungs. This intentional diaphragmatic breathing helps bring emotions to the surface and encourages emotional release. YouTube is a great resource for free, guided sessions.
- **Body scanning:** Lie down and bring your awareness to the top of your head. Slowly scan your body and as you move through each area, gently observe any tension or tightness without judgment. When you notice tension, take a deep, cleansing breath, inhaling calmness and protection, and exhale, releasing stress and tightness from that area. Continue this practice all the way through your body, allowing each part to soften and relax with your breath.

TIP

Begin each practice by tuning into your body and mind, bringing awareness to any areas of tightness or tension. You may find it helpful to journal your observations for deeper reflection. At the conclusion of the practice, take a moment to reassess how you feel, noting any physical or mental shifts. This mindful approach helps you track emotional and physical changes over time. If emotions come up during this practice, stay present with them and allow them to flow without judgment. Emotions are meant to be felt and processed.

Rewiring your brain to boost self-worth

To rewire your brain's neural pathways and strengthen emotional resilience — which directly impacts your hormone balance and nervous system — it's crucial to access your subconscious mind, where your deeply ingrained beliefs and stress responses reside. Techniques such as EMDR, EFT tapping, and hypnosis (all covered in Chapter 9) are highly effective in reshaping these patterns and reducing chronic stress responses. However, you can implement easy and actionable daily habits that will reshape your subconscious gently over time:

TIP

- **Affirmations:** Repeated positive affirmations can create new neural pathways in the brain, replacing negative beliefs with empowering ones. For example, you could repeat, "I am good enough, worthy, and capable," out loud as you drive yourself to work each morning, or you could listen to a free affirmation playlist from YouTube.
- **Visualizations:** Visualizing positive outcomes engages the brain's neural circuits, making it easier to adopt behaviors that align with a confident self-image. Before you go to sleep each night, visualize the highest version of yourself and how you will navigate the following day. Imagine how it feels, focusing on success, ease, and confidence.
- **Challenging negative thoughts:** Reframing negative thoughts disrupts old patterns, encouraging the brain to create new, healthier associations. For example, when a self-critical thought comes up, stop and replace it with, "I'm always learning, growing, and improving. I've got this."
- **Gratitude practice:** Gratitude strengthens positive neural networks and boosts self-esteem. Each evening, write down three things you appreciate about yourself or your day or make it a practice for your family to share one thing you're each grateful when you sit at the dinner table.

Boosting Happy Hormones

When your body's happy hormones — dopamine, serotonin, oxytocin, and endorphins (DOSE) — are balanced, you feel much more positive, motivated, and resilient, both physically and emotionally. Fortunately, they're easily boosted through a variety of simple, accessible activities.

Detoxing dopamine

TIP

The dopamine menu approach — a curated list of healthy, rewarding activities categorized like a restaurant menu — offers a simple, effective solution to resetting your dopamine levels. Take 10 minutes to create your dopamine menu and add some of the habits to your hormone balance action plan. Keep your menu on file somewhere handy (perhaps in a notes app on your phone) so you can refer to it anytime you need to choose healthier, more sustainable sources of dopamine that align with your long-term hormonal and emotional well-being.

Here are the "courses" of the menu:

- **Appetizers:** Quick, easy dopamine hits e.g. stretching, cuddling a pet, drinking a cup of coffee, eating a snack, taking a shower, or listening to your favorite song. These short activities offer a burst of pleasure without drawing you into overstimulation.
- **Mains:** These activities require a bit more effort but provide longer-lasting dopamine rewards e.g. strength training, yoga, journaling, cooking, baking, or taking a walk in nature. They promote a healthier, sustained release of dopamine, supporting emotional resilience and hormone balance.
- **Sides:** These activities add stimulation to boring or mundane tasks, such as listening to music or a podcast while putting together your weekly report for work or turning chores into a game by setting a timer to see how fast you can get them done.
- **Desserts:** These enjoyable but indulgent activities (Netflix bingeing, playing video games, or social media scrolling) should be limited to avoid overstimulation or dopamine crashes.

Asserting your authenticity

REMEMBER

People who live the longest, healthiest lives thrive on a sense of purpose and strong social ties. This purpose is closely linked to authenticity as your nervous system responds not just to what you're doing but to why you're doing it. For example, if you're working for a company with values you disagree with just to meet others' expectations, your nervous system will likely remain in a state of stress. However, if you do the same job at a company with values and mission that align with your own, where you feel valued, seen, and heard as your authentic self, your body reduce stress hormones, and you'll experience more balance and overall well-being.

TIP

Here are some ways to assert your authenticity:

- **Make time for your passions and interests:** Prioritize the activities that light you up, make the time fly, and bring you joy.
- **Honor your values:** Act in line with what matters most to you. When you're living according to your values and principles, it eases internal conflict and reduces nervous system tension.
- **Set clear boundaries:** Boundaries protect your time and energy. Learning to say no is crucial for functioning from a place of calm and empowerment rather than stress and overdrive.

» **Speak your truth:** Expressing yourself honestly even when it's scary or difficult is much less physiologically stressful on the body in the long term than suppressing it.

» **Surround yourself with supportive people:** Authenticity flourishes in environments where you feel seen, valued, and supported. Build a community that encourages you to express your radical authenticity, even if it's people you connect with online to begin with.

» **Listen to your body's signals:** Notice how you feel when you're in alignment with your values and passions. Your body will naturally relax as opposed to feeling tight, tense, or constricted.

Supporting Your Detox Organs

REMEMBER

Researchers from Switzerland and other countries discovered in 2024 that of the roughly 14,000 known chemicals in our food packaging, 3,601 of those — or about 25 percent — have been found in the human body in samples of blood, hair, or breast milk. Many of these chemicals are known to disrupt the endocrine system or cause cancer or other diseases. Unfortunately, we can't eliminate all toxins, but we can absolutely raise awareness in our communities and advocate for larger regulatory changes.

By minimizing your personal toxic load using the advice in this section (as well using suggestions in Chapter 3), you may significantly lower your risk of chronic fatigue, hormone imbalances, dementia, diabetes, autoimmune diseases, and more, as well as reduce your environmental burden. These small individual actions, when combined with broader efforts, will create the meaningful change we need for both our bodies, future generations, and the planet. For a full list of chemicals to avoid you can refer to the online appendix at `www.dummies.com/go/hormonebalancefd`.

Reducing your toxic load

Incorporate the following actions into your life to reduce your toxic load:

TIP

» **Eat organic:** Switching to organic fruits, vegetables, and meats reduces pesticide exposure dramatically. One 2014 study published in *Environmental Research* found a 90 percent drop in urinary pesticides after just one week of eating organic.

- **Choose antibiotic- and hormone-free meat:** Conventional meat often contains hormones and antibiotics that disrupt your endocrine system. Choose pasture-raised, organic meats or wild-caught fish over farmed fish, which can be contaminated with pollutants.
- **Filter your water:** Many chemicals leach into tap water. Use a high-quality water filter to reduce exposure, and avoid plastic water bottles, which can contain harmful chemicals.
- **Avoid all plastics:** Reduce the use of plastics, especially for food storage because chemicals can leach into your food. Great alternatives are glass or stainless-steel containers.
- **Choose natural cleaning products:** Conventional household cleaners and detergents often contain harmful chemicals. Switch to natural, nontoxic alternatives to protect your hormones and reduce indoor air pollution. This doesn't have to be an expensive exercise; you can do a lot with natural ingredients such as apple cider vinegar, which is effective for cleaning surfaces, deodorizing, and even disinfecting. Baking soda and castile soap are other great natural options that clean effectively without harsh toxins.
- **Revamp your beauty routine**: Many cosmetics contain hormone-disrupting chemicals like parabens and phthalates. Choose clean, natural skincare, makeup, and haircare products and ditch standard nail polish for toxin-free versions.

Protecting your kidney and liver

Here are some ways you can protect your kidneys and liver, your detox organs:

TIP

- **Stay hydrated:** Drinking plenty of filtered water aids your kidneys in flushing out toxins. Herbal teas such as nettle or dandelion root are also great options.
- **Eat a liver-supportive diet:** Focus on foods that nourish your liver, such as cruciferous vegetables (broccoli, kale, cauliflower), leafy greens, and foods high in antioxidants, such as berries and citrus fruits. Garlic and turmeric are also excellent for liver health.
- **Avoid processed foods and alcohol:** Highly processed foods and excessive alcohol intake can strain your liver. By minimizing your consumption, you allow the liver to focus on hormone detoxification rather than managing unhealthy external compounds.
- **Incorporate detoxifying herbs:** Herbs such as milk thistle and burdock root are well-known for their liver-protective properties. As always, please consult your healthcare professional before starting any new supplement regimes.

Supporting the lymphatic system

TIP

Your lymphatic system doesn't have a central "pump," so it's up to you to stimulate it to keep your body detoxifying effectively. Here are some ways you can do that:

- **Stay active:** Exercises such as walking, jogging, yoga, or jumping on a trampoline for 10 to 15 minutes daily encourage lymph flow.
- **Dry brushing:** Use a natural bristle brush and start at your feet, brushing upward toward your heart in long, gentle strokes for 5 to 10 minutes before a shower.
- **The Big 6 Lymph Reset by Dr. Perry Nickelston:** This self-massage technique targets key lymphatic areas to enhance flow and detoxification. It's a simple, effective routine you can do at home and easily follow along watching Dr. Nickelston's YouTube videos at `www.youtube.com/watch?v=1T_wW5pNHa4`.
- **Lymphatic massage and acupressure:** Consider scheduling a lymphatic drainage massage or use an acupressure mat at home to stimulate lymph flow and release muscle tension.
- **Hydration:** Hit your water goal each day (2 to 3 liters) to keep your lymphatic fluid moving efficiently. Add a pinch of sea salt or lemon juice for added mineral support.

IN THIS CHAPTER

- » Exporing the dynamic role hormones play during adolescence
- » Empowering teens with education and actionable insights
- » Safeguarding mental and emotional health

Chapter 18 Fostering Hormone Balance in Teenagers

Nothing truly prepares you for the wild ride of puberty — whether you're going through it yourself or witnessing a child or loved one transform into a young adult. Adolescence is a critical period for both hormone and personal development, during which rapid and often bewildering changes shape a teenager's physical, emotional, and mental landscapes. The sentiment that "adults just don't understand" has echoed through generations of teenagers, but today's adolescents truly are facing a new set of challenges. Rising rates of anxiety, the relentless pressures of social media, increasingly sedentary lifestyles, the rise of vaping, and the intensifying demands of academic achievement in a competitive world have added new layers of complexity to an already turbulent time. More than ever, adolescents need deep understanding and unwavering support from those around them.

Understanding the impact of hormonal shifts during this time is not only essential for alleviating the immediate symptoms of adolescence, but it also plays a crucial role in building a healthy hormonal foundation for the future. This chapter explores practical ways to guide and support teenagers through this transition — empowering them to develop a healthy relationship with their hormones with strategies that manage the physical, emotional, and mental challenges to come.

Appreciating the Importance of Hormone Health in Adolescence

The hormonal shifts that define puberty are intricately linked to mood regulation and mental health, influencing energy levels and emotional stability while teens undergo significant physical changes. Indeed, emotional health during this period can significantly impact a teen's life trajectory, affecting their self-esteem, social relationships, and academic performance. For a more in-depth understanding of these hormonal shifts, refer to Chapter 4, which reviews the different stages of male and female sex hormone transformation throughout life.

REMEMBER

It's important to recognize that the experience of puberty is not the same for everyone. For transgender and nonbinary adolescents, this period can be especially challenging as they navigate both the physical and emotional transformations of puberty while grappling with their gender identity. Although this book primarily addresses the hormonal changes typical of cisgender male and female puberty, it's essential to acknowledge that the journeys of transgender and nonbinary adolescents are valid, complex, and deserving of attention.

Estrogen and progesterone's effect on emotional health

Estrogen and progesterone are two of the most influential hormones during puberty when it comes to emotional health, and their effects are most pronounced in females. Estrogen, often referred to as a "mood modulator," plays a crucial role in emotional regulation because of its impact on serotonin — a neurotransmitter linked to mood stabilization. When estrogen levels are at their peak, such as during certain phases of the menstrual cycle, it tends to foster a positive mood. However, as estrogen levels decline, particularly in the latter half of the cycle, serotonin production can also decrease, potentially leading to mood swings, irritability, feelings of sadness, or heightened anxiety.

Progesterone, meanwhile, has a more complex relationship with emotional health. It is known to have a calming effect due to its role in enhancing GABA, a neurotransmitter that reduces neuronal excitability and promotes relaxation. However, when progesterone levels drop abruptly — such as just before menstruation or in response to stress — it can contribute to mood instability, anxiety, and even depressive symptoms.

Men have small amounts of these hormones as well, although the impact on their emotional health is less direct and typically overshadowed by the more prominent effects of testosterone. Nonetheless, the balance of hormones — including the small levels of estrogen and progesterone present in males —still contributes to young men's emotional well-being.

Testosterone: Not just for boys

REMEMBER

While testosterone is responsible for physical changes such as muscle growth, deepening of the voice, and body hair in boys, it also influences mood and behavior. Increased testosterone levels during puberty have been linked to assertiveness, risk-taking behaviors, and, in some cases, aggression. However, low levels of testosterone can result in fatigue and depressive symptoms.

Girls also produce testosterone, though in smaller amounts, and while the research is still evolving, it's clear that testosterone's influence on mood and behavior extends beyond gender boundaries. For instance, higher testosterone levels in girls may encourage assertiveness or risk-taking, while low levels may contribute to lethargy and mood swings.

Sensation seeking and impulsivity

REMEMBER

As we are all aware from countless movies or personal experience, adolescence is a time marked by heightened thrill-seeking and risk-taking. Sensation-seeking, defined as the pursuit of high-intensity and stimulating experiences, increases significantly during this period due to a combination of rising reproductive hormones and social pressures. As puberty progresses, both boys and girls exhibit elevated levels of sensation-seeking, which peaks between ages 13 and 16. This drive often leads to behaviors such as experimenting with drugs, engaging in unprotected sex, and other impulsive actions like driving too fast. This is different from impulsivity that involves acting quickly without considering consequences, a behavior that steadily decreases from childhood into adulthood as the prefrontal cortex continues to develop. This dual pattern of heightened sensation-seeking and still-developing impulse control during early adolescence helps explain why teenagers are particularly prone to risky behaviors, even when they are cognitively aware of potential negative outcomes.

Social dominance and sexual behaviors

REMEMBER

While hormonal changes during puberty certainly contribute to the drive for social dominance and sexual behaviors, peer dynamics, social hierarchies, and prior experiences also play a significant role here. These patterns of behavior differ across genders, with testosterone often driving more aggressive or competitive tendencies in males, and estrogen and progesterone influencing emotional responses and mood regulation in females.

While testosterone in males contributes to competitive and sometimes risk-taking behaviors, the expression of these behaviors is also shaped by social environments, peer pressure, and individual experiences. For females, estrogen and progesterone contribute to emotional regulation, but social factors like peer relationships and perceived social status can further influence how these hormonal changes manifest in behavior.

TIP

Ultimately, the teen push for dominance, social standing, and personal identity is as much about navigating complex social landscapes as it is about hormonal changes, with both factors working together to shape a teenager's transition into adulthood. Encouraging open dialogue, setting healthy boundaries, and providing a stable support system can help adolescents better navigate these challenges.

Social relationships and emotional intelligence

TIP

Because hormones shape physical and emotional development, they also influence social relationships. Increased levels of estrogen and testosterone can intensify feelings of attachment and attraction, making this a time when teens are likely to explore romantic relationships and deeper social connections. However, these same hormones can also lead to jealousy, heartbreak, and social anxiety, which is why developing emotional intelligence — the ability to understand and manage one's emotions — is such a powerful tool. By cultivating self-awareness, emotional regulation, and empathy through practices such as journaling, mindfulness, and active listening, adolescents can start to recognize and regulate their emotions much more effectively.

Educating to Empower

REMEMBER

Strong relationships between adolescents and supportive adults have been consistently associated with numerous positive outcomes, ranging from enhanced psychosocial well-being to better academic performance. For example, a study published in *The Journal of Youth and Adolescence* demonstrated that adolescents with strong connections to parents, teachers, or other caring adults are more likely to experience fewer behavioral problems, exhibit greater self-regulation, and maintain higher levels of self-esteem. This support also correlates with lower rates of depression, anxiety, and substance abuse, underscoring the protective nature of these relationships during a particularly vulnerable period of life.

Encouraging open communication

REMEMBER

Adolescents who feel supported are more likely to seek advice and share concerns about their physical, emotional, and social challenges, including topics like peer pressure, sexual health, and mental health. For instance, research conducted by the Center for Disease Control and Prevention (CDC) found that adolescents with strong connections to at least one trusted adult were more likely to engage in healthy behaviors, such as regular exercise and healthy eating, and were less likely to engage in risky behaviors such as drug use or early sexual activity.

TIP

Open, honest discussions about the body and hormonal changes should also be normalized. Adolescence is an awkward and confusing time, and it's essential to slay any shame that may arise around topics related to the human body. Let your teenagers know that it's completely okay to talk about these things and reinforce that no topic is off-limits. They may resist or say it's "too awkward," and while teenagers may sometimes shy away from discussing sensitive topics with their parents, it's also natural and healthy for them to seek advice or guidance from other trusted adults such as teachers, their friend's parent, an aunt, counselor, or mentor. Encourage them to do so if that makes them feel more comfortable. After all, what matters most is that they feel validated and supported.

Helping teens embrace their hormones

REMEMBER

Hormonal fluctuations are one of the main drivers of mood swings during adolescence, but they are certainly not the only factor. Stress, sleep deprivation, body image concerns, dietary changes, social media use, and social pressures can all exacerbate emotional volatility (and hormone levels themselves), which is why working together to identify specific triggers can help teens and their caregivers navigate the ups and downs with less friction.

Additionally, a holistic, root-cause approach that promotes a hormone-supportive lifestyle will set teenagers up with positive habits they can take forward into adulthood, such as the following:

- **Managing diet and blood sugar regulation:** Ensuring they eat balanced meals rich in whole foods, healthy fats, and lean proteins can help regulate blood sugar levels, which in turn helps stabilize mood, energy, and hormone levels. Encouraging regular meals and avoiding excess sugar or processed foods fosters long-term hormonal balance.

- **Taking care of their nervous system:** Encouraging them to techniques such as deep-breathing exercises, yoga, journaling, or mindfulness can help them manage emotional reactions and build resilience that will serve them well as adults.
- **Encouraging authentic self-expression:** Helping them find ways to express their authentic selves — whether through creative outlets, hobbies, or activities with friends that give them a sense of purpose — can boost crucial "happy hormones" such as dopamine and serotonin to create a positive feedback loop that reinforces emotional stability and supports broader hormone balance.
- **Sleep, sleep, sleep:** Most adolescents rely on the Internet as their primary method of communication; viewing it as essential to their daily lives. However, late-night technology use disrupts sleep patterns, leading to insufficient rest during a critical phase of development. It's important to note that the circadian rhythm naturally shifts later in teenagers, making later bedtimes and rising times a normal part of their development. So, teenagers aren't being lazy when they struggle to get out of bed. It's their natural sleep pattern. Early school schedules, which start as early as 7:00 a.m. in some countries, are completely misaligned with teenage circadian rhythms and contribute to sleep deprivation, impacting learning and overall health. Strategies such as implementing consistent sleep routines, using blue light–blocking glasses, limiting screen time before bed, and emphasizing the long-term benefits of adequate sleep can help adolescents achieve the recommended 8 to 10 hours of rest.
- **Supporting detox organs:** Encouraging teens to support their liver, kidneys, and skin greatly supports hormone health during this period where the body is trying to establish its new rhythms. See the online appendix at `www.dummies.com/go/hormonebalancefd` for more information.
- **Encouraging healthy communication:** Creating a safe space for teens to express their feelings and concerns without fear of judgment or emotional retaliation can help them better understand and regulate their own emotions and feel seen, heard, and supported.

Tracking the menstrual cycle

TIP

Encouraging young women to track their menstrual cycles (whether via an app or calendar) is a powerful way to help them connect with and appreciate their bodies. Though cycles can be irregular during adolescence, tracking provides insight into the four phases described in Chapter 12 — menstrual, follicular, ovulatory, and luteal — and their associated hormonal shifts that impact mood and energy.

It's important to reassure young women that it may take time for their cycles to stabilize and tracking can help them recognize patterns and anticipate changes. Cycle syncing, which aligns lifestyle and activities with each phase of the menstrual cycle, can further support their well-being by encouraging rest during menstruation, more vigorous activity or focused studying during ovulation, and calming practices in the luteal phase. (Read more about cycle syncing in Chapter 12.)

Protecting Mental and Emotional Well-being

Mental health ups and downs are common during adolescence, and hormonal changes can certainly amplify feelings of anxiety or depression. While some level of anxiety is normal, especially in response to school pressures or social conflicts, it becomes concerning when symptoms such as persistent worrying, restlessness, and physical symptoms like rapid heart rate, fatigue, or difficulty concentrating interfere with daily activities. Depression, on the other hand, often appears as persistent sadness, loss of interest in activities once enjoyed, changes in appetite or sleep, feelings of worthlessness, or difficulty focusing. It's normal for teens to experience occasional bouts of sadness, low moods or disinterest, but the persistent presence of these feelings may require professional intervention if support from family and friends falls short.

TIP

Reducing screen time and prioritizing nervous system regulation is crucial. Teenagers are still learning how to cope with big, sudden, and often overwhelming emotional experiences, and teaching them that it's okay to feel stressed, sad, or anxious and showing them effective ways to process, work through, and release those feelings sets them up for long-term emotional resilience that supports hormonal balance. For example, rather than resorting to numbing behaviors such as overeating, excessive screen time, or unhealthy coping mechanisms, adults should model or guide teenagers through activities that help regulate the nervous systems such as talking a walk, practicing deep breathing, exercising, or engaging in creative outlets.

Identifying stressors in teen life

REMEMBER

Today's teens face both traditional stressors and new, often overlooked challenges such as social media, rising concerns around climate change, the pressures of forming gender and sexual identities and exposure to cyberbullying. Academic pressures have also intensified as they prepare for a rapidly evolving and hypercompetitive job market, adding to feelings of uncertainty about the future. Understanding these hidden stressors helps create a safe space for teens to express their concerns, enabling adults to better support and guide them through these challenges.

Cultivating healthy body image and self-esteem

The disorienting physical changes brought about by puberty such as growth spurts, acne, and shifts in body fat distribution, may significantly affect a teenager's body image, self-talk, confidence, and self-esteem. Helping them navigate their concerns and any societal pressures regarding ideal body shapes and sizes with validation, empathy, and support will enable them to embrace their developing bodies with greater confidence. Here are some helpful strategies:

TIP

- **Encourage body positivity:** Highlight the importance of health over physical appearance and foster an environment where diverse body types are accepted and celebrated.
- **Model positive behavior:** Your attitude toward your own body can significantly influence your teen. Show appreciation for your body rather than focusing on physical appearance or perceived flaws, and care for it well with healthy meals and regular exercise. While it may often feel like they're not listening to you, they are.
- **Promote open communication:** Provide a safe space for teens to express their concerns and insecurities about their changing bodies (whether it's with you or members of your wider family/community/support network). Empower them with knowledge about their hormones so that they understand the natural changes their bodies go through during adolescence.
- **Focus on internal attributes:** Remind them that their value isn't determined by their physical appearance (although you recognize that it certainly feels that way as a teen). Praise their resilience, adaptability, effort, confidence, skills, abilities, and commitment to growth.

Sourcing support

REMEMBER

Seeking professional help is not a sign of weakness — rather, it's a compassionate and proactive step forward. Some key signs that indicate it may be time to seek professional mental or emotional help include persistent and intense mood swings, prolonged feelings of sadness or hopelessness, noticeable changes in appetite or sleep patterns, withdrawal from social activities, a sudden decline in academic performance, or engagement in self-destructive behaviors.

Therapists who specialize in adolescent mental health can offer tailored psychotherapy to address their specific challenges. Additionally, school counselors, pediatricians, and family doctors can also be valuable resources, providing guidance and connecting families with mental health professionals. However, child and adolescent mental health services (CAMHS) are often oversubscribed, with long waiting lists, especially in the U.K., which can exacerbate mental health issues before support is accessible. Increased investment in these services is urgently needed but by taking proactive steps, families can create environments that foster resilience.

IN THIS CHAPTER

» Assessing the pros and cons of hormone replacement therapy

» Understanding the impact of diet and lifestyle decisions

» Embracing the power of mental and emotional health

Chapter 19

Maintaining Hormone Balance in Older Age

Think of your hormones as the wind and tides that guide your boat (your body and well-being in this analogy). When you're young, the winds might be strong and steady, making it easier to sail smoothly. But as you age, the winds shift unpredictably, and the tides become more complex. Sometimes the wind is too strong; other times, it dies down completely, and the tides can pull you off course. Although you can't control the wind or the tides, you can learn to navigate them with small adjustments such as changing course slightly, trimming the sails, or shifting your weight to maintain stability and keep your boat moving forward.

Similarly, as your hormones fluctuate with age, you won't always find perfect balance, but you can learn to work with the changes and optimize your body's natural rhythms. By paying attention to your symptoms, practicing good habits, seeking medical support and adjusting as needed, you can keep yourself on course, even as conditions around you continue to shift.

Regardless of whether you're already experiencing these changes, this chapter is crucial reading as humans' natural decline in hormonal function as they age is one of the most significant factors influencing both lifespan and health span, contributing to chronic issues such as atherosclerosis (where the arteries become narrowed and hardened), diabetes, osteoporosis, and even cognitive decline — particularly for those with metabolic problems. Alzheimer's, for instance, is increasingly referred to as "type 3 diabetes." However, with the right knowledge and proactive strategies, you can mitigate these risks and support a healthier, more vibrant life at every stage.

The following pages explore the potential benefits and risks of hormone replacement therapy (HRT), delve into essential diet and lifestyle strategies that promote optimal hormonal health, and uncover the critical role that mental and emotional well-being plays in the aging process.

Understanding Hormone Replacement Therapy

Thanks to wonderful advances in medicine, people now live longer than ever before in history, with the U.S. population aged 65 and older projected to exceed 83 million by 2050. Similar trends are in effect worldwide as global life expectancy continues to rise. As the world population ages, there's an increasing focus not just on living longer but living well by preserving vitality and supporting both physical and mental health.

From a medical perspective, supporting the hormone health of older adults presents two primary challenges: accurate interpretation of diagnostic tests and the implementation of personalized treatment plans. Unfortunately, clinical trials tend to under enroll older participants, meaning much of what is recommended is based on studies in younger populations. The aging process is highly complex, with individual factors such as gender, nutrition, medication use, and comorbidities (the presence of two or more diseases) complicating the interpretation of hormone levels, and there is an urgent need for specific diagnostic thresholds in older populations to accurately assess and manage these changes.

TIP

Effectively managing hormonal health in older adults requires a very nuanced understanding of the physiology of aging to avoid misdiagnosis. A thorough assessment of nutritional and functional health and social, factors such as feelings of loneliness or fulfillment, are also valuable. While personalized treatment protocols tailored to the needs of older adults are on the horizon, they are not yet mainstream practice, which is why it's so important to take individual responsibility and educate yourself on the shifts that are occurring. Proactively monitoring your symptoms, exploring supportive interventions, and engaging with healthcare professionals who understand the complexities of aging hormones can all help to enhance your quality of life.

Endocrine system changes in older age

REMEMBER

Although changes to hormone secretion patterns, receptor sensitivity, and hormone metabolism remain relatively underexplored, what is clear is that aging impacts several hormones that play crucial roles in maintaining physical performance, body composition, metabolic health, and cognitive function.

Testosterone, estrogen, progesterone, dehydroepiandrosterone (DHEA), and growth hormone/insulin-like growth factor 1 (GH/IGF-1) all decline naturally with age, and symptoms show up differently in men and women. Understanding these intricate hormonal shifts is essential when weighing the benefits of emerging and evolving treatment options such as hormone replacement therapy (HRT), which I discuss in the next section, so here's a closer look at what they entail:

- **Menopause:** Marked by gradual fluctuations in estrogen and progesterone levels during midlife, leading to physical and emotional changes and eventually resulting in the permanent cessation of menstruation. For many women, hormone levels fluctuate over several years before stabilizing at lower levels once menopause is complete. Read more about menopause in Chapter 4.
- **Andropause:** Refers to the gradual decline of testosterone levels in men and begins around 30 years of age. (For more information, refer to Chapter 4.) While women also experience decreased testosterone levels with age, their levels are approximately 10 times lower than in men.
- **Adrenopause:** Refers to the reduced secretion of DHEA, which is referred to as the "mother" of all hormones because of its critical role as a precursor (building block) to the production of key sex hormones and its sulfate (DHEA-S). These hormones, which are produced by the adrenal glands, play important roles in metabolism, energy levels, and immune function. As levels decrease over time, you may experience reduced vitality, increased fat accumulation, and a weaker immune response. The gradual decline of these hormones is closely linked to the overall slowing of your body's metabolic processes as you age.
- **Somatopause:** Characterized by a decline in the production of growth hormone (GH) and insulin-like growth factor 1 (IGF-1) levels. Both are essential for maintaining muscle mass, bone density, and metabolic function so as their levels diminish, the body experiences muscle loss (sarcopenia), reduced bone strength, and a general decrease in physical resilience. This decline contributes to the frailty and reduced mobility that often accompany aging, making it a significant focus for those interested in promoting healthy aging strategies.

TECHNICAL STUFF

Table 19-1, based on Mayo Clinic research, highlights some potential shifts that occur with declining levels of testosterone, DHEA, and growth hormone as we age. Please keep in mind that these changes are often subtle and typically fall into the subclinical range — meaning they're part of a complex, natural process that doesn't always result in clear-cut symptoms or require intervention. I'm including this table to give you a general sense of what can happen, not to overwhelm you with details. It's more complex than you probably need to know, but I want to reassure you: These gradual shifts are part of the body's natural aging process, and there's no need to panic. By focusing on holistic hormone-balancing practices outlined in this book such as nutrition, exercise, and stress management, you can help maintain your muscle mass, bone density, and metabolic health. The aim here is to empower you with knowledge, not create unnecessary worry or complexity.

TABLE 19-1 **Potential Age-Related Consequences**

Hormone	Consequences
Testosterone	Increased subcutaneous and visceral fat
	Increased risk for obesity
	Decreased insulin sensitivity
	Increased risk for type 2 diabetes
	Increased high blood pressure
	Increased triglycerides
	Increased risk of metabolic syndrome
	Decreased muscle mass
	Decreased strength
	Decreased bone density
Reduced DHEA	Increased body fat mass
	Increased waist to hip ratio
	Decreased lean body mass
	Decreased VO_2 max
	Increased risk of cardiovascular disease
	Increased risk of heart disease
	Decreased bone density

Hormone	Consequences
Growth hormone	Increased risk for obesity
	Increased visceral adipose tissue
	Decreased lean body mass
	Decreased strength
	Increased risk of metabolic syndrome
	Increased risk of cardiovascular disease
	Decreased bone density

Hormone replacement therapy (HRT)

REMEMBER

HRT has long been considered a potential solution to addressing the symptoms associated with the decline in hormone production associated with aging. The aim of HRT is to improve quality of life and mitigate the age-related and end organ effects (the specific tissues or organs that respond to hormonal signals). Common examples include estrogen and progesterone therapy for women moving through menopause, and testosterone replacement therapy for men with hypogonadism (when they can't produce enough testosterone or sperm or both); the latter helps to restore energy, mood, muscle mass, and overall well-being. Studies are also being conducted on the potential benefits of DHEA and GH replacement therapy for mitigating age-related changes higher up in the endocrine system.

Women

HRT is clearly indicated for women with significant hormone deficiencies, such as those with premature ovarian insufficiency (very early menopause) or menopause induced by medical or surgical interventions. However, for most women who undergo natural menopause, which involves a more gradual and fluctuating decline in hormone levels, HRT can also offer significant benefits — for example, relief from hot flashes, night sweats/improved sleep quality, emotional roller coasters, vaginal dryness; protection of cardiovascular health; prevention of osteoporosis; and, possibly, protection of memory/cognitive function. The way you feel on HRT is the most important factor in determining how effective it is, so if your HRT treatment is optimized but symptoms persist, a further evaluation for other medical conditions or a change in your HRT regimen may be necessary.

Hormone blood testing may be offered to help diagnose perimenopause and menopause. However, in perimenopause, hormone levels can vary significantly — even within the same day — making results challenging to interpret. As a result, diagnosing perimenopause, depending on age group, is typically based on symptoms and quality of life, with a collaborative decision between the individual and their doctor on whether hormone therapies may be beneficial

Before starting an HRT regimen, it's essential to consider other potential causes of and contributors to symptoms, such as thyroid dysfunction, lifestyle factors, or chronic stress. A comprehensive initial assessment often includes blood tests, such as cholesterol levels, blood glucose, thyroid function, and other health markers like blood pressure, height, weight, and assessments for osteoporosis and fracture risk. Some specialists may also recommend further blood tests tailored to individual needs and circumstances, as well as potential follow-up testing to monitor HRT response.

TIP

Lifestyle and environmental factors should always be addressed from the outset because they can play a significant role in ameliorating menopause symptoms either alongside or independently of HRT. Indeed, lifestyle modifications alone or in combination with HRT can offer substantial benefits, particularly in supporting bone and muscle strength, cardiovascular health, and brain function.

WARNING

Our understanding of HRT and its benefits, risks, and side effects for women continues to evolve as more research emerges. Recent studies show that when HRT is initiated in women under 60 or within 10 years of menopause, the benefits tend to outweigh the risks for many health outcomes, including a reduction in cardiovascular events — especially with estrogen-only therapy, which is used in women who have had their uterus removed. Additionally, the risk of breast cancer, once a major concern, has been shown to be much lower than previously thought, particularly with transdermal estradiol (a type of estrogen delivered through the skin via a patch or gel), and in some cases, estrogen-only therapy, which may even reduce your breast cancer risk. However, combined estrogen and progesterone therapy has been associated with a slightly higher risk of developing breast cancer, although it does not seem to increase mortality from the disease. The progesterone component of HRT makes a difference too; for example, using bioidentical options such as micronized progesterone (processed into tiny particles for better absorption by the body) reduces this risk. There is a similar relationship between your choice of progesterone and a reduced risk of blood clots in the veins. Overall, the effect of HRT on breast cancer risk is a modest one and is far outweighed by the increased risk from other factors, such as being overweight, lack of exercise, and alcohol intake greater than recommended levels. Of course, a history of breast cancer or a strong family history of certain types of breast cancer will affect any decision to begin HRT.

While caution is still advised in older postmenopausal women or those more than 10 years past menopause, emerging data suggests that HRT, even in these populations, may not carry as much risk as previously thought. That said, careful consideration of individual risk factors, lifestyle, and alternative treatment options remains important in these cases.

WHEN SHOULD WOMEN STOP TAKING HRT?

A crucial point to consider is the fact that women are now living longer than ever, with many experiencing low sex hormone levels for over three to four decades. This prolonged hormonal deficiency can significantly affect various aspects of health, including cardiovascular, musculoskeletal, mental, cognitive, sexual, and urogenital (genitals and urinary tract) health. While lifestyle and environmental factors certainly influence the experience of menopausal symptoms, HRT can play an important role in managing symptoms and improving quality of life for women during the menopause transition and post-menopause. In fact, current prescribing advice is that there need be no arbitrary end date to HRT prescriptions if the woman is deriving benefit and the benefits continue to outweigh the risks. Unlike hormonal contraception, where high doses of synthetic hormones are introduced, HRT replaces deficient hormones, offering a different risk-benefit profile.

CAN WOMEN USE HRT FOR DISEASE PREVENTION?

Although there is promising data showing reduced all-cause mortality and improved health outcomes in women who begin HRT within 10 years of menopause, HRT is currently not recommended solely for disease prevention, with the focus remaining on symptom relief. One exception to this is osteoporosis; HRT is now recognized as a suitable first-line option for the prevention and treatment in women with very early menopause (POI) and those under 60. Thinking about HRT as a form of preventative medicine continues to evolve, and recommendations may change in future.

Men

As discussed in Chapter 12, although testosterone replacement therapy continues to gain popularity, it's not the most appropriate solution for the vast majority men. In fact, only a small percentage of those reporting symptoms of andropause have a significant testosterone deficiency. Age-related declines in testosterone levels occur in men slowly from their thirties, and many of the symptoms can be prevented or ameliorated with healthy lifestyle interventions. TRT (testosterone replacement therapy) comes with potential risks, including mood swings, cardiovascular complications, and disruption of reproductive hormone balance. Consequently, it's necessary for the decision about whether to pursue TRT to be made carefully and under professional guidance, particularly for older men.

However, one big exception is the increasing rates of testosterone deficiency in younger men, where the impact is often more pronounced than the gradual loss associated with age. Factors covered in Chapters 6 and 11, such as lifestyle, obesity, medicines/illicit drugs, and exposure to endocrine disrupting chemicals (EDCs), can contribute to this early decline, making TRT an appealing option when lifestyle interventions fail to restore hormone balance. Any decision to pursue TRT should, of course, be made carefully and under professional guidance to ensure safety and effectiveness.

I cover this in more detail in Chapter 4, but the decline in testosterone is a normal part of aging and serves important biological and sociological functions, such as helping to reduce impulsive and risky behaviors and promoting a shift toward more cooperative and socially attuned roles within families and communities. These changes give men exactly what they need to thrive in this next phase of life, such as enhanced reading of social groups and providing wise counsel. The healthiest conclusion in the research, therefore, is that the best approach to managing andropause is following a healthy lifestyle and the guidance provided in this book about nutrition, weight, stress, trauma, and emotional management. However, further correlational research is needed to optimize the balance between lifestyle adjustments and chemical interventions. Additionally, improving access to information and education will empower individuals to make informed choices regarding their health.

REMEMBER

Clearly, HRT is a highly nuanced field, and the future of hormone therapy will depend on personalization — fine-tuning formulations, adjusting dosages, and carefully monitoring individual risk factors. The key to success lies in continuous dialogue between patients and healthcare providers to ensure that treatment strategies are both effective and safe, evolving in response to new developments and individual health changes. As more advanced therapeutic options continue to emerge, this personalized approach will be essential to optimizing outcomes and minimizing potential risks.

Powering Up with Diet and Lifestyle Interventions

REMEMBER

Emerging evidence strongly supports lifestyle interventions as safer and more effective strategies for maintaining hormone balance and overall health in aging populations, with three of the most effective being regular exercise, caloric restriction, adequate protein intake, and other positive lifestyle habits. All help to prevent fat accumulation and support muscle mass, which are critical for avoiding age-related frailty and reducing cardio-metabolic risk. They also boost sexual health and positively regulate GH, IGF-1, and testosterone with minimal side effects, unlike HRT. Hormone health really is all about the fundamentals, so let's take a closer look at how they combat the effects of hormonal decline.

Exercise

As people get older, it's common for their physical activity levels to decline, perhaps because they no longer have the same work-related activities, and they don't replace them with other forms of exercise or movement — especially after retirement. Although some people worry that exercise may lead to injuries as they age, research shows that older adults are not significantly more prone to exercise-related injuries than younger people.

REMEMBER

There are many benefits of exercise, but its importance in maintaining hormone balance as you age — particularly in boosting testosterone and growth hormone (GH) — is especially noteworthy. In particular, strength or resistance training helps improve muscle strength, bone density, and overall metabolic health without the risks associated with HRT. In fact, research indicates that resistance training is more effective in improving metabolic health in older adults than combining testosterone therapy with exercise. Likewise, GH levels naturally rise during physical activity, aiding metabolism and muscle function, while studies show that adding GH replacement to exercise doesn't provide significant additional benefits. Therefore, regular exercise remains the most dependable and effective way to maintain hormone balance and promote overall health as we age.

TIP

Importantly, exercise also plays a key role in protecting brain health. Aging is associated with declines in brain glucose metabolism, oxidative damage, and mitochondrial dysfunction, which all contribute to cognitive decline. But studies continue to demonstrate that older adults who maintain an active lifestyle, particularly with regular aerobic or resistance exercise, show improved cognitive function compared to their sedentary counterparts.

Caloric restriction

In overweight older male individuals, reducing caloric intake has been shown to increase testosterone levels and improve testicular function. However, in healthy male individuals, prolonged caloric restriction was shown to have the opposite effect and reduce testosterone production. Similarly, studies have shown that caloric restriction has little to no impact on GH and DHEA levels in individuals of normal weight, making it less effective than exercise in promoting hormone balance. I know, it gets a little bit complicated as we age. Hence the need for personalized and tailored approaches!

Where caloric restriction truly shines, is in its potential to protect against cognitive decline. Research shows that it can enhance brain function by improving metabolic efficiency, upregulating autophagy (the process of removing damaged cellular components), and reducing oxidative stress in the brain. Nevertheless, although it may offer significant benefits for cognitive function, its overall impact on hormone regulation remains less potent than the effects of regular exercise.

WARNING

Women and men, however, need to approach fasting and caloric restriction differently — a topic I cover in detail in Chapter 17. Women's hormone balance, particularly estrogen, can be more sensitive to caloric deficits, which may disrupt menstrual cycles, stress responses, and overall metabolic health if not carefully managed. Tailored fasting protocols are essential to support each gender's unique hormonal landscape effectively.

Adequate protein intake

Every person, no matter their age, should be prioritizing adequate protein intake. It plays a vital role in maintaining muscle strength and physical function, preventing frailty, and supporting overall metabolic health, which becomes increasingly important in older adults to reduce the risk of sarcopenia (age-related muscle loss) and associated health problems.

TIP

How much protein should you be consuming? Protein needs differ based on size, age, activity level and lifestyle, but a general recommendation for women is 20–30 g of protein with each meal, three times a day aiming for a total of 60–100 g protein daily. Then for men, 30 g of protein with each meal is the general recommendation. Experts at the forefront of this conversation, such as Dr. Gabrielle Lyon, recommend aiming for about 1.2–1.6 g of protein per kg of body weight (or approximately 0.54–0.73 g per pound) for optimal levels.

Other lifestyle habits

Maintaining optimal hormone health as you age involves several key lifestyle practices that go beyond exercise and caloric intake. Managing chronic inflammation is essential because unchecked inflammation can disrupt hormone balance and contribute to a range of health issues. A diet rich in anti-inflammatory foods, such as leafy greens, berries, nuts, and omega-3-rich fish, can help support this balance along with reducing your consumption of processed foods and sugar. Gut health also plays a crucial role because an unhealthy gut can interfere with hormone production and metabolism. Eating prebiotic and probiotic foods, like garlic, onions, yogurt, and sauerkraut, can foster a healthy gut microbiome. (Refer to Chapter 10 for more tips on taking care of your gut.)

TIP

In addition, ensuring sufficient vitamin D levels is vital for both sex hormone and thyroid hormone support because low vitamin D has been linked to hormone imbalances. Spending time outdoors, eating vitamin D–rich foods (such as fatty fish, eggs, and fortified products), or considering supplements can help maintain adequate levels. Lastly, quality sleep cannot be overstated. During sleep, the body regulates and produces essential hormones. Creating a restful bedtime routine, avoiding screens before bed, wearing blue light blocking glasses in the evenings, and keeping a consistent sleep schedule are all steps that support hormone health.

Protecting Mental and Emotional Well-being

Mental health concerns such as anxiety, depression, and cognitive decline become increasingly prevalent with age, yet these challenges are often overlooked or misinterpreted. Anxiety, in particular, is frequently dismissed as a natural consequence of aging, which can exacerbate feelings of isolation, stress, and emotional distress. Many older adults may mistakenly attribute symptoms such as irritability, restlessness, or disrupted sleep to the aging process rather than recognizing them as indicators of underlying anxiety. Additionally, physical manifestations such as dizziness or chest pain can often obscure the psychological roots of the issue, complicating the diagnosis.

This section explores how mental health concerns intersect with hormonal changes because age-related hormonal shifts can influence the DOSE neurotransmitters — dopamine, oxytocin, serotonin, and endorphins — which play vital roles in mood regulation, motivation, social bonding, and stress resilience. Reduced levels of these neurotransmitters can lead to a more reactive nervous system, increasing stress hormone levels such as cortisol, which, as a tier 1 hormone, affects every tissue in the body and can significantly disrupt overall hormonal balance. Chronically elevated cortisol is associated with increased inflammation, weakened immune function, and impaired cognitive and emotional health.

To counteract these effects, promoting the release of oxytocin, another tier 1 hormone, is essential. Oxytocin, which is often called "the bonding hormone," not only fosters social connection and emotional warmth but also helps regulate cortisol, reducing its harmful effects on the body and supporting a calmer, more balanced state. By understanding these connections, we see how managing mental health and nurturing social bonds can promote hormonal resilience, stability, and vitality in later life.

Social isolation and loneliness

REMEMBER

One of the most significant factors contributing to declining mental health in older adults is social isolation. As friends and family members pass away and physical limitations make it more difficult to engage with community, many older adults experience heightened feelings of loneliness. This isolation can negatively impact the key DOSE neurotransmitters (read more in Chapter 2), which are essential for emotional well-being.

Social engagement helps boost dopamine, supporting motivation and pleasure; oxytocin, fostering feelings of bonding and stress relief; serotonin, enhancing mood and resilience; and endorphins, reducing stress and physical discomfort. Without regular interaction, lower levels of these neurotransmitters can lead to increased feelings of sadness, anxiety, and even physical pain (yes, loneliness really does hurt!). Staying connected — whether through family, friendships, community programs, senior centers, social clubs, or even digital tools such as video calls and social media — offers essential opportunities for older adults to thrive. These connections also activate the parasympathetic (rest-and-digest) nervous system, promoting relaxation, resilience, and a reduction in the body's reactivity to minor stressors.

Resilience and emotional flexibility

Older adulthood brings profound life transitions — retirement, the loss of loved ones and friends, and shifts in physical health — that can present deep emotional challenges. Cultivating resilience and emotional flexibility becomes essential in adapting to these changes with grace and maintaining both mental health and self-worth. Hormones play a critical role in supporting this adaptability. For instance, cortisol, can heighten feelings of anxiety and tension when elevated, while balanced levels promote a calm, steady response to life's challenges. Oxytocin then strengthens feelings of connection and emotional support, which are essential for resilience.

Practices that support the nervous system outlined in Chapters 9 and 17, such as mindfulness, breathwork, and gentle movement, can help ease stress, grounding you through periods of uncertainty. Engaging in regular physical activity, nurturing meaningful social connections, and embracing a daily gratitude practice are other powerful ways to foster adaptability and well-being. Together, these practices build inner strength, creating a foundation of calm and flexibility that allows you to navigate life's transitions with greater ease, and in a way that won't erode your mental, physical, or emotional health.

Nutrition

TIP

Diets rich in omega-3 fatty acids, antioxidants, and vitamins (such as the Mediterranean diet) have been linked to lower rates of depression, anxiety, and cognitive decline in older age. In particular, omega-3 fatty acids are known to support brain health by reducing inflammation and promoting the production of neurotransmitters such as serotonin.

Support for happy hormones

The neurotransmitter systems that play a key role in mood, motivation, and cognitive function undergo significant changes as people age. Often, these changes manifest as emotional difficulties and cognitive impairments. Here are some examples:

- Dopamine, the neurotransmitter essential for motivation and reward pathways, declines steadily over time, which can impact both mood and motor functions.
- Serotonin, which helps regulate mood and sleep, tends to decrease — potentially increasing vulnerability to depression and anxiety.
- Acetylcholine is crucial for memory and learning, so when levels diminish with age, it contributes to cognitive decline and memory challenges.

TIP

However, thanks to the brain's incredible capacity for neuroplasticity (its ability to adapt and form new connections), there's significant potential to slow, or even counteract, some of these age-related declines. Positive lifestyle changes, such as regular exercise, social engagement, and proper nutrition, can stimulate neurotransmitter production, helping to maintain emotional well-being and cognitive function.

Wisdom From the Blue Zones

To cultivate a truly happy, healthy, and thriving older population, we collectively need to overcome pervasive ageism, a deep-seated stigma that diminishes the value of aging. Society often views aging as a list of inevitable declines — such as loss of productivity, independence, or relevance — rather than recognizing the wisdom, resilience, and valuable contributions that come with it. This negative perception affects not only how society views older adults but also how older adults perceive themselves, which can lead to feelings of isolation, worthlessness, loneliness, anxiety, and depression. Such emotions can dysregulate the nervous system and trigger a rise in cortisol, a tier 1 hormone that affects every single tissue in the body. Chronically elevated cortisol disrupts hormone balance, weakens immune function, slows wound healing, and can accelerate physical decline over time.

Research in the world's Blue Zones — regions where residents live longer, healthier lives — shows how a sense of purpose, fulfillment, and social integration is essential for thriving in older age. In these communities, older adults maintain significant roles in family and community life, with their wisdom and life experiences seen as vital to the social fabric. This purpose-driven life has a powerful influence on hormone health: engaging in meaningful, socially connected activities helps keep cortisol levels in check and boosts oxytocin, another tier 1 hormone that mitigates cortisol's effects. Oxytocin promotes feelings of connection and calm, directly counteracting cortisol's impact and supporting emotional resilience and physical well-being.

The desire for a purposeful life among older adults presents an enormous opportunity for individual and societal benefit. For instance, if the 69-plus million retirees in the United States each volunteered just 3.3 hours per week over the next 20 years, they could contribute 238 billion hours to their communities, valued at approximately $6.8 trillion. This engagement not only enriches communities but also provides essential hormonal and mental benefits for individuals, helping to reduce stress, boost "feel-good" neurotransmitters, and promote overall health.

TIP

To combat ageism, we must continue to highlight and reinforce the positive aspects of aging, such as resilience, wisdom, and prosocial behaviors, both to ourselves and to those around us. Research in the field of positive psychiatry of aging reveals that focusing on strengths rather than deficits can mitigate the effects of neurocognitive disorders, major depression, and even conditions like schizophrenia in later life, positively influencing both mental health and hormonal balance.

The power of purpose

TIP

The purpose-driven lives of people in the Blue Zones offer a valuable model for addressing mental and physical health challenges associated with aging. Research shows that having a strong sense of purpose is linked to decreased mortality from all causes. Engaging in meaningful activities — whether through community involvement, mentorship, volunteering, or familial roles — helps older adults deepen their sense of self-worth and fulfillment, which in turn promotes physical, cognitive, and emotional well-being. Purpose-driven engagement is powerful as it regulates the nervous system, supporting balanced levels of cortisol, and enhancing oxytocin release. This combination contributes to resilience, mental clarity, and a sense of calm, reinforcing both hormone health and overall vitality.

For those who experience reduced mobility, chronic pain, frailty, dementia, or other health challenges that require long-term care, purpose can still play a pivotal role in well-being. Activities such as cognitive exercises, reading, creative hobbies, setting small goals, maintaining daily routines, and engaging in faith-based practices can offer comfort, stability, and a sense of connection, all of which help support mental and hormonal balance.

5

The Part of Tens

IN THIS PART . . .

Take control of your hormones by implementing key lifestyle adjustments, such as improving your diet, reducing toxic exposure, and building a resilient nervous system.

Break free from common myths and misconceptions about hormone health and make confident, empowered decisions about your body.

IN THIS CHAPTER

» Knowing the essential diet and lifestyle foundations for balanced hormones

» Mastering the art of nurturing your endocrine system

» Elevating your mental and emotional well-being

Chapter 20 Ten Essential Habits for Hormone Health

This chapter is going to help you kick-start your new hormone-supportive lifestyle and familiarize you with a root-cause approach. The ten essential habits in this chapter are a great place to put things in motion for better sleep, greater metabolic flexibility, more energy, a higher libido, higher sperm count, a greater sense of happiness and fulfilment, and easier periods.

REMEMBER

It can take 30 to 40 days for new habits become second nature to you, so refer to Chapter 15 if you would like tips and tricks on how to create effective habits that stick. Remember that you're overhauling major processes in your body, and that can take some time. You're in a marathon, not a sprint. Hormone balancing is about transforming your lifestyle, not going all in on a short-term diet or protocol that you forget about in a few months. You might see instant change, or it might take you a little longer. Celebrate your progress, no matter how small, and trust that your body is working hard in the background. All you need to do is keep going.

Setting Up Your Hormonal Clock

Synchronizing your "hormonal clocks" is the first habit I encourage all of my clients to follow because it's foundational to resetting your hormonal balance. (Read more in Chapter 2.)

The first step is prioritizing 10 to 15 minutes of morning sunlight exposure. Blue light (a type of light within the visible spectrum) plays a crucial role in regulating your circadian rhythm, which governs sleep-wake cycles, hormone release (such as cortisol in the morning to wake you up and melatonin in the evening to induce sleep), and other vital bodily functions.

As an Australian who endured brutally dark London winters for 6 years, I learnt a thing or two about how important it is to have exposure to sunlight in the mornings. A great solution is to buy a sunrise alarm clock, which wakes you up with the light and helps you maintain a rhythm of morning sun exposure!

TIP

The next step is limiting your exposure to blue light in the evenings. Although blue light exposure is something you want in the mornings, you're probably also exposed to artificial blue light from screens and electronic devices throughout the evening, which keeps your cortisol levels elevated when what you want them to decline. A great solution is to buy some groovy blue light–blocking glasses and pop them on two to three hours before you go to bed in the evenings. They filter out the blue light, allowing your body to produce melatonin naturally and prepare for a restful night's sleep.

Eating Adequate Protein

As covered in Chapter 2, proteins are the building blocks for hormones, and amino acids are the building blocks for proteins. Hormones can't communicate across the body or have their desired effects without these essential amino acids. There are 20 of them, 9 of which are essential, meaning that your body can't make them and you need to get them through your diet.

Protein is also essential for blood sugar balance, helping to keep your insulin levels in check, positively benefiting the rest of your hormone hierarchy. Protein also decreases the hunger hormone, ghrelin, and increases hormones that help promote a feeling of satiety or the feeling of being full after a meal, which reduces cravings.

TIP

But how much protein should you consume? Protein needs will differ based on size, age, activity level, and lifestyle, but a general recommendation for women is 20 to 30 grams of protein with each meal, for a total of 60 to 100 grams of protein daily. Men should have 30 grams of protein with each meal. Experts at the forefront of this conversation, such as Dr. Gabrielle Lyon, recommend aiming for about 1.2 to 1.6 grams of protein per kilogram of body weight. Additionally, older adults may require a higher proportion of protein in their diet to maintain muscle mass, which naturally declines with age.

WARNING

Quality matters when it comes to protein, and it's important to include a variety of sources. Animal-based proteins typically provide a complete amino acid profile, whereas plant-based proteins may require a greater variety or quantity to meet your needs. However, some experts suggest the source may not matter as much as once thought because both animal and plant proteins are broken down into essential amino acids during digestion. Choose what works best for you and refer to the online appendix at `www.dummies.com/go/hormonebalancefd` for a list of protein sources.

However, please be cautious with protein powders. Many contain added sugars, calories, and potential contaminants linked to inflammation and hormonal imbalances. For help sourcing healthy protein powder options, check the online appendix.

Getting Off Blood Sugar Rollercoasters

Tweaking your diet and lifestyle to support healthy blood sugar/glucose and insulin levels is absolutely crucial. Excess glucose in your body and the spikes and dips it causes changes you on a cellular level and throws off your entire hormonal hierarchy. Weight gain, sleep disturbance, cravings, anxiety, and fertility and reproductive hormone issues are some of the many symptoms of blood sugar rollercoasters. I go through solutions in much more detail in Chapter 17, but the following three habits are a fabulous place to start:

TIP

- **Eat a savory, high-protein breakfast:** In the morning, you're in a fasted state and most sensitive to glucose. An ideal first meal of the day includes a good amount of protein, fiber, fat, and optional carbohydrates or fruit. Think an egg muffin rather than a chocolate croissant, cereal, granola, or jam on toast.
- **Eat fiber first, carbohydrates last:** Fiber creates a viscous (sticky) mesh in your small intestine, which makes it harder for glucose to get into your bloodstream. Eating vegetables at the start of your meal, then protein and fats, and then your carbohydrates or sugars significantly changes what happens in your body. So if you're out for pizza, order a side salad and eat that first.
- **Move after your meals:** Every time your muscles contract, glucose molecules burn up. You have 70 minutes after the end of your meal to reduce a glucose spike, so try walking, doing push-ups or, squats, a planking, or weight lifting. Resistance exercise (weight lifting) is especially good because it's been shown to reduce the glucose spike by 30 percent.

Reducing Your Toxic Load

REMEMBER

Nobody is certain of the extent of the harmful effects hormone disruptors have on our bodies, or how much it takes to cause a harmful impact. The latest evidence shows that it only takes miniscule amounts, and we're exposed to many of them on a daily basis. Your daily choices have an enormous impact on reducing your daily toxin exposure, so here are three things you can do reduce your toxic load. (For more tips, refer to the online appendix.)

TIP

- **Go natural:** Transition all cleaning, personal care, and make-up products to natural equivalents. Use natural air fresheners and perfumes.
- **Pass on plastic:** Store and heat all food in glass or stainless steel containers. Don't use plastic water bottles. When drinking tea, opt for brands with compostable tea bags.
- **Opt for organic:** Consume organic meats and produce when possible or avoid foods on the EWG Dirty Dozen list, the produce that is most heavily contaminated (`www.ewg.org/foodnews/dirty-dozen.php`).

Supporting Your Lymphatic System

You can think of the lymphatic system as the body's drainage system; congestion or blockages in these pathways can cause swelling, cellulite, brain fog, stubborn weight gain, bloating, and generally put greater strain on your body's ability to detox and support healthy, balanced hormones. Because the lymphatic system doesn't have a central pump to move the fluid around (like your heart moves blood around for your circulatory system), you need to incorporate daily practices to boost its circulation and give it some support. Here are some ways to do that:

TIP

- **Dry brushing:** This practice is most frequently used for exfoliation but is also helpful in encouraging proper lymphatic flow.
- **Exercise:** Any movement is helpful in encouraging lymphatic drainage. Some of the most effective exercises for lymph support include yoga, Pilates, strength training, rebounding (yes, jumping on a trampoline!), and running.
- **Breathwork:** Abdominal (diaphragmatic) breathing exercises are a valuable tool in stimulating deep lymphatic structures.

Meeting Your Inner Voice

Your inner voice plays a significant role in how you perceive and respond to stress, obstacles, relationships, or challenges. When left unchecked, negative self-talk can lead to increased cortisol levels, disrupting your hormonal balance and impacting your physical health. It can also lead to self-sabotaging behaviors such as over- or under eating, over- or underexercising, substance abuse, lashing out, or numbing through late-night Netflix sessions. These behaviors can pull you off the path of progress with your health over and over again.

By meeting and transforming your inner voice, you can reduce stress, improve emotional regulation, stay consistent with your healthy habits, keep the promises you make to yourself, and support a balanced hormonal system. Use these steps:

TIP

1. **Recognize its presence.**

   Understand that the inner critic is an adaptative or survival part of you that stems from pain, shame, past experiences, traumas, societal conditioning, or learned behaviors. It's just trying to keep you "safe." It's not who you really are authentically.

2. **Label the critic.**

   Give your inner critic a name or identity. This can help you separate it from your true self and make it easier to address.

3. **Question its validity.**

   Ask yourself if the negative thoughts are based on facts or assumptions. Are they rational or irrational? Is it someone else's voice you're hearing? Perhaps a parent? Childhood bully? A dismissive teacher?

4. **Reframe the thoughts.**

   Replace these negative thoughts with positive perspectives. For example, if you think, "I always mess things up," reframe it to, "I am learning and growing from my experiences." With repetition over time, this new way of thinking will feel more natural to you.

5. **Seek support.**

   Consider seeking professional help from a therapist or counselor. They can provide valuable tools and strategies for understanding and managing your inner critic.

Doing More of What You Love

As people get older and the responsibilities pile up, one of the first things people often do is sacrifice sour passions and hobbies. You'll find the best results on your hormone healing journey when you bring more fun, joy, creativity, silliness, ease, and relaxation into your life. So, let your inner child have some fun! When you engage in activities that you deeply enjoy, your nervous system takes a big exhale, and your whole body relaxes. Boosting your happy hormones, reducing inflammation, turning down cortisol, promoting relaxation, and improving your sleep.

Working With the Nervous System

REMEMBER

If you have any sort of hormone imbalance or related symptoms, it's essential to give your nervous system some love (refer to Chapter 9 for a deeper exploration). It's responsible for 80 percent of the signals in your body (only 20 percent go from the brain down) and operates with a binary programming language, constantly asking itself, "Am I safe or unsafe?" This determination significantly influences your hormonal activity, especially tier 1 hormones (see Chapter 3).

While traditional talk therapy is certainly helpful and can cultivate awareness of your inner critic and inner voice, along with your patterns, habits, or coping mechanisms such as people-pleasing, perfectionism, numbing, self-sabotaging, or being a "control-freak," hormone specialist Dr. Sara Gottfried found that it's only about 30 percent effective for trauma or post-traumatic stress disorder (PTSD). In my opinion, talk therapy alone is not enough when you're treating hormone imbalances and want to support your nervous system for a couple of reasons. For one, traditional talk therapy can sometimes retraumatize the nervous system by revisiting painful memories that engage the conscious mind — which is responsible for only 5 to 10 percent of our mental activity — without addressing the subconscious, which controls 80 to 90 percent of our experiences. Additionally, talk therapy often fails to release the emotions that get trapped in the body's muscles, tissues, and fascia, adding further pressure on the nervous system.

Here are some incredible tools you can check out as alternatives to talk therapy:

TIP

- **Somatic work:** You can find a somatic practitioner, move through one of my ThetaSomatics courses (`https://isabellamainwaring.com`), make dancing or somatic shaking part of your daily routine, or incorporate practices like yoga or other body-focused therapies such as tai chi that help release stored tension and emotions.

- **Eye movement desensitization and reprocessing (EMDR):** This incredible therapy helps process and integrate traumatic memories (whether big or small), rewiring the brain and body to feel safe and resilient.

Harnessing the Power of 30 for Gut Health

REMEMBER

As covered in Chapter 10, the microorganisms in your gut microbiome play a crucial role in hormone regulation and balance. Research shows that by eating a wide variety of plant-based foods — 30 a week — you introduce the optimal range of fibers and nutrients that help different types of beneficial bacteria thrive. Trust me, it's a lot cheaper, easier, and tastier than you might think. Here are some tips:

TIP

- **Add nuts and seeds:** Incorporate a mix of nuts and seeds like almonds, walnuts, chia seeds, flaxseeds, and sunflower seeds into your diet. Sprinkle them on your breakfast, salads, or sandwiches. Easy peasy!
- **Herbs and spices:** Season your protein and add ingredients such as basil, cilantro, rosemary, turmeric, and ginger to your meals.
- **Mix up your vegetables:** Rotate your greens (like spinach, kale, and arugula), cruciferous vegetables (like broccoli, cauliflower, and Brussels sprouts), and root vegetables (like carrots and sweet potatoes).
- **Incorporate fruits:** Berries, citrus fruits, apples, and tropical fruits all offer different fibers and nutrients beneficial for gut health.
- **Experiment with whole grains:** Add variety with whole grains such as quinoa, farro, barley, and oats.
- **Use legumes and pulses:** Beans, lentils, chickpeas, and peas are excellent sources of fiber and plant protein.

Detoxing from Dopamine

While a complete dopamine detox isn't going to be possible because your brain constantly produces dopamine, you can reset your brain's reward system to help you feel more fulfilled each day, reduce addictive behaviors, and help rebalance hormones such as cortisol, serotonin, oxytocin, melatonin, and insulin.

TIP

If you find yourself constantly seeking quick hits of pleasure, whether through social media, junk food, or binge-watching TV, it could be a sign that your dopamine system is overloaded. Other signs include struggling to concentrate on tasks that require sustained attention, feeling unmotivated, increased anxiety, sleep disturbances, overeating or emotional eating, and reduced enjoyment of simple pleasures. Here's what you can do:

TIP

- **Identify addictive behaviors:** Recognize activities that overstimulate your brain's reward system.
- **Set clear goals:** Decide whether you want to avoid specific activities for a day or abstain from all forms of technology for a more extended period.
- **Create a plan:** Replace addictive behaviors with healthier alternatives, such as reading a book or going for a walk.
- **Start small:** Begin with a short detox period, like a day or a weekend, and gradually increase the duration as you feel more comfortable.
- **Stay mindful:** Pay attention to how you feel during the detox. Notice any changes in your mood, focus, and overall well-being.
- **Reintroduce activities gradually:** After the detox, reintroduce previously addictive activities in moderation. Set boundaries to prevent slipping back into old habits.

IN THIS CHAPTER

» Uncovering the truth about your genes and the aging process

» Empowering yourself to transform your metabolism and fertility

» Discovering the true and devastating impacts of stress and birth control

Chapter 21
Ten Myths about Hormone Health Debunked

While hormone health and balancing have become hot topics in recent years, with increased attention comes a flood of information — not all of it accurate. Misconceptions and myths about hormones are everywhere, leading to confusion, overwhelm, "analysis paralysis," and misguided health decisions.

This chapter reveals the truth behind ten common myths about hormone health and balancing. You'll explore the influence of genetics, the impact of stress, your ability to manage your health naturally, and holistic solutions. By separating fact from fiction, you'll feel much more empowered and better equipped to make informed decisions about your health and overall well-being. Remember, this isn't a diet or short-term trend; it's a way of life.

Genetics Determine Your Destiny

Genes are remarkable, but the idea that your biological makeup (as opposed to your environment or personal decisions) is the dominant determinant of your health or behavior just isn't true. It's not that genes don't matter; they do. It's that they do not and cannot determine even simple behaviors, let alone the extremely complex process that is a human life. Genes also don't provide complete answers or cures for most illnesses, nor do they fully explain them.

What science shows us is that while genes play a significant role, they are not the definitive script of our lives. The reality is far more empowering and dynamic, involving the fascinating relationship between our genetics and our internal and external environments. This new and rapidly growing field of science is called epigenetics, and it shows there is a clear relationship between our genetics, environment, and the function of our endocrine (hormone) system (you can explore this further in Chapter 8.)

REMEMBER

What epigenetic researchers have found is that while our genes provide the basic blueprint, environmental factors such as diet, stress, trauma, emotions, toxin exposure, and lifestyle choices significantly shape how your genes are expressed. Think of it like a series of light switches: environmental factors can "switch on" or "switch off" certain genes, influencing how your body functions. This means your hormonal health is not determined by your genetic makeup alone but is influenced by how you interact with your environment and the choices you make each day.

While some people have genetic predispositions, such as for developing type 2 diabetes, this doesn't mean that the condition is inevitable or that it can't be managed effectively. Lifestyle factors significantly influence whether the disease manifests and how well it can be treated (or even reversed). You always have the power to make changes that can improve your health.

Stress Doesn't Impact Your Hormones

This myth likely originated from a lack of understanding about how interconnected the mind and body's systems are. While Western medicine overlooked this relationship for a long time despite decades of research, ancient medical systems like traditional Chinese medicine and Ayurveda have recognized it for centuries. In fact, this mind-body connection is at the center of their healing philosophies.

In the past, Western medicine viewed stress as a purely mental or emotional issue, separate from physical health. However, modern science is revealing that mental and emotional states are closely linked to physical health, particularly through the endocrine system.

TIP

Stress isn't just feeling anxious or agitated. It triggers changes throughout your body, especially in the endocrine system. These responses are linked to the sympathetic (fight or flight) and parasympathetic (rest and digest) nervous systems, which are covered in Chapter 9. By managing stress effectively using the tips and tools I share in Part 4 of this book, you can support hormonal balance, improving both your mental and physical health.

You Can't Fix Your Hormone Levels Naturally

The idea that you can't fix your hormone levels through natural or holistic interventions is one of the most persistent and disempowering myths out there. It was certainly one I believed for far too long before the side effects of birth control paired with mental health struggles, acne, lack of sleep, and weight gain became so frustrating I had no choice but to take things into my own hands.

Many of us are told that once are hormones are out of balance, the only solution is medication (such as birth control pills) or hormone replacement therapies. Alternatively, many of us know we need to overhaul our lifestyle but instead look for a "quick fix," hoping to ignore or delay the inevitable changes we need to make by relying on medication. While these treatments can absolutely be necessary and effective for some individuals on the hormone healing journey, it's important to understand that holistic solutions are an essential ingredient to improving your hormone health long term. You can start today using the tips I've outlined for you in Part 4 of this book, as well as the 10 habits outlined in the preceding chapter.

REMEMBER

Our bodies all have a natural self-repair and healing system that we can tap into. If you can heal from a cut or bruise, you can certainly help guide your body back to hormonal balance. Listening to your body's signals and making small changes will lead to big improvements over time.

You Can't Fix Your Metabolism Naturally

Do you know people who complain about having a slow metabolism? Who say they barely eat anything and still gain weight? Or have you met people who can seemingly eat whatever they want without gaining weight due to a "fast metabolism"? While it's true that your metabolism can be fast or slow, it's not true that you are powerless over speeding it up.

It's also important to note that there are significant differences in male and female physiology when it comes to how people use, store, and access energy in their bodies. Historically, much of the research on diet and metabolism has been conducted on men, often overlooking the unique metabolic needs of women. So while we often describe metabolism as "burning body fat or glucose for energy," the actual processes are more nuanced and complicated than that. For example, the thyroid gland plays a significant role in regulating your metabolic rate through the release of hormones like T3 and T4, and for women, hormonal fluctuations throughout the menstrual cycle, pregnancy, and menopause can significantly influence thyroid function.

REMEMBER

What's important to understand is that the complex process of having a fast or slow metabolisms encompasses how metabolically flexible or inflexible you are — meaning how efficiently your body can shift between fuel sources such as glucose or body fat, depending on its needs. Consider our hunter-gatherer ancestors who faced food shortages. Their bodies needed to be able to store glucose both in the short and the long term, giving them energy when food was limited. Your metabolism is actually a really intelligent system that keeps you alive, so there is no reason to hate or shame your body!

Today, most people are not this metabolically flexible. As explored in Chapter 7, our modern lives have not been designed to support our metabolic flexibility. Many of us are eating multiple carbohydrate-heavy meals a day without enough protein or fiber to prevent glucose rollercoasters. We also aren't building muscle (where the body loves to store excess glucose) or moving our bodies after we eat because we spend our day sitting in an office and driving to and from work. This means the body generally has an abundance of glucose available at all times and doesn't readily switch from burning glucose to burning alternative fuel sources such as body fat.

Signs of a slow metabolism or metabolic inflexibility include insulin resistance; weight gain; weight that is stubborn and won't shift; mood swings; trouble sleeping; hormone imbalances such as PCOS, painful periods PMS, or infertility; hunger after meals or cravings; and a sense of sluggishness or fatigue.

TIP

A key ingredient to becoming metabolically flexible is stabilizing your blood sugar and therefore insulin levels. This means you can easily shift between burning glucose (from your last meal) for energy, and burning stored fat for fuel. A second key ingredient is to manage stress, which can lead to high blood sugar levels. You can refer to the Chapters 16 and 20 for tips on how to tweak your lifestyle and level of stress to support metabolic health.

Lastly, despite our advanced understanding of our metabolism and how it works, the myth that you can't fix it naturally continues to be perpetuated by the increasing reliance on GLP-1 receptor drugs like Ozempic. While certainly necessary for some people, these medications and the way they are marketed are cultivating the belief that holistic or natural methods are ineffective or too difficult. Although these drugs can be part of a treatment plan when appropriate, if you want sustainable, long-term results (without negative side effects), you need to work on your metabolic flexibility.

Birth Control Fixes Hormone Imbalances

Here I'm talking about synthetic (hormonal) birth control, as opposed to natural methods such as condoms. The introduction of oral contraceptives in the 1960s was certainly a major breakthrough for women, giving us more autonomy, freedom, and reproductive choice. A woman's choice to go on or off synthetic birth control is her own, and I support all women and believe they know what's best for them. But, do we know the true effects that it's having on our hormones and overall balance?

In medicine there's a concept called informed consent, meaning that your healthcare should give you information on the benefits and the risks of the option that they are recommending, as well as all the other existing options. With regard to birth control, what most women aren't told is that while synthetic hormones are unlikely cause serious harm in most women who use it, these options (especially the pill) are associated with a long list of mild to severe side effects, such as an increased risk of anxiety and depression. Additionally, the pill is linked to lower levels of essential vitamins and minerals like B6, B12, C, zinc, selenium, magnesium, and folate, and some research suggests they even negatively alter your gut microbiome (you can explore the pill's impact on the immune system, brain health, mental health, and your stress response in much more detail in Chapter 12).

What's often overlooked is that these contraceptives don't address some of the root-cause drivers and contributory factors of hormonal issues, such as poor gut health, high toxin exposure, or chronic stress. Instead, they work as a bandage solution, masking symptoms. This means you need to be extremely mindful of your diet and lifestyle while on these contraceptives to prevent more severe hormonal imbalances developing if and when you decide to transition off them.

REMEMBER

Of course, there are instances where your symptoms are so severe that you might use these options under the supervision of a healthcare professional who can help you bridge a natural, root-cause and hormonal approach. In fact, there are plenty of valid reasons a woman would use hormonal contraceptives or other medical interventions as part of her health journey. I encourage you to research, experiment, and troubleshoot until you find the solutions that work the best for you.

You Can't Fix Infertility

If it's taking longer than you thought it would to get pregnant, or if you've been told you have a fertility problem, you might be starting to feel anxious. What's reassuring to know is that the majority of couples struggling with infertility do eventually get pregnant. Please don't lose hope or confidence in your body and know that both men and women contribute pretty equally to infertility. There's a lot we can all do to enhance fertility, whether you're still trying to conceive the old-fashioned way or you've started on a fertility treatment journey.

While it's a complex and very individual journey, there is hope. The tips and tools outlined in this book will help reduce inflammation, boost sperm count, and rebalance your hormones — all factors that can impact fertility, conception, and prenatal health. I've worked with women who have been trying to get their period back or conceive for years and by addressing nervous system regulation, boosting their self-esteem, and making lifestyle and dietary shifts, they were able to conceive.

Why? Well, let's take a step back and think about the broader, evolutionary picture. We are animals, after all. Why would your body want to create life when it's in a state of chronic stress? That would put you and your potential child in danger. Unfortunately, our mind, body, and nervous system can't tell the difference between being chased by a lion and facing a big work deadline. Stress is stress. Whether stress comes from work, lack of sleep, blood sugar fluctuations, the pressure to get pregnant quickly, fears about parenthood, the fear of childbirth, or high exposure to environmental toxins, your body will always prioritize your survival over reproduction.

TIP

With rising rates of obesity, insulin resistance, poor gut health, chronic stress, reproductive hormone imbalances, plus exposure to environmental toxins, and all sorts of other stressors discussed throughout this book, our bodies are getting pretty overwhelmed. Add in the daily mental and emotional juggling act of modern life — career ambitions, family goals, keeping up with the Joneses, climate change, long commutes, sedentary lifestyles, social media addiction, financial worries, and unprocessed trauma — and it's easy to see why our bodies might say, "We're in survival mode right now — reproduction needs to wait!"

TIP

Statistically it takes 12 to 24 months to conceive, and while it often happens incredibly quickly, I usually ask my clients to give it 12 months of trying. It can take a while to restore or boost fertility with a natural, root-cause based approach. You're overhauling major systems in the body and your way of life, after all! That being said, not everyone can get pregnant even with medical interventions, and it doesn't mean you're to blame, broken, or aren't trying hard enough. Sometimes it's just not in the cards. While many interventions can significantly enhance fertility, it can also be caused by a variety of factors such as blocked fallopian tubes, severe endometriosis, or low sperm count due to genetic factors. That's why it's essential to work closely with healthcare providers to understand your underlying causes and to develop a custom, comprehensive plan that includes medical and holistic approaches.

Hormone Imbalances Are a Natural Part of Aging and Can't Be Treated

While hormonal transitions are a fact of life, it doesn't mean that you can't manage or treat them effectively. There are more medical and holistic options available for you than ever before, which can dramatically increase your quality of life mentally, emotionally, and physically in your later years.

TIP

As women age, they transition through perimenopause and menopause, leading to changes in estrogen and progesterone levels. Similarly, men experience a gradual decline in testosterone, leading to changes in mood, weight and sexual function in both sexes. (Read more in Chapters 4 and 12.) However, age isn't solely to blame — lifestyle factors, diet, stress, unresolved emotions, and your environment play significant roles in how you experience these shifts as well.

These transitions can be the ultimate portal to personal growth and transformation if you let them be. Learning to say "no"; doing more of what lights you up; and protecting your time, stress levels, and energy will be essential. By combining the diet and lifestyle modifications outlined in this book along with medical treatments such as hormone replacement therapy (HRT), you can absolutely improve your experience of this transition and thrive in later years. (To find out more, refer to Chapter 19.)

You Can Fix Cortisol Levels with Supplements

Pretty-looking "evening adrenal tonics," cortisol balancing supplements, and adaptogens such as Ashwagandha continue to surge in popularity. While some supplements can absolutely deliver on their promises and support adrenal function or stress management, they cannot address the root-cause drivers of elevated stress hormone levels. Yes, they may provide temporary relief and can serve as a useful tool on your hormone balancing journey, but you certainly don't want to rely on them forever. (Please note that I'm not referring here to serious medical conditions such as tumors or diseases that can disrupt cortisol levels.)

TIP

As I like to tell my clients, "You can't supplement your way out of survival mode." If you have high or low cortisol levels over a sustained period of time (not just a shorter burst like finishing a work project), it's pointing to deeper issues that need to be resolved. By focusing on building confidence, delegating tasks, addressing big *T* and little *t* trauma, releasing suppressed emotions, boosting your self-worth, and making healthy lifestyle choices (as outlined in Chapters 10 and 16), you can heal the key drivers of your imbalanced cortisol levels. Supplements should complement, not replace, the deeper work required for lasting change.

Only Women Need to Worry About Estrogen Levels

This misconception stems from the fact that estrogen is often labeled as a "female hormone," but as you now know, estrogen is crucial for both male and female health. Indeed, imbalances (particularly elevated levels) are increasing at rapid rates in men, causing an array of health issues such as low moods, anxiety, infertility, low sperm count, and sexual dysfunction.

TIP

There are three key reasons for this:

- **Chronic stress:** Elevated cortisol levels can lead to a decrease in testosterone production. Since testosterone is a precursor (building block) for estrogen, when its levels drop, it can create an imbalance where estrogen becomes relatively higher.
- **Environmental factors:** Exposure to xenoestrogens — chemicals that mimic estrogen in the body — found in plastics, personal care products, and other everyday items can increase estrogen levels in both men and women.

These endocrine (hormone) disruptors can interfere with the body's natural hormone balance, leading to elevated estrogen levels.

- **Diet, lack of exercise and obesity:** Consuming a diet high in refined carbohydrates and unhealthy fats can increase fat tissue (which contains aromatase, an enzyme that converts testosterone into estrogen) and leads to higher overall levels of estrogen in the body. Maintaining a healthy weight, eating a balanced diet, and engaging in regular physical activity can help regulate hormone levels and prevent imbalances.

You Need a Diagnosis in Order to Act

This final myth is the most problematic of them all, and I want to be very clear here: You absolutely do not need to wait for a diagnosis or test to start taking care of your hormones. While medical professionals and diagnostics play a crucial role in identifying and managing hormonal issues, let's be honest, most of the time testing leaves us with more questions than answers, and you'll feel better much faster if you're taking action daily rather than waiting for more tests, results, and explanations to confirm what you already feel.

Ultimately, you are the only expert in you, so even if your tests come back normal or in a "healthy range," it doesn't mean you shouldn't be taking care of your hormones. Hormone balance is complex and highly individual. You and I could have the same hormone levels and feel completely different because we each have unique hormone sensitivity and our bodies, lifestyles, and experiences are different. Following the steps outlined in this book will positively benefit your health whether a test tells you it's time for change or not.

REMEMBER

Trust in your ability to understand and respond to your body's signals. Making simple, consistent adjustments to your lifestyle and diet can lead to significant improvements in how you feel that might not be reflected on a test.

Index

A

F

G

H

I

J

K

L

M

N

O

P

Q

R

S

T

About the Author

Isabella Mainwaring is a leading educator in hormone balance, feminine vitality, and trauma healing. As the creator of the ThetaSomatics method, she's pioneered an innovative approach to healing the endocrine system by rewiring the nervous system and subconscious mind to promote hormone balance, resilience, emotional well-being and consistency in sticking to healthy habits.

Isabella's personal journey of overcoming a battle with hormone imbalances that lasted more than a decade began at age 13 and culminated during her high-pressure role as a strategy consultant for one of the world's leading academic and scientific publishers in London. It was there she experienced the devastating effects of chronic stress, unprocessed emotions, and the demands of modern living. Determined to restore her own health and revolutionize the lives of others facing similar challenges, Isabella left the corporate world behind to retrain.

Aside from authoring *Hormone Balance for Dummies*, she also contributed several chapters to *Women's Health All-In-One For Dummies*. She's a sought-after speaker, podcast host, and visionary leader who has a social media audience of over 260,000 and helps individuals worldwide to unlock their full potential by taking back control of their hormone health. Her larger mission is to create a global movement of women creating success in a way that nourishes their bodies, working with their unique hormonal profile to create a life that radiates confidence, freedom, and purpose.

You can learn more about Isabella's work, share your comments about this book, and join her community by visiting her website `https://isabellamainwaring.com`, on Instagram @isabella.mainwaring, or on TikTok @isabella.mainwaring or tuning into her podcast, *Breakthrough*.

Author's Acknowledgment

I would like to thank Dr. Jenny Fildes for her support and generosity in serving as the technical reviewer for this book and contributing her expertise. At Wiley, I want to thank Tracy Boggier for being so warm, enthusiastic, and a pleasure to work with. I'm also extremely grateful for the guidance of Charlotte Kughen, a brilliant and efficient editor who ensured we packed as much valuable information into this book as we could.

While it's impossible to acknowledge every individual and organization that has generously supported my education and advocacy, I must give special thanks to my parents, Paul and Sarah; my brother, Jasper; and my extraordinary teachers at Geelong Grammar School who taught me to how to think outside the box, trust myself, and find solutions. A thousand thank-yous to Emily Pollock for helping me find my voice and to Helen Donoghue for the gift of her beach house, where so much of this book came to life. And to my wonderful partner, Andrew — your unwavering belief in me, constant encouragement, and endless stream of herbal tea deliveries have been my greatest support.

Finally, I'm deeply grateful to the wider community of practitioners, researchers, and pioneers across Eastern, Western, functional, and integrative medicine. Your dedication to advancing our understanding of hormone health and healing has been an inspiration, and I am honored to contribute to this growing body of knowledge. This book is as much a reflection of your work as it is mine.

Dedication

This book is dedicated to the readers. Your devotion to improving your hormone health is a powerful act of self-love and strength, one that ripples out to positively impact the well-being of those around you, and future generations. May this journey of self-discovery inspire you to trust your body's innate wisdom and step into your full potential.

Publisher's Acknowledgments

Senior Acquisitions Editor: Tracy Boggier

Project Editor: Charlotte Kughen

Technical Editor: Jenny Fildes

Senior Managing Editor: Kristie Pyles

Production Editor: Saikarthick Kumarasamy

Cover Image: © PeopleImages.com – Yuri A/ Shutterstock